Ayurvedic Tongue Diagnosis

by

Walter 'Shantree' Kacera, D.N., Ph.D.

Preface by Dr. David Frawley &
Foreword by Dr. Gabriel Cousens

LOTUS PRESS

P.O. Box 325
Twin Lakes, WI 53181 USA

This book is not intended to treat, diagnose or prescribe. The information contained herein is in no way to be considered as a substitute for a consultation with a duly licensed health care professional.

Page Design / Layout: Paul Bond, Art & Soul Design

Cover Design: Susan Tinkle

Reprinted, 2012, 2023

First Edition, 2006

Printed in the United States of America

Ayurvedic Tongue Diagnosis

ISBN: 978-0-9409-8577-3

Library of Congress Control Number: 2006925367

Published by:
Lotus Press
P.O. Box 325
Twin Lakes, Wisconsin 53181 USA
web: www.lotuspress.com
e-mail: lotuspress@lotuspress.com
800-824-6396

Dedication

This book is dedicated to my cherished Lorenna, who is my inspiration, companion, a gifted healer and Shamanu teacher, best friend, a creative chef, and resident goddess, my beloved soul mate — in essence, pure magic.

Table of Contents

List of Illustrations, Charts and Tables

Acknowledgments

It is a beautiful gift for me to honor publicly those who have inspired me, taught me, supported me and stood by my side.

My first thanks goes to my parents, Anna and Andrew Kacera, whose union provided the spark and love that created me. Thank you for your unceasing love.

To my wife Lorenna for her hours of dedicated support as editor of this book, and for the nourishment of her Shamanu Practices that kept me connected, healthy and strong.

To all my students who asked just the right questions to keep me on my path. To all my patients and clients who keep reminding me of my purpose.

To Gabriel Cousens for his wisdom and leading edge thinking, and who continues to be a guiding light for me.

To David Frawley for many years as a wonderful and inspirational teacher and many more to come.

My gratitude goes out to all the teachers of Ayurveda and the Healing Arts: especially Dr. Vasant Lad, Dr. Robert Svoboda, Michael and Leslie Tierra, Dr. Deepak Chopra, Dr. Bernard Jensen, Farida Sharon, Maya Tiwari, Bob Lewanski and Bob Zuraw.

Other inspirational teachers for awakening my mind to the power of living foods: Victoras Kulvinskas, Dr. Bernard Jensen, Dr. Ann Wigmore.

I wish to thank Lotus Press for their enduring support for the creation of this book. And also to thank Yvonne Stapleton, Gabriel Bousquet from PC Tantrum and Graham from A&B Printing.

To Earth Gaia for her unending nourishment and love.

To the Five Sacred Elements for their continuous teachings both in Canada and in Costa Rica.

To my sacred home 'Spirit of the Earth, 'The Living Centre' for holding me and providing the teachings and beauty of nature.

Peace Be With You.

— *Walter 'Shantree' Kacera*

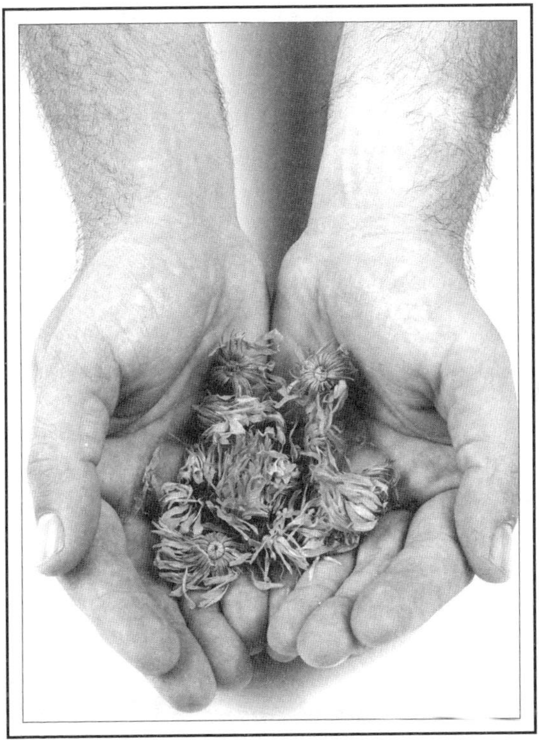

Foreword

Dr. Gabriel Cousens

Ayurvedic Tongue Diagnosis is a book that is about much more than Ayurvedic tongue diagnosis. It is one of the best books ever written on the relationship of Ayurvedic medicine to modern nutrition. I say this from a variety of perspectives: as a holistic physician for over 30 years, as a Diplomat in Ayurveda and a student of Ayurveda since 1979, as a homeopathic physician, as the Director of the Tree of Life Rejuvenation Center, where we actively practice the principles of Ayurveda, Panchakarma and Rasayana, and also as the author of *Spiritual Nutrition and the Rainbow Diet, Conscious Eating* and *Rainbow Green Live Food Cuisine,* all books dealing with the different subtle levels of live foods and nutrition for spiritual life. This book, which is quite excellent, touches on all of these levels in an in-depth way and was a joy to read.

Because of my interest in re-introducing live foods into Ayurveda, I particularly appreciated the in-depth understanding that Walter 'Shantree' Kacera has shown in this area. His understanding of life force and the importance of life force in food is an important part of Ayurveda. He defines life force as the ability to create life. What he points out very clearly is that cooked seed, when you replant it in the ground, does not germinate. Live food seeds do.

In *Ayurvedic Tongue Diagnosis,* Walter brings in the importance of life force foods on our tongue, through our taste, through the shape and size and color and patterns on the tongue. One particular insight that I found most exciting is the understanding of the subtle levels of Kapha, Pitta and Vata as Ojas, Tejas and Prana. Vata correlates to Prana, which is, in essence, the Chi in the food and also the oxygen in the food.

Live food has a significantly higher amount of oxygen and Prana. The ancient Rishis primarily ate live food, as pointed out by Dr. David Frawley. The reason they ate this live food is because they knew it had more Prana and Prana helps to expand consciousness.

The principle of Tejas in essence is the Fire Element in food. Tejas relates to the amount of electricity that is in the food, as well as the amount of enzymes. Cooked food has significantly diminished Tejas because the metabolic power of the food, which is the enzymes, is destroyed when you cook the food. As I point out in great scientific detail in *Conscious Eating* and also *Spiritual Nutrition and the Rainbow Diet,* live food has considerably higher electrical, enzymes and life force energies. These are disrupted and minimized when the food is cooked. Therefore, live food has more Tejas.

Ojas is the third element, and Ojas relates to Kapha and also relates to, in a sense, the lubricating nectar of the water current as it serves the subtle structure of the system. Walter describes it as the fluid essence that has been digested. The process of cooking does, in essence, destroy the structured quality of water. It disrupts the internal structure of water that is important for, not only bringing energy into the body through the structured water, but is also, according to the latest research, important for maintaining the subtle structure of the DNA. When we think about food in terms of the way that Walter Kacera has described it, as carriers of its subtle elemental essences, Prana, Tejas and Ojas, we have a much deeper understanding of the importance of live food in Ayurveda. Unfortunately, cultural programming for those who are traditional Ayurvedic is strong, and has obscured the ability to truly understand the importance of live food as it once was used by the Rishis for spiritual development, health and vitality.

Walter provides a good explanation of how we can, indeed, incorporate the foundational principles of Ayurveda into a balanced, health promoting, longevity promoting and rejuvenating way of life. I am absolutely delighted to see this work because of this point alone.

Ayurvedic Tongue Diagnosis makes the point that Ayurveda is about trusting nature and following the rules of nature, as we are a part of nature, so that we can reach a place of complete balance and health. In essence, Walter talks about Ayurveda as not just a medical system, but as the science of life; and that we are a part of nature, and because of that, we need to live by the subtle laws of nature, in order to create health, harmony and balance in our own being. It is from this point of view that we can best understand the importance of live food. If we are trusting in nature, since nature gave the food to us as a gift from God in its live form, perhaps we should accept the gift in the way that it came to us, rather than wanting to alter it to meet our own ego needs and particular tastes. This is not to ignore the fact that, at a certain time in India, because of parasites, because of poor modes of sanitation, that it was relevant and necessary to cook the food. At this point in time, particularly in the United States, these are lesser concerns, and using food with the highest amount of life force, Prana, Tejas and Ojas should take more precedence.

Vatas clearly have the potential to be unbalanced on a poorly organized live food diet. Walter is able to point out that if we follow these basic Ayurvedic guidelines and understand how they apply to the different types of live food, we can eat live foods and not really have a problem keeping the Vata balanced. Of course, we must define live foods and understand that live foods are more than a salad or some sprouts. It is the whole vegetable kingdom. It is the soaked nuts and seeds that bring the water that balances the normal drying of Vata that you get with nuts and seeds. It is the blending of the nuts and seeds and the blending of some of the vegetables that creates the smoothness and sweetness that allows us to balance the Vata. It is the use of high mineral content foods and Celtic salt that brings the salt taste. Again, once we understand these qualities, we can really appreciate the point that Walter makes, which is that "if it's not broken, don't fix it."

As a student of Ayurvedic medicine since 1979, I have had an opportunity to read a variety of Ayurvedic books that have been translated into English and am impressed with the depth of understanding that Walter discusses as he explains the doshas, the dhatus and the scrotas. His descriptions bring a new level of interest in terms of understanding that we eat as part of a way of not only maintaining our health, but also rejuvenating our health. At the Tree of Life, we have actually worked out a system of live food Panchakarma and we are presently more deeply trying to work out formulas of Rasayanas that do not involve white sugar or animal products, including ghee. This is not only because of the new phase of world health issues, which include Candida, fungus and prions, made worse by animal products and by all sorts of sugar including fruit sugars. Walter's Ayurvedic understanding leads the reader very gently into understanding how to activate these nutritional forces.

This book speaks to the layperson as well as the trained healer, as it delves deep into the art and science of conscious living, which is, indeed, the systematic approach to Ayurveda. This art and science is primarily to continually strengthen ourselves so that we can overcome the imbalances that cause what we call chronic disease. As Walter points out, the Ayurvedic principles create a strong body, clarity of mind and tranquility of spirit.

This book goes one step deeper than the usual Ayurvedic books, into the subtlety of the philosophy of Ayurveda, particularly in the issues related to the relationship of nutrition and the subtle elements in the food to rejuvenation. Walter has created a particularly interesting questionnaire, which is the elemental body / mind / nature questionnaire.

The educational foundation of the book prepares us to really understand the meaning and use of tongue diagnosis. The ancient art of tongue diagnosis, as this book defines it, is "the science of the shape, shadings and markings of the tongue, which describe the current state of an individual's health, as well as their inherited constitution." The potential of tongue diagnosis is that it gives a non-invasive way to measure the tissue integrity of the body, especially the Agni of the digestive system or the Fire or strength of the digestive system. This can be assessed by simply observing the color and structure of the tongue, then we have a very simple way to take preventive steps to correct those imbalances, and we have a very simple feedback system, meaning the tongue's color, size, shape and shading, to let us know how successful our approach has been.

Tongue diagnosis gives us an opportunity to have a very low tech, but effective feedback system of how we are doing. Tongue diagnosis is also an effective way of assessing an individual's genetic constitution and thereby understanding the sort of healing forces, lifestyle habits and diet needed for healing. Walter Kacera also points out, both metaphorically and practically, that tongue diagnosis gives us an idea of which healing tastes will bring us back to our optimal level of health, and also the healing tastes we need to stay at our peak quality of health. *Ayurvedic Tongue Diagnosis* makes the point that these foods for healing are Sattvic foods. The main Sattvic diet at this time in our history, not a thousand years ago, not a hundred years ago, is at least an 80% live food diet, because it contains more life force than any other diet on the planet. Sattvic foods are those foods that give us life force and support peace of the body, mind and emotions and also maintain peace with the environment and expand consciousness. A healthy tongue is a wonderful indicator that we are on a healthy path of optimizing our constitution. In essence, the tongue lets us taste our way to health, and Mother Nature, through the live foods that she offers us, gives us the highest essence of the Ojas, Tejas and Prana to do that.

The benefits of tongue diagnosis are one of the many reasons to read this book. Its greatest advantage is its value in self-diagnosis and the monitoring of one's state of health in a simple, non-technical, self-healing manner. Tongue diagnosis helps us determine our unique constitution and our current state of health, which we also know as Prakruti and Vikruti. It can be used as an early detector for imbalances in the body and a clue to the underlying cause of disease.

One of the most important advantages is that it tells us the state of the Agni, the power of digestion, and of the whole digestive system including the liver, stomach, spleen and the small and large intestines. It also can be used to reflect the quality of the circulation of Prana, blood and bodily fluids. The color of the mucous of the tongue gives us a feeling for the acid / alkaline balance, which is very important, and also helps to mirror the condition of the bodily fluids and the function of the organs. This is a wonderful, simple, effective, age-old way to make self-treatment, which I believe is somewhat the foundation of Ayurvedic medicine, functional for those people who are committed to taking responsibility for their own health.

I honor Walter0 'Shantree' Kacera for the excellent work he

has done in this book and I strongly recommend this book for both lay people and trained healers as a way to increase their depth of understanding and knowledge. This book introduces us to the philosophy of the tongue, which takes us deep into the philosophy of Ayurveda, and helps us merge, in wonderful ways, with the healing powers of Ayurvedic principles as they are applied to the use of high vitality foods.

— Gabriel Cousens, M.D., M.D. (H), Diplomat in Ayurveda
Author, *Spiritual Nutrition and Conscious Eating*, etc.

Preface

Dr. David Frawley

The tongue shows us the nature of Agni, or the digestive fire, and after the pulse, is the most important tool of diagnosis in Ayurvedic medicine. The tongue, however, is easier to read than the pulse and so is often a good place to start learning the art of diagnosis. Learning to examine it properly is one of the main clinical skills in Ayurveda and a good means of self-examination as well. Ayurvedic Tongue Diagnosis is the first book on Ayurveda published in the West that focuses on this vital subject. It is an important new addition to Ayurvedic literature that is useful both for those who already know Ayurveda and also for those who want to learn about it.

The author, Walter Shantree Kacera, presents a broad view of the entire system of Ayurveda, including its relationship with Chinese medicine and western nutritional and herbal approaches. This provides the reader with the necessary background to understand the Ayurvedic view of tongue diagnosis and how it compares with other systems.

The book is detailed, well-illustrated and well-referenced, making it a good desk-top guide for serious students and practitioners alike. We look forward to future books by this author, who displays both deep knowledge and original insight in his approach to Ayurveda and to healing as a whole.

— Dr. David Frawley (Pandit Vamadeva Shastri)
Author, *Yoga and Ayurveda, Ayurvedic Healing* etc.

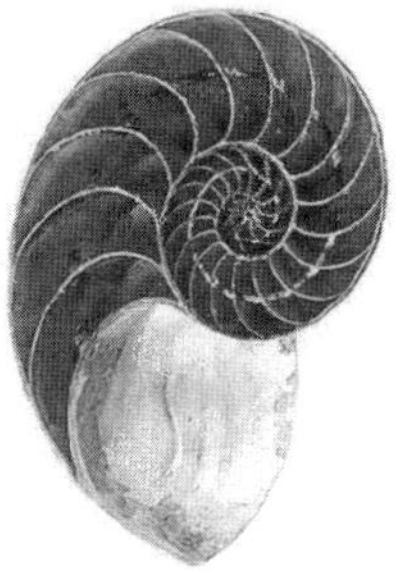

PART ONE

The Introduction

1 Introduction

- An Overview: Tongue Diagnosis
- Inspirations for this Book
- What is Ayurveda?
- The Fundamental Principles
- Signs of Health
- The Benefits of Ayurvedic Tongue Diagnosis
- Ayurvedic and Chinese Systems in Comparison

An Overview: Ayurvedic Tongue Diagnosis

The Art and Science of Ayurvedic Tongue Diagnosis

Tongue diagnosis is a vital instrument used in Ayurvedic medicine both for assessing a person's current state of health and for providing a basis for prognosis. Ayurveda, the oldest known healing modality in the world, describes tongue diagnosis as a technique to determine a person's state of physical, mental and emotional health. This diagnostic technique informs the practitioner of underlying challenges and strengths in organs and body systems. Imbalances and potential disease can be detected in their early stages, giving the person an opportunity to bring balance before disease manifests. With regular practice and guidance, one can acquire the proficiency to use the knowledge contained in this book to heal oneself and others.

While Ayurveda draws on a variety of diagnostic tools and treatments, tongue diagnosis is revered as one of the most important, especially in conjunction with pulse diagnosis. The purpose of this book is to provide you with the knowledge and understanding needed to incorporate this easy to learn yet extremely effective diagnostic tool. This book is for professionals and laypersons alike. As well as gaining a comprehensive understanding of tongue diagnosis, this book includes ancient and modern healing practices based on the Healing Tastes, Herbal Therapies and Diet.

Who Should Read This Book?

Everyone who is health conscious and concerned about their health, both in prevention and treatment, can benefit from reading this book. This information is appropriate for the layperson who wants to take charge of their own health and well-being as well as that of their families and loved ones. All health care providers: acupuncturist, herbalist, homeopath, nutritionist, naturopath, colon therapist, Iridologist, Ayurvedic practitioner, natural health care counselors and practitioners can benefit from this book.

What is Tongue Diagnosis?

The ancient art of Tongue Diagnosis may be defined as the science of the shape, shadings and markings of the tongue to describe the current state of an individual's health, as well as their inherited constitution.

Tongue diagnosis is a way of viewing inherited tendencies and illnesses that could occur, depending upon the person's lifestyle. It reveals existing disease processes and is a means of health evaluation that is accurate. While there are degrees of complexity, overall, the basis of tongue diagnosis is easy to learn. This form of diagnosis can give important information on systemic pathology and is a valuable tool for health practitioners.

An Energetic Model

Like most constitutional diagnostic techniques in Ayurvedic medicine, the knowledge, perception, and intuition of the practitioner will determine the accuracy of diagnosis. Tongue diagnosis reveals energetic as well as physical imbalances. The energetic condition of the individual is visible in the tongue's body shape and color, and a developing pathology is reflected by a change in these characteristics. Changes in the tongue can take weeks to years, giving the practitioner information about the depth and length of the illness.

The excitement and potential of tongue diagnosis stems from the thought that if the tissue integrity of the body, especially the digestive system, can be assessed by simply observing the color and structure of the tongue, then preventative steps can be taken. You can easily learn to correlate the appearance of the tongue with problems in the body long before the diseases strike.

You don't have to be a health-care professional. You don't have to be a college graduate. And you don't have to be an expert to prove to yourself the validity and the benefits of reading the tongue. The pages of this book will guide you step-by-step to the place where you, with no special equipment, other than good natural lighting or a flashlight, a simple magnifying lens or mirror, can examine yours or another's tongue and gain valuable information. How you utilize this information can be instrumental for you in attaining and maintaining health.

Studying the art and science of tongue diagnosis means learning the language of the tongue. These pages will help you to explore this fascinating territory by learning the tongue's unique landmarks and practicing the principles of diagnosis. This will give providers an inexpensive, non-invasive alternative and complementary approach to the medical model. Tongue diagnosis, as an alternative screening method, can make a significant difference to the prevention and treatment of chronic disease.

Tongue diagnosis does not stand alone. It is part of a larger family. Its close relatives are the many branches of Ayurveda 'the art of living in harmony with life'. Its marriage partner is the science of nutrition, to which it is joined for all time.

The tongue is a universal language, true of all ages, cultures and races. The tongue reveals its mysteries to those who learn the language and observe the unique patterning of each person. The language of the tongue can reveal the cause of illness so that the practitioner can act quickly and wisely with treatment protocols. The right thing at the right time is powerful medicine.

If you have ever wondered about the secrets the tongue can reveal and wanted to learn a simple diagnostic barometer to help yourself, family or incorporate into your healing practice, here it is. In part one of this book you will learn the history, tools, language and major signs of tongue diagnosis. In layman's terms, you will discover how and why it works. If you are a practitioner, you will learn tools to support your already existing practice and how to apply these tools through constitutional nutrition, herbal protocols and the healing tastes. It is my hope that this book will contribute to a deeper understanding of Ayurvedic diagnosis and nutritional medicine.

Now, let's take a closer look. Open wide and look closely in the mirror. Discover the meaning of the tongue shape, color and markings of your own unique tongue spirit. Come with me and discover how your interior life affects the tongue patterns and thus the absorption of your food, world, emotions, thoughts and life. The tongue, as a mirror of the body, reflects back to us the health and integrity of our internal state.

Inspiration for this Book

The inspiration for writing this book arose from the passion I have for my work as a student and practitioner in the natural healing arts for the last 30 years. During these years, I have integrated the healing practices of the East and the West in the understanding of nutritional medicine and Ayurvedic medicine. The 1970's saw an explosion of interest in the whole area of consciousness and healthful living, and me along with it. Since the early 1980's, when I was first exposed to Ayurvedic constitutional healing, my personal and professional journey turned to understanding the true meaning of nourishment. In Ayurvedic medicine, the understanding of constitution is the most complete system I have been exposed to. I was fascinated by the thoroughness of this approach both in dietary and lifestyle protocols.

Tongue diagnosis is about understanding nourishment and how we absorb and balance nourishment from the elemental forces of nature. The tongue lets us taste our way to health and Mother Nature gives us the best life-giving elements to do just that, through clean air, sunlight, pure water and the fertile soil.

From diagnosing an individual's constitution, we will know which healing tastes you will need to bring back good health and keep it optimal. The foods that will keep us at our peak are foods that are called Sattvic foods. These are the foods that give us life and support peace of body, mind and emotions while also supporting our environment.

In my 30 years of exploring the natural healing arts, both as a student and as a teacher, I have learned positive ways to integrate whole-food nutrition. I have evolved a deep understanding of how to select foods that support speedy recovery, maintenance and prevention. Having taught and trained thousands of students and worked with tens of thousands of patients, I have come to the conclusion, both from the Ayurvedic and modern nutritional science perspective that the closer we eat from Nature's garden the healthier and happier we become.

The tongue is an excellent indicator that we are on a healthy path for our own constitution. As I have applied these principles to myself, my loved ones and then shared them with thousands of patients and students over the years, I have observed amazing results. I continue to fine-tune my knowledge by supporting individuals to be in touch with their inner nature through harmonious living.

My deepest desire is that tongue diagnosis will support both students and practitioners in achieving a higher level of consciousness.

What is Ayurveda?

Ayurveda (pronounced eye-yer-vay-duh) is the art of healthy living, supporting a person to create harmony in body, mind, emotions and spirit. The word Ayurveda comes from Sanskrit, an ancient Indian language, and literally means *"Knowledge of Life"* or *"the Art of Conscious Living"*. Ayu means "life", and Veda, means "the knowledge of". To know about life is Ayurveda. However, to fully comprehend the vast scope of Ayurveda let us first define "Ayu", or life. According to the ancient Ayurvedic scholar Charaka, "ayu" is comprised of four essential parts - mind, body, senses and the soul. Inherent in Ayurvedic principles is the concept that you are capable of taking charge of your own life and healing. Ayurveda is a wholistic system that uses a constitutional model. Its aim is to provide guidance regarding food and lifestyle so that healthy people can stay healthy and those with health challenges can improve their health.

Ayurvedic Medicine: An Integrative Approach

A Biochemical, Bioenergetic and Biospiritual System

Ayurveda is mainly a bioenergetic and a biospiritual system. However it does integrate a biochemical understanding of healing. This is brought into the practice of understanding how foods, herbs and essential oils work in supporting healing. This is not through the way modern pharmaceuticals approach it, which isolates chemical constituents and nutrients and uses them in isolation. Through the biochemical system we can understand the natural world through different eyes. This is valuable as long as we integrate it with the bioenergetic and biospiritual approaches as well.

As a bioenergetic system, it utilizes the principles of classifying plants and herbs according to their tastes, energy, post-digestive effects and specific action (rasa-virya-vipaka-prabhava), relative to the elements that compose them. The most essential aspect is the effect of substances on the whole body, as outlined in Ayurvedic physiology according to the doshas, bodily tissues, systems and waste-materials (dosha-dhatu-mala-srotas).

In the biospiritual aspect, it classifies plants and natural substances according to the three primary qualities of Nature; Sattva (clarity), Rajas (agitation) and Tamas (darkness). It observes the effect of plants upon the mind and consciousness, and their ability to either enhance or diminish awareness. The biospiritual approach relates to ones spiritual life. Ayurveda encourages a 'Sattvic', or peaceful lifestyle and diet. The core principle in Ayurveda is to raise consciousness on every level of life.

The Art & Science of Conscious Living

Ayurveda is a systematic approach that utilizes all that nature provides to not only overcome illness but also continually strengthen oneself. Ayurveda evolved in an ancient culture that understood the human condition to be limitless. The day-to-day implementation of Ayurvedic principles creates a strong body, clarity of mind and tranquility of spirit so the individual may move closer to realizing her/his true potential.

There are several aspects to Ayurveda that are quite unique:

- Each person is regarded as unique. Food and lifestyle recommendations are determined through a constitutional model according to the person's unique constitution.
- Everything in Ayurveda is validated by observation, inquiry, direct examination and knowledge derived from the ancient texts.
- It understands that there are energetic forces that influence nature and human beings. These forces are called the Tridoshas.
- Ayurveda sees a strong connection between the mind and the body, and provides us with a huge resource of information regarding this relationship.

Ayurveda: Medicine of the Gods

The Development

Ayurveda, the oldest system of medicine in the world, traces its roots to the Vedic period in ancient India (1500 B.C.). The *Rig Veda*, a compilation of verse on the nature of existence, is the oldest surviving book of any Indo-European manuscripts (1500 B.C.). The *Rig Veda* refers to the cosmology known as Sankhya, which lies at the base of both Ayurveda and Yoga. In it are verses on the nature of health and disease, pathogenesis and principles of treatment. The *Atreya Samhita* is the oldest medical book in the world. It survived from Takashila University, which was operating as early as 800 B.C. The *Atharva Veda* (800 B.C).lists the Eight Divisions of Ayurveda: Internal Medicine, Surgery of Head and Neck, Ophthalmology and Otorinolaryngology, Surgery, Toxicology, Psychiatry, Pediatrics, Gerontology or Science of Rejuvenation, and the Science of Fertility. In 500 B.C. at the University of Benares, Sushruta, a surgeon who developed the operative techniques of rhinoplasty (plastic surgery), wrote the *Sushruta Samhita* that describes a highly developed surgery. In 100 A.D., the physician Charaka revised and supplemented the *Atreya Samhita*. The *Charaka Samhita* is a major work on internal medicine.

Influence of Ayurveda on East and West

By 400 A.D., Ayurvedic works were translated into Chinese. By 700 A.D., Chinese scholars were studying medicine in India at Nalanda University. Indian thought, as well as influencing Chinese spirituality and philosophy through Buddhism, greatly influenced Chinese medicine and herbalism. In 800 A.D., Ayurvedic works were translated into Arabic. A century later, under physicians such as Avicenna and Razi Serapion, both of whom quoted Indian texts, Islamic medicine became very influential in Europe, helping to form the foundation of the European medical tradition. In 16th century Europe, Paracelsus, who is known as the father of modern Western medicine, practiced and propagated a system of medicine that borrowed from Ayurveda.

Ayurveda Today

In the modern world, Ayurveda is becoming increasingly popular because it speaks to those elementary concepts of (1) contact with nature, (2) wholism and (3) we are what we eat. Ayurveda forms an integral part of the daily regimen of hundreds of millions of people worldwide. Its principles are utilized not only to treat persons who are ill but it also teaches how to prepare a balanced meal and to construct a harmonious environment. Ayurveda brings to life the concepts of preventive health care and health promotion. The goal of Ayurveda is to help the individual discover a personal knowledge of living.

Most people feel isolated from their own bodies and nature. We live in a world that promotes the acquisition of wealth above all else. The consequence of this path has been a separation from each other and from nature. The Vedic view is that the human condition is limitless and that we have a deep desire to realize unity with nature and the divinity within all of life and ourselves. Ayurveda holds knowledge of what nature in her generosity provides.

We are a part of nature. Just as all creatures and plants live by the Laws of Nature to create health and balance within their beings, we too must adhere to these same Laws if we desire health. Ayurveda draws on the inherent principles of nature for its foundation and guiding principles to help us maintain balance and maintain connection with the spirit of ones essential self.

Overview

The linking of the Sanskrit words ayur (life) and veda (knowledge) aptly describes the essence of this ancient Indian system of medicine. The foundations of Ayurveda lie in the meticulous observation skills of the ancients. They observed and recorded the relationship between themselves and their environment. A distinct clinical system was then formulated. Through observation and constitutional knowledge an Ayurvedic practitioner can diagnose patterns of imbalance and, hence, is able to deduce inherent strengths, weaknesses and tendencies. An Ayurvedic physician is trained in the use of diet, food preparation, breathwork, meditation and a vast herbal pharmacopoeia. Ayurveda brings to life the concepts of preventive health care and health promotion.

Ayurveda recognizes that there are three main energy processes that combine to form the universe: growth, maintenance and decay. Their actions are named anabolism, metabolism and catabolism in the western sciences. Life, light and love exemplify all these energies and are found in our environments at every moment on every level.

These energies combine in limitless ways to create the unique qualities of each individual. When you become aware of these qualities within yourself, you take the first step toward creating a healthy life. Ayurveda assists you in identifying these energies in your body and shows you how to more fully experience their gifts and to gain freedom from their limitations. By working with the body's unique nature, you are able to create true health. Ayurveda names these basic energies Vata, Pitta and Kapha – the three Doshas.

Everyday Ayurveda can assist you on this healing journey through a wise understanding of the foods you eat and how you eat them, daily practices including exercise, rest and massage, and the five-sense therapies utilizing color, aroma, taste, touch and sounds.

The Fundamental Principles

Mind, Body and Senses

We tend to identify most with our physical bodies; yet, in actuality, there is more to us than what meets the eye. We can see that underlying our physical structure is the mind, which not only controls our thought processes, but also helps assist us in carrying out day-to-day activities such as respiration, circulation, digestion and elimination. The mind and the body work in conjunction with one another to regulate our physiology. In order for the mind to act appropriately to assist the physical body, we must use our senses as information gatherers. We can think of the mind as a computer and the senses as the data that gets entered into the computer. For example, smell and taste are two important senses that aid in the digestive process. When the mind registers that a particular food is entering the gastrointestinal tract, it directs the body to act accordingly by releasing various digestive enzymes. However, if we overindulge the taste buds with too much of a certain taste, such as sweet, we may find that the ability of the mind to perceive the sweet taste is impaired; and thereby the body becomes challenged in its ability to process sweet foods. Maintaining the clarity of our senses is an essential aspect in allowing the mind-body connection to integrate and keep us healthy and happy.

Principles

Let's look at some of the principles of Ayurveda and how they might affect us.

In Ayurveda we view a person as a unique individual made up of five primary elements: Air, Fire, Water, Earth and Ether /Space. These elements have an ability to combine to create various physiological functions. Ether and Air combine to form what is known in Ayurveda as the Vata dosha. Vata governs the principle of movement and therefore can be seen as the force that directs nerve impulses, circulation, respiration and elimination. Fire and Water are the elements that combine to form the Pitta dosha. The Pitta dosha is the process of transformation or metabolism. The transformation of food into nutrients for assimilation is an example of a Pitta function. Pitta is also responsible for metabolism in the organ and tissue systems, as well as cellular metabolism. Finally, it is predominantly the Water and Earth elements that combine to form the Kapha dosha. Kapha is what is responsible for growth and adding structure unit by unit. Another function of the Kapha dosha is to offer protection. Cerebral-spinal fluid protects the brain and spinal column and is a type of Kapha found in the spinal chord. We are each made up of unique proportions of Vata, Pitta and Kapha. The ratios of the doshas vary in each individual. This accounts for the enormous diversity of individuals.

When a dosha is out of balance, Ayurveda provides us with specific lifestyle and nutritional guidelines to assist in bringing that dosha back into balance. Herbal supplements may also be suggested to hasten the healing process. If toxins in the body are abundant, Ayurveda offers a variety of cleansing treatments called Pancha Karma to eliminate these unwanted toxins.

1.1 Ayurvedic Principles

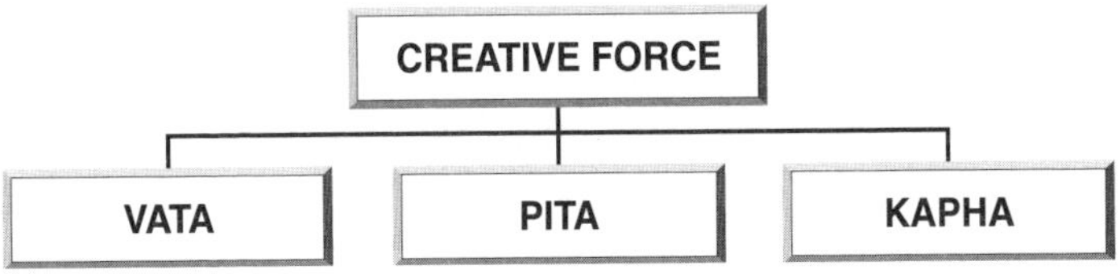

The Three Forces:

Vata the force symbolized by AIR

Pitta the force symbolized by FIRE

Kapha the force symbolized by WATER

The quality and the relative balance of these forces determine health and disease. When these forces act harmoniously, the functions of digestion, absorption and elimination (physically and mentally) create health. Since these three forces are responsible for specific areas of body / mind function, the symptoms of imbalance indicate which of these forces is deficient or excessive.

Treatment

A disease will manifest in different constitutions in different ways. An individual with a predominantly Vata constitution, for example, will experience symptoms that are different than those for Pitta or Kapha, even though they all have been diagnosed with the same disease. Constitutional treatment of the individual is a priority since the constitution helps in understanding how a particular illness will move in an individual.

Signs of Health

Ayurvedic Definition of Health

In Ayurvedic medicine, health is defined as soundness of body, mind and Spirit. Each of these must be nurtured if the individual is to create health. Ayurveda offers a wholistic approach based upon the understanding that no single agent by itself causes disease or brings health.

The following factors portray a state of health:

- Desire for nourishing food.
- Comfortable assimilation of the food eaten.
- Comfortable passing of urine and feces.
- Lightness of body after eating.
- Very favorable sensory capabilities.
- Easy and sound sleep.
- Easy awakening.
- A good source of energy, strength and endurance.
- Good complexion.
- A positive and cheerful spirit.

The objective of Ayurveda is to preserve and support health in the present and to prevent diseases from occurring in the future. If one is already suffering from a disease, Ayurveda teaches how to heal ourselves with the aim being to get to the cause.

Ayurveda advises following a daily routine, seasonal regimen, the cycles and rhythms of nature and a balanced behavior to evade the excitation of Dosha and prevent advance development of a pathogenesis.

When control or regression of the doshic disturbances takes place, the regression of cellular changes, for example, natural recession of diseases is automatic.

The Benefits of Ayurvedic Tongue Diagnosis

Assessment Benefits

Tongue diagnosis is an important health assessment tool used by many systems of traditional medicine, including Ayurvedic and Traditional Chinese medicine. At one time, both pulse and tongue assessments were important diagnostic techniques used in the Western medical tradition, particularly by the Physio-medicalist and Eclectic physicians of the late 19th century. The tongue indicates not only the state of digestion but also the health of the various organ systems.

Benefits of Tongue Diagnosis

- The greatest advantage is its value in self-diagnosis and monitoring one's state of health on a daily basis.
- The beauty of Tongue Diagnosis is in its simplicity and immediacy.
- Determines one's Unique Inherited Constitution.
- Assesses a person's current health.
- Used as an early detector for disorders in the body.
- Informs the practitioner about the underlying cause of disease.
- Is an accurate way of determining what is happening in the digestive system: liver, stomach, spleen, small and large intestines.
- Reveals the stage and progression of a particular illness.
- Shows the quality of the individual's energy production.
- Reflects the quality of the circulation of Prana, blood, bodily fluids and essence.
- Reveals the quality and balance of the five elements as revealed within the organs and overall body chemistry.

- Determines the acid-alkaline pH balance.
- Mirrors the condition of the bodily fluids, function of the organs, strengths and depth of the pathogenic factors in the body.
- Assists in determining the cause of illness.
- Reveals the emotional aspects relative to the condition.
- Pathological processes for disorders that are full of contradictions are quickly clarified.

Ayurvedic and Chinese Systems in Comparison

The Traditional Chinese Medical System (TCM) and Ayurvedic Medicine have a great deal in common. They contain a wealth of knowledge and wisdom that has been passed down for thousands of years by both traditions. These two energetic models of natural healing have many similarities when it comes to understanding tongue diagnosis. One of the greatest mysteries is why two great systems should appear simultaneously, in different corners of the world, each a unique expression, yet possessing numerous similar characteristics. Some scholars theorize that their fundamental vision and insights came about from humanity's collective unconscious. However this exchange happened, this we do know; at the very core of both of these healing traditions there is a world view that sees the deep connection between humanity and Mother Nature.

There is much knowledge that has been generously passed down to us from the ancient wise men and women. Much of the knowledge that has been translated into English on tongue diagnosis comes to us from the Chinese System. I have drawn on some of this wisdom and integrated it with Ayurveda to give you a comprehensive understanding of Tongue Diagnosis. It has been stated by teachers and authors of both traditions that perhaps one day, in the not too distant future, these two systems will more openly draw on the knowledge and wisdom of the other. It is a time of integration in our world. Let us continue to expand our borders of consciousness by including all that is available to us from the many traditions, both ancient and modern.

Both systems concentrate on the energetic aspects of physiology and value the vital aspects of life force. These systems describe the existence of pervasive life force, called Chi by the Chinese and Prana by the Ayurvedic tradition. The concept "life-force energy" includes the belief that this substance flows through subtle channels or pathways, called Meridians by the Chinese and Nadis and Srotas by the Ayurvedic model.

Another similarity in these two systems is that all life is composed of the five elements. It is the five elements that provide and maintains life and from which all tissues are derived. The primary substances in the Ayurvedic system are Life Force (Prana), Subtle Fire (Tejas) and essence (Ojas). These are seen as being pure expressions of the Five Elements within the body. From these three subtle quintessential elements comes the action of digestive and metabolic activity that creates the seven substances that maintain the body. These seven substances are lymph, blood, tissue, fat, bones, marrow and reproductive tissue. The three doshas of Vata, Pitta and Kapha are seen as the fuller expressions of the qualities of Prana, Tejas and Ojas.

Similarly, in the Chinese system the body is composed of the five basic substances called Chi, Blood, Fluids, Essence and Spirit. These are the energetic reflections of the Five Elements with each dependent upon the others. The Five Elements play an interactive and energetic role in linking substances with specific tissues, organs and structures.

Both Ayurveda and Chinese medicine utilize a Five Element model to diagnose a constitution and organize the internal terrain. In Ayurveda, the Five Elements are a way of understanding the human physiology and energetic associations and the theory of the three doshas. This is very similar to the Chinese System of Yin, Yang and Chi. Vata, which is primarily associated with the Air Element in Ayurveda, is in charge of all forms of circulation including that of Prana. This is similar to the Chinese idea of Chi. Pitta, which displays the qualities of the Fire Element corresponds to that of Yang. Kapha most closely relates to the qualities of the Element of Water and is seen in the Chinese model as Yin.

1.2 Five Element Correspondences

Radical Healing, Rudolph Ballentine, M.D. page 187

INDIAN CHINESE	EARTH EARTH	WATER WATER	FIRE FIRE	AIR METAL	ETHER WOOD
Ayurvedic Chakras	Root	Genital	Solar Plexus	Heart	Throat
Chinese Yin Organs Yang Organs	Spleen Stomach	Kidney Bladder	Heart Sm. Intestines	Lungs Lg. Intestines	Liver Gall-Bladder

Both the Ayurvedic and the Chinese system agree that disorders and illness can occur either from within the body or from the external environment the individual lives in, as well as the constitutional precipitating factors. According to Ayurveda, most illness can be traced to the weakness of the digestive fire as can be seen in tongue diagnosis. This does not have as much emphasis is Chinese medicine because this system puts more emphasis on the external climatic and endogenous organ causes for disease.

1.3 Ayurvedic AND Chinese Climatic Factors

Tao and Dharma- Svoboda and Arnie Lade, page 103

AYURVEDIC SYSTEM		CHINESE SYSTEM	
DOSHA	CLIMATIC FACTOR	SUBSTANCE	CLIMATIC FACTOR
Vata	Wind & Cold-Dryness	Chi	Wind & Dryness
Pitta	Heat & Humidity	Yang	Heat & Summer Heat
Kapha	Cold- Dampness	Yin	Cold- Dampness

In Ayurveda, physiology the three doshas are divided into five aspects each. The five aspects of Vata divide the body into five influences, similar to the Chinese system of the Triple burner. The five aspects of Pitta appear as five transformative substances and the five forms of Kapha appear as special body lubricants.

1.4 Five Forms of Vata and Triple Burner

Tao and Dharma- Svoboba and Arnie Lade, page 97

PRANA	ACTIVITY	LOCATION	BURN-ER	CHI TYPE	EFFECT
PRANA	Forward	Chest	Upper	Ancestral	Dispersion Absorption
SAMANA	Equalizing	Upper abdo-men	Middle	Nutritive	Assimilation
APANA	Downward	Lower abdomen	Lower	-----	Elimination Storage
VYANA	Pervasive	Upper	Systemic	Defensive	Protection Warmth
UPANA	Upward-moving	Head	-----	-----	-----

The forward-moving Prana, Vata, is situated between the throat and diaphragm where it takes in and circulates the life force similar to the function of the ancestral Chi within the Upper Burner in the Chinese System. The harmonizing aspect of Samana Vata is located between the diaphragm and the navel and takes care of the digestive and assimilation process similar to Nutritive Chi that's located within the Middle Burner. The Apana Vata is located in the lower trunk between the navel and diaphram and has the function of pushing things downward and out of the body similar in action and location to the Lower Burner. There is also the descending function which is specific to the Stomach's Organ Chi. The fifth, the upward-moving Udana Vata, extends from the throat to the top of the head and is the only part of this model that does not have a similar counterpart in the Chinese system.

Regarding the emotional correlation to the various organs, both models assign the same emotional effects. From an Ayurvedic perspective, imbalanced emotions will disturb the corresponding dosha; however, the manifestation of the imbalance may occur in another area of the body. In the Chinese system, specific imbalanced emotions generate directional changes in the flow of Chi, thus creating an imbalance.

One thing that both systems agree upon is that, once the healing process has been initiated, they both endeavor to retrace the causes of the disease so as to re-route the imbalanced energies through the opposite pathway.

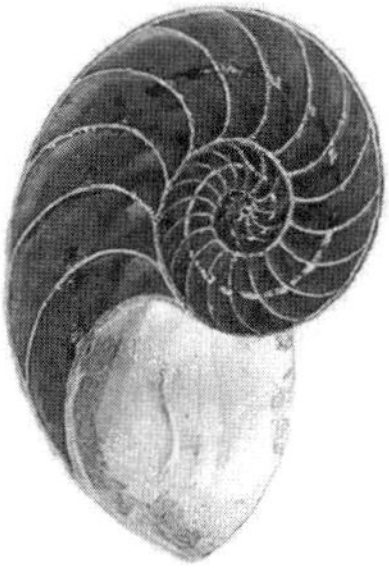

PART TWO

The Seed

The seed is the beginning. Each of us is born as a seed - this determines our constitution. The constitution that we are born with is our Prakruti. This is our baseline. Knowing what kind of seed we are helps us to know how to tend to our health in body, mind and heart. If you don't know your Prakruti it is like trying to grow a plant without knowing what kind of seed it is. How successful will you be in supporting that plant to grow to its fullest potential? You will not know what kind of soil, water or sun it needs. This is the first step on our journey of discovery, finding out what kind of seed you are. This is also the first step in constitutional tongue diagnosis.

Tongue diagnosis is one way of determining what you inherited from your family tree, your traits, tendencies and dispositions. These inherited qualities are referred to as your Prakruti constitution. The tongue body color and shape is the indicating factor for determining your Prakruti. This provides you with a map from which to start because knowing your Prakruti is knowing who you really are. It points towards your inborn gifts and tendencies, both physically and psychologically. What you do with these gifts is your choice.

Once we have determined the Prakruti constitution, you can go beyond just treating symptoms into prevention. This is the value of knowing what seed you are. To know your constitution – the unique seed that you are – gives you the advantage of understanding. With understanding comes wisdom, and with wisdom comes the ability to care for yourself and your loved ones in practical and effective ways.

2 The Constitution: Your Inherited Genetic Blueprint

The Constitution: The Seed

Constitutional Medicine Quotes

"Never regard study as a duty but as an enviable opportunity to learn to know the liberating influence of beauty in the realm of spirit for your own personal joy and to the profit of the community to which your later works belong."
— Albert Einstein

"Those who are accomplished in application, theory and knowledge of allied sciences and success of treatment are the true healers. In them is the glory of the physician fully manifested."
— Ca. Su. 11:53

"We all yearn deep within our hearts:
- to know who we are &
- why we are here."

"He who knows others is learned.
He who knows himself is wise."
— Lao Tzu

"The constitution helps us by giving us a direction in which to work, but only as long as we remember that it is not only telling us who we are, but how we have limited who we are.

Knowing your constitution is the first step. Constitutional knowledge empowers the individual to take control of their health, happiness and destiny. What you do with this knowledge is what matters".
— Lorenna Bousquet-Kacera

Understanding our constitution and its dynamics, therefore,
offers an especially potent approach to the unconscious,
To our wounds and compensations,
And ultimately,
To our healing and transformations.
— Krishnamurti

"Learn what you are and be such."
— Pindar

Tongue Diagnosis and Constitutional Understanding

According to Ayurveda, the most essential component in understanding this system of natural healing is recognizing the value of the constitution. The constitution is the foundation. It determines the core, or blueprint of the individual. The constitution is the beginning. The uniqueness of Ayurveda is that there are two constitutions, the Prakruti and the Vikruti. Prakruti represents our starting point, what we are born with, and Vikruti is where we are today.

The tongue reveals Prakruti through its body color, shape and size. Vikruti is seen more through the changeable signs, such as the tongue coating, markings and moisture.

Prakruti and Vikruti

Prakruti (hereditary factors) is the term used in Ayurveda to describe one's genetic constitution. The Prakruti indicates the specific tendencies and predispositions of tissues, organ and structural imbalances in an individual. The Prakruti also indicates the primary and secondary traits, or problem areas, that are manifesting at present and are primarily due to a person's ancestral heritage. The Vikruti may modify Prakruti inheritance, within limits.

Vikruti (environmental factors) is the term used to describe how the environmental influences have shaped who the person has become today. Some of these factors are climate, home, diet, nutrition, social life, etc. Prakruti determines the substance, which we are given to work with in our lives - physically, mentally, emotionally and spiritually. Vikruti reflects how we have used that substance.

These two complementary forces represent our outer and inner worlds and their interaction. Together they determine the quality of a person's health. When imbalance is experienced, an appropriate nutritional, cleansing and therapeutic regime can return the body to its original constitutional balance.

Prakruti: Your Permanent Constitution

> *"The basic constitution of the individual remains unaltered during the lifetime, as it is genetically determined. The combination of elements present at birth remains constant. However, the combination of elements that governs the continuous physio-pathological changes in the body alters in response to changes in the environment."*
>
> — Dr. Vasant Lad

The Seed that You Were Born As

The Five Great Elements - Air, Fire, Water, Earth and Ether - manifest in the human physiology and psyche as three fundamental bio-energies known as the three doshas. From Ether and Air comes Vata, which regulates our energies and movements. From Fire and Water comes Pitta, which gives us warmth and perception and the capacity to transform substances within our bodies. From Water and Earth comes Kapha, which makes up our structure, our flesh and secretions, and creates solidity and cohesiveness.

Through the action of the tridosha, we replicate the great Cosmic Forces in our own bodies and participate in the eternal cosmic dance of creation, maintenance and destruction. The ancient sages observed that although every individual is constituted of the three doshas, each of us inherits them in differing proportions. This accounts for our differences in appearance, preferences, aversions, behavioral patterns and emotional tendencies. The proportion of the three doshas present in an individual at birth will determine his or her essential constitution or Prakruti. Prakruti comes from two Sanskrit roots, which mean "the initial creation", or alternatively this interesting word can also mean, "to come forth into creation." It represents how we initially come into life before any deviations took place.

The Prakruti remains unchanged during the course of one's lifetime and is genetically determined. Prakruti represents the proportion of the doshas, which represents the ideal state of balance, and it serves as the goal for us to strive towards. It will manifest in us throughout our lifetimes through our physical characteristics, natural urges, likes and dislikes and psychological predilections as we have stated above. However, one's Prakruti will also determine, to a great extent, how one will develop the highest order of human qualities: love, compassion and pure consciousness. Thus, the proportion of the three doshas that a person inherits will be at the foundation of his or her experience and existence. From the perspective of the Ayurvedic physician, precise determination of the Prakruti is absolutely mandatory as the first step in formulating a course of action for each patient. Knowledge of an individual's Prakruti will instruct the physician of the following:

- Most effective means to prevent diseases from arising.
- Prognosis of both simple and complex diseases.
- The most effective treatment.
- The recuperative capacity of an individual.
- The best dietary regimen for that individual.
- How to compound herbal formulations to the best advantage.
- The most beneficial rejuvenative program.

What Determines The Prakruti

There are five factors that influence the Prakruti constitution of an individual.

1. The state of the doshas in the body of the mother and father at the time of conception is the most influential factor.

If the father has an excess of Kapha dosha, sperms, which flourish in a Kapha environment, will predominate in the ejaculate. If the mother happens to have an excess of Vata dosha at the time of intercourse her vaginal and uterine environments will produce ova with Vata-dominant energies. Thus, the resulting child will inherit a Vata-Kapha or Kapha-Vata Prakruti.

2. The mental state and intentions of the mother and father at the time of conception.

The reproductive tissues of human beings are the most highly evolved in the entire physical body and, as such, are most affected by the subtle energies of thought and emotion. Changes in the chemical environment, pH, viscosity, temperature and blood flow of the genitalia and their respective seeds will occur due to psychological effects. Sexual intercourse for pleasure (Kapha), out of "duty" (Pitta), with a stranger (Vata), out of fear (Vata), in anger (Pitta), for money (Kapha), or for any intention will have a corresponding effect on the dosha pattern in the child.

In fact, Ayurveda recommends that all couples contemplating having a baby first undergo a complete purification therapy. This would eliminate any Doshic excesses and make it more likely that the parents will be healthy during the succeeding sexual activity. Dietary regimens and restrictions are also recommended for prospective parents. Men should avail themselves of Ashwagandha root, licorice root and raisins while avoiding red meat, very spicy foods, eggplant, and cold drinks. Women should have basmati rice, sesame oil, mung dal, Amalaki and asparagus while avoiding poultry, game, red meat and garlic. Ayurveda compares the creation of a new human life to the creation of a new universe, and to maintain this perspective is an important step to preserving the sanctity of the act of sex. This can have an enormous benefit to the mental characteristics of the child.

3. The familial hereditary characteristics.

There are certain tendencies that run in families such as the tendency to obesity, tendency to athleticism or artistic or scientific aptitude. This can exert an effect on the Doshic combination of entire family trees.

4. The diet and daily activities of the mother during pregnancy.

The strange food cravings that develop during pregnancy are well documented. The predominance of one specific taste or food, (for example, sardines with vanilla ice cream seems to be popular!), can certainly influence the developing child. If the mother is working, attending school, staying home, or living with her parents during pregnancy, this will also register on the Doshic pattern of the newborn. The home climate, weather, exercise, rest and sleep patterns and recreation will similarly have an effect. Any arguments or negative emotions should be avoided if possible.

5. The conditions dominate in the uterus during pregnancy.

Any trauma to this area of the mother's body will be detrimental to the developing baby. Conversely, loving attention to the womb, such as talking to the baby, stroking and touching the area by both parents, and soothing Sattvic music can be balancing influences.

The Tridosha

The Five Elements, Air, Fire, Water, Earth and Ether (Space), can be seen to exist in the material universe at all scales, both organic and inorganic, from peas to planets. When they enter into the biology of a living organism, man for example, they acquire a biological form. According to Ayurveda, the Five Elements are coded into three biological forces that govern all life processes. These three forces are known as the three doshas, or simply, the tridosha. The tridosha regulates every physiological and psychological process in the living organism. The interplay between these three doshas determines the qualities and conditions of the individual. A harmonious state of the three doshas creates balance and health; an imbalance, which might be an excess or deficiency, manifests as a sign or symptom of disease. The three doshas are known as Vata, Pitta and Kapha.

These three doshas are the fundamental biological energies that regulate all the life processes of an individual. While everyone is made up of these same three energies, each person has them in unique proportions. The doshas obtain their qualities by virtue of their elemental composition, as we can see in the simple diagram below.

2.1 The Tridosha

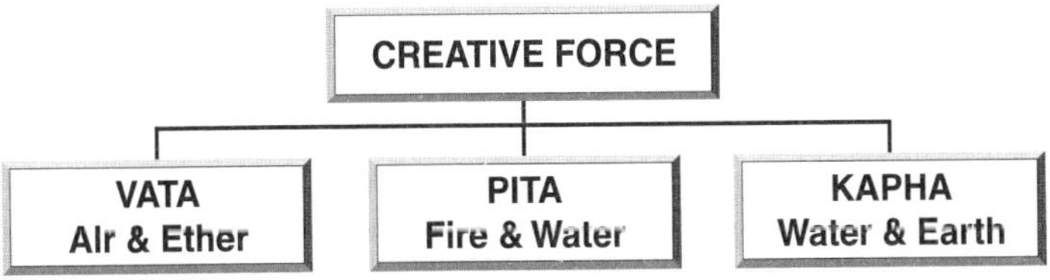

Elements Composing the Tridosha

Each of the three doshas is composed of two elements:

Vata is composed of Air and Ether

Pitta of Fire and Water

Kapha of Water and Earth

The Vata dosha has the mobility and quickness of Air and Ether; the Pitta dosha the metabolic qualities of Fire and Water and the Kapha dosha the stability and solidity of Water and Earth. When these forces are in balance we experience their life-supporting qualities; when out of balance they become agents of disease and suffering.

Your Constitutional Blueprint

Constitutional medicine is a means of determining the combination of principles or forces that determine your individuality. Your constitution reveals the blueprint outlining the innate tendencies that have been built into your system. It shows functional habits of the body as determined by the genetic endowment of the individual and modified by environmental factors. It reveals your uniqueness and your hidden potentials, your challenges and lessons along with your gifts. Your personality, body and mind are direct reflections of your constitution.

The ratio of the Elements in a person's constitution and the qualities expressed by them are as unique to the individual as is one's fingerprint. The degree to which the Elements interact with one another is what gives a person their unique characteristics. Everything is composed of antagonistic and complementary factors and everything operates due to the change of relationships between these opposing factors and tendencies. Human physical and mental manifestations are also constituted and function according to these factors and tendencies. A person's constitution stays the same throughout their life. This is, however, not a static event, as there is a constant ebb and flow of the elements. This flow is governed by physio-psychological and personal choice.

The ancient wisdom of constitutional medicine provides specific guidelines to help us identify our constitutional nature. Knowing your constitution is the first step to anticipating the type of disorders and imbalances that can create disease. Equally, this knowledge enables you to adjust your life to maintain health.

> *"In the constitution, one has inherited something that is unassimilated, conflicting or unresolved from past generations. This can serve as an obstacle or as a stimulus to greater effort and a new possibility of achievement. We must recognize constitutional tendencies as focal points we should not wish to do without; they are signposts on the road to healing that we cannot evade. They direct us toward the unfinished business of past generations."*
>
> — Harri Wolf "The Iris and the Constitution"

Ayurvedic Constitutional Medicine

The concept of constitutional medicine is the main framework of most ancient and modern healing modalities. As mentioned, each person has an inborn genetic code, the constitution, which sets physical, emotional and mental patterns. The constitution determines one's susceptibility to certain diseases, the patterns and the course that these diseases will most likely follow, the complications that may arise and the prognosis of the disease. An individual's inborn constitution, or Prakruti, determines how that individual will instinctively react when exposed to a stimulus. The constitution helps us to understand and explain responses to treatments. Constitution indicates which foods, medicines and lifestyle will keep the individual healthy.

Constitution - The Beginning

> *"The basic constitution of the individual remains unaltered during the lifetime, as it is genetically determined. The combination of elements present at birth remains constant. However, the combination of elements that governs the continuous psycho-pathological changes in the body alters in response to changes in the environment."*
>
> — Dr. Vasant Lad

Your Prakruti is determined by:

- The parents and ancestral conditions.
- The quality of the reproductive cells.
- The condition of the uterus.
- The date of conception and birth.
- The place of birth and growing up.
- The dietary and nutritional intake of the mother both during and after pregnancy.
- Emotional and mental influences of the parents during the pregnancy period.
- The present lifestyle, family, social and cultural influences.
- Environmental conditions.
- The five elements that make up the fetus.

Prakruti is derived from particular combinations and permutations of the five elements in the sperm and ovum at the time of conception. While we may be influenced by our culture, society, and environment, our basic nature is established from the interlacing of the elements. Once the elements have made their imprint, we cannot alter it to suit our needs without adversely affecting our well-being. The life-giving elements are at the very core of our numinous nature. They are the organizing forces that maintain or disrupt health.

We are composed of a constitutional inheritance with the

strengths and weaknesses of our ancestors. While we cannot change our Prakruti, we can, through healthful living, alter genetically inherited effects and transform the cycle of genetics so as to not pass the same patterns onto our children.

HEREDITARY INFLUENCES

Our genetic composition is pulled together from a familial gene pool that reaches back for generations. What a person is today is rooted in their past, but it is our parents who have the greatest influence on our own constitutional makeup. The ancient Hindus likened one's mother to the earth and one's father to the seed, symbolically demonstrating the beautiful and essential role of each parent.

A disease does not run in a family, an inherent trait does. However, a disposition or an inherent trait does not necessarily have to pass from generation to generation. Through purification and regeneration processes one can rise above the influence of constitution.

An inherent disposition or trait is not a disease; it is an expression of our uniqueness and shows our potentials. If we learn to see it as an opportunity rather than an obstacle, or as a challenge that can raise us to a higher level of functioning, then it can guide us to reach our fullest potential.

Environmental Factors

Dr. Bernard Aschner states that:

> *"The constitution is a genetically programmed state which may be modified by environmental influences acting on the individual by his reaction to these influences."*

There are numerous environmental factors that can contribute to disease. Our genetic makeup is definitely affected by the effects of acid rain, the burn of the sun, harmful pesticides, industrial fumes and drugs. Alcohol and smoking, two common drugs used in society today, have been linked to harmfully affecting the genetic structure of an unborn child. There are now thousands of chemicals, herbicides and pesticides released into the atmosphere that our bodies don't know how to deal with. Pollutants affect the air we breathe and the soil in which we grow our food. Commercial processing and packaging devitalize the foods we eat resulting in toxicity and chemical imbalances in the body.

It is important to understand how the environment can alter or enhance one's genetic material. For instance, 1,000 meters above sea level metabolism speeds up and thyroid function improves. The differences of climate, altitude, geography, soil and mineral composition, wind patterns, water quality, etc., molds a person's physical, mental and emotional traits to such an extent that, over time, we see many races and ethnic groups being formed.

What is Ayurvedic Constitutional Medicine?

Simply put, understanding one's constitution is a means of determining what one is born with and the combination of principles or forces that determine individuality. Constitution reveals the blueprint outlining the innate tendencies that have been built into a person's system. It shows functional habits of the body as determined by the genetic endowment of the individual and modified by environmental factors. It reveals uniqueness and hidden potentials, challenges and lessons along with gifts. One's personality, body and mind are direct reflections of one's constitution.

Dorland's medical dictionary defines constitution as:

> *"The makeup or functional habit of the body determined by the genetic, biochemical and physiological endow of the individual and modified in great measure by environmental factors."*

Taber's Medical Dictionary defines constitution as:

> *"the physical makeup and functional habits of the body."*

A constitutional disease is defined as:

> *"one that is dependent upon an individual's hereditary make up."*

According to European Iridology, Dr. Josef Deck, one of the world's most respected authors on the subject of Constitutional Iridology:

> *"The constitution is the product of the creative principle of the soul as a unit of existence: anima + animus = corpus (female + male = body)." -statement written in 1936 by Dr. Deck*

"The constitution is a product of somatic, psychic, manifest or latent characteristics which are a result of endogenous factors (mostly hereditary) and which decide and regulate the ontogenetic development." - *statement written in 1956 by Dr. Deck*

Another definition by Harri Wolf's in his book *Iridology: A Modern Perspective, Vol. II* says:

"Human constitution is the totality of physiological, emotional, and mental properties that function to keep everything in a balanced order to help the individual merge with the surrounding activities."

Our present health status is conditioned by the effects of external events upon the "Constants of the Constitution," or "Constitutional Terrain." Since the external factors are a continuous influence, it is most advisable to discover and acknowledge our potential challenges and gifts. This places the individual in a position to maneuver around environmental influences.

According to Ayurveda, every person's ultimate nature is both unified and whole. While the elements and doshas help us to grasp the concept of self, it is understood that the individual is much more than body type. Constitutional medicine provides guidelines to identify our innate nature so that we may use this wisdom to better ourselves and reach fulfillment.

2.2 Elements of the Three Doshas

VATA	PITA	KAPHA
Ether + Air	Fire + Water	Earth + Water

As a general rule, the strongest element in a person's constitution has the highest tendency of increasing; therefore, that person will be most susceptible to illnesses associated with an increase of that element.

The outstanding homeopath, Grauvogel, empathically claims "acute diseases run their course in the track marked out by the bodily constitutions". Our dominant miasm (inherited traits from ancestral disease) waits for stress, shock or fatigue to lower immune resistance so that it can rise up and pull us down.

> *"In the constitution, one has inherited something that is unassimilated, conflicting or unresolved from past generations. This can serve as an obstacle or as a stimulus to greater effort and a new possibility of achievement. We must recognize constitutional tendencies as focal points we should not wish to do without; they are signposts on the road to healing that we cannot evade. They direct us toward the unfinished business of past generations."*
>
> — Harri Wolf "The Iris and the Constitution"

We are born into this world with an innate constitution. What we do with what we have is totally up to us. Knowing our constitution is like a gardener knowing the seed he is planting so that he can best determine the type of soil and nutrients to use so the seed can grow to its fullest potential. Constitutional knowledge informs us of which cleansing regimes would be best for us, which organs and systems need most attention, what fuel the body uses most efficiently and what the maximum speed our bodies and minds are able to run at. In other words, constitution is our source book for health, vitality and well being. In Ayurvedic medicine, the main focus is to recognize and understand the essence of temperament and physiology, the basic ways individuals relate to their environment and deal with life. Meeting one's physical and psychological needs assures good health and peace of mind, offering informed choices regarding the health care methods that are most appropriate.

> *"In constitutional medicine the aim is to understand the unique, individual flow of internal energy resulting from the merger of physical and mental energetic patterns."*
>
> — Harri Wolf

Ayurveda does not work on a symptomatic level, but rather goes to the root cause of a disorder. The purpose is to bring each individual to his or her natural harmonious self. To only treat the disease disregards the very foundation of constitutional Ayurveda, which works on the basis of preventative medicine.

"Will supersedes structure." What this means is that, at some point in life, there may be a conflict between a requirement to adapt and the individual's constitutional ability to meet the challenge. Our constitutional tendencies can be interpreted with a positive and encouraging outlook without sacrificing acknowledgment and an understanding of the person's restrictions and limitations.

Advantages of Ayurvedic Medicine

1. The seeds of disease are sown early. Even young children are prone to hay fever, asthma, obesity, chronic disorders and skin problems, to name a few. At an early age when incipient disease is easiest to treat and prevent, symptoms are usually difficult to read. By understanding one's genetic blueprint, preventative steps can be taken at a time when they will have the best long-term effect.
2. Constitutional typing makes prevention more specific. Understanding the constitution can help create a program to prevent genetically inherited conditions from arising.
3. Knowing your constitution makes treatment more specific once an illness appears. Generalization treatment is a hit-and-miss form of therapy. It assumes that a given disease is the same in all people. Constitutional typing helps us to identify the genetic disadvantages within the individual. Ten people may suffer from a similar disease. The cause, however, may be totally different in each case. According to your constitution, an accurate treatment can be pinpointed.
4. Constitutional medicine is not overly concerned with the symptoms of disease but rather with eliminating the imbalance in the doshas that is causing the symptoms. The main advantage is that the health achieved through balancing the constitution is permanent and will often eliminate other seemingly unrelated symptoms or illnesses.
5. With the constitutional system, you are diagnosed and treated as an individual. In other words, you are treated according to your personal needs rather than as a percentage. The knowledge you learn helps you to take control of your health. This is the best insurance against illness.
6. Constitutional diagnosing is inexpensive and relatively easy to learn. It is completely non-invasive to the body and reveals

the interrelationship of body, mind and spirit.

7. Constitutional medicine values the senses of sight, smell, sound, taste and touch as valuable diagnostic tools. Constitutional Ayurveda is a medical system that still trusts the human senses. It's through our senses that we experience the world around us, so the more awakened the senses are, the more alive we feel.
8. Ayurvedic Medicine is a natural, holistic medical system encompassing the whole person from the physical to the spiritual. A core philosophy is the idea that the universe, as macrocosm, and man, as microcosm, are directly related. They reflect one another, and one is always present in the other.
9. Knowledge of our inherited constitution is essential to the experience of enlightenment.

"Remaining stable in one's own state of being, the soul (Purusha) perceives the nature (Prakruti) as the witness observer."
— San. Ka. 65

Constitutional Nature

"We live in a soft, vulnerable, transparent body. The world within, in all its pulsing, vibrant tapestry of dynamic action, the living, chemistry in motion, the miraculous processes of cellar metabolism, and the waves of absorption and elimination, harbors so much life, so much energy and so much power. This body that we live in is a miracle. It is the temple of our life and our spirit, our home while we are in this world. It is truly the crown of creation.

We have this incredible opportunity to discover the world within the body in which we live. We can understand it. We can listen to it. We can give it what it needs. We can work with it instead of against it. We can treasure and protect our inheritance, making the most of what we have, instead of wasting it and waking up to the cold realities of ill and weakness only when it is too late. This heightened consciousness and respect will not only help us to appreciate the body we have been given, but it will encourage respect and responsibility towards the world of nature in which we live and the forces which nourish and protect us."

-Farida Sharon "Iridology"

Like the environment, our bodies have numerous different climates. These are referred to as our constitution, indicating general function of reactive patterns.

"...disease in general is due to some basic error in our constitution...to discover the wrong within ourselves, work to eradicate this fault by developing the virtue which will destroy it, not by fighting wrong, but by bringing in such a flow of its opposing virtue that it will be swept from our nature."

— Dr. Edward Bach, "Heal Thyself"

The true goal or vision of Constitutional Medicine is to break from the disease orientation of various medical models and to address each individual's search for personal growth, well being and transpersonal assessment. It seeks to understand the unique, individual flow of internal energy resulting from the merger of physical and mental energetic patterns.

A patient receiving a consultation is given the understanding of their constitutional type and how their body proceeds towards disease. The foundational level of treatment should activate all the eliminative channels (bowel, skin, lungs and kidneys). By maintaining a fluid system, stagnation of impurities and toxins will not develop and cause disease. Constitutional knowledge combined with treatment of body systems and organs will manifest into a healthier, happier organism.

We all need to know how to take charge of our own body to stay healthy. As more of us take responsibility for our health, we support the industry of "wellness." In this day and age, the body does not need to be a mystery; a miracle, yes always, but not a mystery. Enlightenment is all around us waiting to be tapped into. By living consciously and treating our body with utmost respect and love, we recognize it as the sacred temple for our life; it is, after all, the only body we have. Constitutional medicine can provide us with the keys for preventing diseases from developing and also the means of reaching higher levels of consciousness and health.

Constitutional Understanding - Microcosm Holding Macrocosm

> *"Everything that exists in the external universe has its counterpart in the internal universe of the human body."*

The Law of the Macrocosm and Microcosm states that every natural force and object, the elements, the sun, moon, stars, the whole universe, is present in the body in a modified form. This is the reason why even the most insignificant of disturbances in the external cosmos will induce a like disturbance internally in the body.

> *"If there is to be health, the vibratory conditions of the organism must be in harmony with nature's established harmonic relations in the physical, mental and psychical realms of human life and action. Everything that is to be normal, natural, healthy, good, beautiful, must vibrate in unison with its correlated harmonics in nature."*
>
> — Dr. Henry Lindlahr's Vol. I of "Natural Therapeutics"

How these two forces interrelate and how the part affects the whole is a concept that is in all fields of science, medicine, psychology, ecology and religion. This concept is essential if we are to survive and preserve the balance of nature so that we can, not only avoid catastrophe, but also maintain quality of life.

"Everything affects everything else" is one of the laws of nature. Every part of our body has an affect on the function of the whole body. Treatment needs to address the whole person. Treatment may start with one specific area of need but must then work towards the whole. Our body is constantly transforming and adjusting to maintain harmony between inner and outer ecology. When treating an individual, their total lifestyle must be considered in order to create total health.

By attuning ourselves to the laws of nature we reawaken the instinctive knowledge of what is true and right. Then, and only then, can we uphold universal truths through our own effort, discipline and a loving desire for following the "path of heart."

> *"These highest and purest attainments of the human soul are*

not the results of mere physical well being, but of the peace and harmony which come only through obedience to natural law."
— Dr. Henry Lindlhr's Vol. 1 of "Natural Therapeutics"

Fruit of Our Past Actions - Seeds of Our Future

The seeds of our future are held in the actions of our present and our past. This means that each of us has the freedom to create our future. Through conscious living, we have a choice to break free from identification with disease patterns from our past and recreate new ways of being in life. This may not always be easy, but, with desire and the application of knowledge, it is possible. Direct change for the future can take place when we empower ourselves to take charge of the present. We have the ability and opportunity to transform the present by clearing the past and creating new causes for the future.

"No knowledge is perfect unless it includes an understanding of the origin - that is, the beginning; and as all man's diseases originate in his constitution, it is necessary that his constitution should be known if we wish to know his disease."
— Paracelsus

Inner Ecology and Outer Ecology

Our constitution reveals to us where we've come from and what is taking place within us now. Health is not static, just as the elements in nature are not static. Just as the elements of nature manifest through winds, rains, earthquakes, volcanoes and gentle summer days, we can see how the elements manifest in our own organism. A constitutional health practitioner is really an interior ecologist, determining the excesses, deficiency and probable movement of the elements in our bodies. When the elements are dancing in harmony, the body will take care of illness. We are a beautiful expression of nature. When we live in accordance with nature's laws, we know abundance.

2.3 Constitutional Vitality – The Fabric of Life: The Elemental Forces

What creates vitality and what creates disease? The following factors contribute in creating disease in our bodies:

Earth	Poor nutrition, inorganic minerals, improper eating habits, pesticides, drugs, chemicals
Water	Water contaminates, chemical poisoning, pollution in swimming pools, lakes and oceans
Fire	Alcohol, shock, trauma, radiation, toxins, denatured foods, lack of passion and exercise
Air	Extreme emotions, mental obsessions, depression, extreme anxiety, poor breathing and air
Ether	Vaccines, famine or war, deprivation during poverty, sedentary living, lacking spirituality

The following factors support constitutional vitality:

Earth	Organic food, nutrition, herbs, spices, natural minerals, vitamins and supplements
Water	Pure spring water, fresh juices, bathing in clean springs, lakes and oceans, purification
Fire	Digestive enzymes in fermented foods, passion, love, joy and positive emotions for all life
Air	Deep breathing, fresh air, positive thoughts, accepting life's ups and downs, holistic medicine
Ether	Purity, simplicity, attitudes of mind and spirit, balanced and natural living, love of spirit

Constitution: The Nutritional View

We are today what we ate and absorbed yesterday. The body is molded by the food we eat. Whatever we choose to eat today will build a certain kind of body and mind. Understanding an individual's chemical, mental and physical constitution avoids the guessing games, experimentation and side effects that occur from an improper diagnosis and treatment plan.

How do we select the best natural treatment program? Why is it that one individual can thrive on stressful challenges whereas another individual can't? Why can one person smoke and abuse their body and suffer no noticeable symptoms, whereas another person would develop bronchitis, emphysema or even cancer? Why is it that a particular virus produces a disease in one individual but not in another? The answer is simple; we are all unique. Each of us has different physical and emotional qualities. The virus or germ is not the determining factor in the disease; the determining factor is you, your constitution and the state of your immune system at that particular time. Once again, if you know your constitution you will know the appropriate course of action to take.

Vital Principles of Constitutional Medicine

The science of constitutional medicine can assist practitioners in the natural healing arts as well as conventional medical practitioners. No other analytical method offers such an immediate, practical and reliable means of determining the genotype and predisposition of an individual. No other approach lends itself as well to the goal of prevention.

The desire is to identify problems as early as possible to allow for minimal therapeutic intervention. The ultimate goal of every health professional should be:

1. To use minimum therapeutic intervention to restore the health of the patient.
2. To educate the patient in preventative health care practices.

Conclusion

Ayurvedic Constitutional Medicine has sustained the test of time providing mankind with an approach that allows the individual the opportunity to fulfill his or her goals and destiny. Its teachings go well beyond physical health and it recognizes that a human's destiny is rooted in their spiritual evolution. The practice of Constitutional Medicine is not a path of selfish pursuit for pleasure, wealth or fame. The true path is of service, healing, knowledge and liberation for all.

This knowledge that has been passed forward to us from our ancestors is given to us as a gift. What we do with this gift is up to us. We have, in this model of healing, everything we need to live our lives in perfect and absolute harmony with all of life.

2.4 Constitution Chart

This chart, in combination with tongue diagnosis, will help you to determine your constitution. The table below has been adapted from *Ayurvedic Healing* - Dr. David Frawley and *Ayurveda: Life, Health and Longevity* - Dr. Robert Svoboda.

Attributes	**Vata**	**Pitta**	**Kapha**
Built/frame	Thin, tall, short	Medium	Stout, broad, heavy
Weight	Hard to gain, low	Moderate	Gains easily, heavy
Skin	Thin, dry, tans deeply, cold, rough	Light, freckles, acne, warm, sunburns easily	Soft, smooth, cold, thick, medium tan
Complexion	Dull, dark	Red, flushed	White, pale
Hair	Dry, coarse, wavy, dark, scanty	Fine, gray or goes bald easily, straight, soft	Oily, luctrous, brown, thick
Head	Small	Moderate	Large
Forehead	Small, narrow	Moderate with folds	Large
Eyes	Unsteady, small dull	Piercing, medium	Wide, watery
Eye color	Violet, gray tones	Green, blue, hazel	Brown or blue
Eyebrows	Fine, thin	Moderate	Thick, bushy
Eyelashes	Dry, firm, short	Short, thin, fine	Long, thick
Nose	Small, crooked, thin	Medium	Oily, thick, big
Lips	Thin, small, dry	Soft, red, medium	Thick, firm, large
Teeth and gums	Small, crooked	Medium, pink, bleeds easily	Thick, firm, large
Shoulders	Thin, small	Medium	Broad, firm
Chest	Narrow, small	Medium	Broad, firm
Arms	Thin, small	Medium	Well developed, thick
Hands, feet and joint	Small, dry, cold, thin	Warm, medium	Large, firm

Attributes	Vata	Pitta	Kapha
Calves	Small	Loose, soft	Round, firm
Nails	Small, dry, rough	Soft, pink	Thick, smooth, white
Urine and feces	Erratic, colorless, gas, constipation	Regular, loose motion, burning sensation	Slow, whitish, solid, mucus in stool
Sweat/body odor	No smell	Strong body scent	Cold, pleasant smell
Appetite	Variable	Medium	Regular
Energy/ stamina	Poor, over exert	Medium	Good, under exert
Voice/ speech	Low, weak/quick, erratic, talkative	High, sharp/ argumentative	Pleasant, good tone, slow, not talkative
Weather	Likes warm	Likes cool	Likes seasons
Mental	Quick, indecisive	Intelligent, critical	Slow, emotional
Memory	Poor, learns easily but forgets quickly	Sharp, good memory	Learns slowly & forgets slowly
Emotions	Fearful, nervous	Irritable	Calm, sentimental
Sleep	Variable, often light	Moderate	Deep
Faith	Erratic	Determined	Constant
Dreams	Restless, nightmares	Colorful, passion	few dreams
Sex drive	Variable	Intense	Steady
Resistance to disease	Poor	Medium	Good
Disease tendency	Nervous system, mental, arthritis	Infections, inflammatory	Respiratory
Side effects of medications	Quick, nervous reaction	Medium	Slow, reacts to high doses usually
Pulse	Rapid, irregular	Moderate	Deep, slow or steady

A person can be a combination of two humors with one predominating.

Understanding Your Constitution and Your Current Condition

In counseling, two specific aspects of your health are paid especially close attention to: your constitution, Prakruti and your present condition, Vikruti.

Your Prakruti constitution is what you were born with and primarily refers to your physical make up. Your parents' genetic contribution, the season in which you were born, the geographical and environmental conditions you were surrounded by during pregnancy and, particularly, the quality of the food your mother ate while pregnant are the primary influences on your constitution. In addition, the quality of your parents' relationship immediately preceding conception, as well as during the entire pregnancy, and the parents' individual mental and emotional health during pregnancy, significantly influenced the development of your constitution.

Although most of the constitutional characteristics are established during utero, the development of the constitution does not end at birth. The constitution continues to be established until approximately the age of five. The food most regularly eaten during the first years after birth and the early childhood environment are the main factors contributing to the further development of the constitution.

A person's constitution can range from strong or resilient to delicate. This does not mean "good" or "bad." It depends entirely upon how one cares for oneself.

The benefit of a resilient constitution is that it provides one with a deep inner reserve of energy. This can be drawn upon in times of illness and used for recovery. The drawback to a hardy constitution is that often these people do not take the time to listen to their body's messages. They often push through life, overworking, overeating, over-doing until it is too late and the body collapses with illness. People with resilient constitutions often have great difficulty accepting the challenges of illness or dietary changes because they have usually been very strong and hard working. They have generally lived with a "damn the torpedoes, full speed ahead" attitude. The resilient constitution is truly wonderful, but it can be accompanied by an open or hidden arrogance that says, "I'm as strong as an ox; I can eat, drink and do whatever I choose to."

The obvious drawback to a delicate constitution is that the individual may not have deep reserves of physical energy to draw on in times of need. However, on the positive side, individuals with delicate constitutions often outlive those with resilient constitutions because they usually come to terms with their physical limits earlier in life. They learn to listen to their bodies and take care of themselves. They often cultivate a deeper spiritual reserve since they may have had to deal with illness and physical weakness. This has given many of them a stronger will and sometimes a wider view of life than those with very a hardy constitution.

What Does All This Mean?

Generally, if a person has a resilient constitution, health is easier to establish or recover and maintain. However, as is typical of those with resilient constitutions, they may not see the real need or value of taking the time and effort to make changes in their lifestyle and food choices. On the other hand, they may very well be the kind of person who can use their strong qualities to quickly change and make choices that will support them in the long run.

The delicate constitution will have a few more challenges in establishing and maintaining their physical health. They may have to be more careful and more aware of how to eat and live. Over time they can create lasting health. A delicate constitution doesn't mean a delicate personal character. They may discover deep resources of spirit as a result of their challenges.

Keep in mind that the constitution is like the structure of a building, once it has been built, it doesn't change much over the years. The tenants may change, paint color, rugs, windows, etc., may change, but the structure of a building stays the same. Your Prakruti does not change. What you have at birth in the form of your physical constitution is pretty well in place - this is your seed.

Current Vikruti Condition

On the other hand, conditions and circumstances in life change from day to day. This is our Vikruti. Some days we feel good, other days tired. Some days we are ill, other days healthy. The condition is constantly changing because the factors that influence our condition are also constantly changing.

Here are the main factors that influence our day-to-day condition:

- Blood quality
- Acid or alkaline state of your body fluids
- Weather conditions
- Climate / Season
- Geographical location
- Atmospheric conditions
- Environmental conditions
- Internal energy circulation
- Social surroundings
- Current housing
- Breathing pattern
- Past and present eating and drinking patterns
- Education / Family / Parents
- Work / Career
- Physical and mental activity
- Personal happiness

Blood Quality

The quality of our blood is the main factor affecting our day-to-day energy and internal physical condition. Fortunately, blood quality is one thing over which we do have control. Through a healthy, vital diet we can control our blood quality; from our blood all of the rest of our body is produced. All of our cells are created from blood and these cells gather to form tissue and tissue gathers to form organs. Out of blood, cells, tissue and organs comes our overall physical condition; from our overall physical condition our moods, emotions, thoughts, judging ability, mental state and behaviors emerge.

The Ayurvedic constitutional view is that to change cells, tissue, organs, overall physical conditions, moods, thoughts, behavior, etc., we have to go back to their source, the blood, and change it. In order to change the blood, we have to go back to the blood's source, our daily food.

Daily Food - Blood Quality

Changing our daily food will do more than anything else to change the quality of our blood.

The life of a red blood cell is 120 days. What we eat and drink today will determine the quality of our blood for the next 120 days. If our food choices are poor: cells, tissue, organs, bones, nerves, hormones, immunity, endocrine glands, internal functions, moods, thoughts, emotions, behavior, attitude, etc., blood and therefore health declines. Of course, if our food choices are healthy, the opposite happens.

From a constitutional view, the main factors determining our blood quality are as follows:

- pH: blood acidity or alkalinity
- Na (sodium) / K (potassium) mineral balance
- Blood sugar balance
- Water balance
- Healthy functioning of the stomach
- Healthy functioning of the small intestine
- Healthy functioning of the liver
- Healthy functioning of the spleen

Current and Recurring Physical Signs

Listed below are just a few of the ways that a current condition expresses itself physically and psychological. Each person's unique condition will reveal itself in ways that are specific to that person:

Physically

- Changes in normal urination
- Functions of elimination
- Infections

- Weak immune function
- Fevers
- Headaches
- Weight gain
- Level of vitality
- Great appetite or no appetite
- Fatigue
- Skin troubles
- Congestion
- Vision problems
- Rashes, warts, moles, calluses

Psychological

- Mood
- Attitude
- Quality of relationships
- Social skills
- Emotional expression
- Thoughts
- Treatment of others
- Obsessions and phobias

The current Vikruti state is an expression of the physical and psychological harmony or disharmony present in a person's life. It is an expression of excess, deficiency or stagnation. The condition reveals the current internal environment of the blood, other body fluids, cells, nervous system, tissue, organs and the mind. By understanding the current condition, we can determine what actions and choices are necessary to properly practice an Ayurvedic lifestyle in order to re-balance the condition.

The Twenty Attributes

To fully understand the constitution of an individual we need to take a look at what is called the twenty attributes. These twenty main attributes, or ten pairs of opposites, are a way of describing the seed and its make-up. It is also a way of understanding the terrain or the soil that the seed is growing in, which we will explore in the next section.

According to Ayurveda, these attributes are the fundamental qualities. They are positive and negative, the yin and yang of all forces of the universe. They are the basis for the properties of all objects in nature both material and mental. We experience everything through these ten pairs of fundamental qualities. These attributes are also called Gunas.

Ayurveda recognizes the whole universe, both the internal and external, as a manifestation of opposites. In this way, it is possible to understand the universe in terms of the interactions of opposing forces that manifest as the basic attributes.

Understanding the attributes is essential for creating healing and preventative protocols based on the action and reaction of the twenty qualities to and upon one another. If a person repetitively takes substances with qualities that are opposite to those in their body, these opposite qualities will become dominant and result in illness.

The relationship between a pair of qualities is the basis of two of Ayurveda's fundamental rules. These principles are a key to healing with Ayurveda.

These qualities are found in the world around us and in our bodies. Today's weather may feel light or heavy, liquid or dry, mobile (windy) or stable, hot or cold, cloudy or clear. The food we eat can be comprised of a number of these qualities. Ice-cold tea for example, is wet, cold, soft and liquid. Our skin may be oily or dry, rough or smooth. Our moods, too, can be heavy or light, cloudy or clear; our mind quiet and stable, slow or sharp, mobile and hyperactive, clear or cloudy. We are constantly affected by changes in these qualities. Cold, windy, clear, dry weather aggravates Vata dosha and may lead to colds and any number of Vata ailments such as insomnia, constipation or arthritis. Hot, humid weather aggravates Pitta and may lead to outbreaks of irritation and anger as well as physical complaints like acne, eczema or skin rashes. Cloudy, gray, humid or rainy weather can aggravate Kapha, leading to colds and coughs, depression, lethargy, overeating, oversleeping and weight gain.

When an imbalance has manifested, successful treatment

requires increasing opposite qualities. For example, if there is too much heat such as excess Pitta, a cool drink, a swim or some herbs with cooling properties will greatly help pacify Pitta and reduce the heat. A person suffering from too much heat will not be helped by being active in the sun, eating spicy foods or taking a hot shower. Similarly, if you are cold and shivering from exposure to cold windy weather, have a bowl of warm soup, wrap up in a blanket or take a hot bath. These simple remedies immediately make sense to us because they are so natural.

Ayurvedic practitioners have carefully observed nature and located these qualities within all things, both organic and inorganic. Ayurvedic treatment consists, to a great extent, in identifying a person's disorder in terms of these qualities and setting right any imbalances.

How is this done? In general terms, excessive dryness in the body such as constipation, dry skin, emaciation, etc., is frequently associated with aggravated Vata. Excessive heat, burning urine, irritated eyes, fever, inflammation, anger or a critical attitude is associated with aggravated Pitta. Undue heaviness, lethargy, overweight, congestion and excess mucus is associated with unbalanced Kapha. Once you have an understanding of which dosha is out of balance and the corresponding attribute, it is a matter of making some simple adjustments to your lifestyle diet, exercise, etc., and balance will be restored.

2.5 Principles of the 20 Attributes

Like increases like.
A quality is decreased by its opposite quality

The first column of the attributes relates to the water element and is more contracting in nature. The second column relates to the fire element and is more expansive in nature.

1. COLD / HOT
2. WET / DRY
3. HEAVY / LIGHT
4. GROSS / SUBTLE
5. DENSE / FLOWING

6. STATIC / MOBILE
7. DULL / SHARP
8. SOFT / HARD
9. SMOOTH / ROUGH
10. CLEAR / CLOUDY

COLD relates to all elements except Fire increases Kapha and Vata decreases Pitta	HOT relates to Fire increases Pitta decreases Kapha and Vata
WET relates to Water increases Kapha decreases Vata	DRY relates to Air increases Vata decreases Kapha
HEAVY relates to Earth & Water increases Kapha decreases Vata	LIGHT relates to Fire, Air & Ether increases Vata and Pitta (slightly) decreases Kapha
GROSS relates to Earth & Water increases Kapha decreases Vata and Pitta (slightly)	SUBTLE relates to Fire, Air & Ether increases Vata and Pitta (slightly) decreases Kapha
DENSE relates to Earth increases Kapha decreases Vata and Pitta	FLOWING relates to Water & Fire increases Pitta decreases Vata and Kapha
STATIC relates to Earth & Water increases Kapha decreases Vata and Pitta	MOBILE relates to Air & Fire increases Vata and Pitta decreases Kapha
DULL relates to Earth & Water increases Kapha decreases Vata and Pitta	SHARP relates to Fire, Air & Water increases Pitta and Vata decreases Kapha
SOFT relates to Water increases Kapha and Pitta decreases Vata	HARD relates to Air & Ether increases Vata decreases Pitta and Kapha
SMOOTH relates to Water increases Kapha and Pitta decreases Vata	ROUGH relates to Air & Earth increases Vata decreases Kapha and Pitta
CLOUDY/DARK relates to Water & Earth increases Kapha decreases Vata and Pitta	CLEAR/LIGHT relates to Fire, Air & Ether increases Vata and Pitta decreases Kapha

2.6 Attributes of the Biological Humors

VATA	cold, dry, light, subtle, mobile, sharp, hard, rough, clear
PITTA	hot, slightly wet, light, subtle, flowing, mobile, sharp, soft, smooth, clear
KAPHA	cold, wet, heavy, gross, dense, static, dull, soft, smooth, cloudy

By knowing these attributes we can begin to recognize and differentiate the humors.

2.7 Attributes and the Gunas

SATTVA	light, subtle, mobile, sharp, soft, smooth, clear.
RAJAS	hot, slightly wet, slightly heavy, gross, mobile, sharp, hard, rough, cloudy
TAMAS	cold, wet, heavy, gross, solid, static, dull, hard, rough, cloudy (dark)

The attributes arise from the Gunas.

Sattva is subtle and balanced in qualities.

Raja is imbalanced, agitated and aggressive.

Tama is heavy, gross and generally stagnant in energy.

2.8 Attributes of the Elements

ETHER	cold, dry, light, subtle, liquid, mobile, sharp, soft, smooth, clear
AIR	cold, dry, light, subtle, mobile, sharp, rough, hard, clear
FIRE	hot, dry, light, subtle, mobile, sharp, rough, hard, clear
WATER	cold, wet, heavy, gross, liquid, static, dull, soft, smooth, cloudy

Treatment According to the Attributes

Each and every day factors are increasing or decreasing the twenty attributes. An increase of like attributes is the causative factor in an increase of the humors. The general rule of thumb is that "like increases like". Applying the opposite attributes will reduce tendencies toward imbalance and illness. Another useful rule is to treat one attribute at a time, especially when a person is showing extreme imbalance.

3 The Three Doshas

- Attributes of the Dosha
- Doshas and their Location in the Body
- Understanding the Doshas
- Doshas and their Attributes
- Functions of Vata, Pitta, Kapha
- Effects of Vata, Pitta, Kapha
- Characteristics of Vata, Pitta and Kapha Types
- Signs of Vata, Pitta and Kapha Imbalance
- The Ten Constitutional Types
- Sites of the Doshas

Since the human body and nature are in a state of continuous flux, Ayurveda maintains that a dynamic equilibrium of all the body's constituents is imperative for perfect health.

When any of the three doshas become excessively agitated or increases disproportionately in relation to the others, an imbalance is created and disease results. The loss of dynamic equilibrium may be due to the excessive or deficient use or misuse of the five sense organs - the ears, skin, eyes, tongue, and nose; as well as the body-mind action, speech, and the time of year or season.

Restoration of health equals regaining the balance of the three doshas. When the Ayurvedic practitioner knows the nature of the imbalance of the doshas, he may prescribe remedies, nutritional program, lifestyle changes and psychological counseling.

Nature provides us with a vast array of natural substances for healing and Ayurveda has collected a fund of data on their therapeutic effects integrating them into a complex theory of physical health.

3.1 Doshas, Attributesand the Six Tastes

Dosha & Attributes	Increased by:	Decreased by:
Vata Dry, Cool, Light	Astringent Bitter Pungent	Sweet Sour Salty
Pitta Hot, Light, Wet	Pungent Sour Salty	Bitter Astringent Sweet
Kapha Heavy, Wet, Cool	Sweet Salty Sour	Bitter Pungent Astringent

3.2 Doshas and Their Locations in the Body

VATA	PITTA	KAPHA
Brain	Skin	Brain
Heart	Eyes	Joints
Colon	Liver	Mouth
Bones	Brain	Lymph
Lungs	Blood	Stomach
Bladder	Spleen	Pleural Cavity
Bone Marrow	Endocrine	Pericardial Cavity
Nerve Function	Metabolic Function	Bodily Fluid Function
Large Intestines	Small Intestines	Stomach

Body Constitutions

The theory of Tridoshas has led the ancient teachers to make a classification of human constitutions. The predominance of one dosha determines the constitution of a person. In other words, if there is an excess of Vata, if the air element is dominant, it results in a person having a Vata constitution. Likewise, the predominance Fire and Water gives rise to Pitta. Constitutions depend on the vitiation of more than one dosha. The Prakruti is pre-determined at the moment of conception and there is no change in its basic structure until a person dies.

Each constitution has peculiar to itself dietary and other habits as well as a predictable response to drugs. It is one of the cardinal rules of Ayurveda that medicine cannot be prescribed for a patient unless the physician has taken into account the type of constitution the patient has. This is because a drug that may help one type of constitution may not help another. It is imperative to understand that, in Ayurveda, the true drug is the one that cures a patient without producing any side effects.

Let us now take a closer look at each of the body constituents.

Understanding the Doshas

3.3 Understanding the Doshas

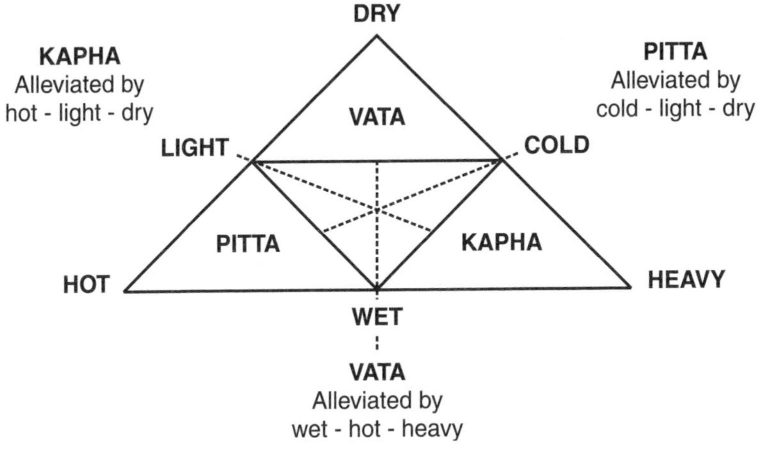

"Dosha" is a Sanskrit word meaning "blame" or "fault." This is the literal meaning but in the context of health care it would be more appropriate to translate "Doshas" as "forces in the body that easily go out of balance."

The Three Doshas Are: VATA, PITTA, KAPHA

VATA means a force that generates and possesses the qualities of Air & Ether.

PITTA means a force that generates and possesses the qualities of Fire & Water.

KAPHA means a force that generates and possesses the qualities of Water & Earth.

Each one of us is made up of all three Doshas. At the time of conception, Nature decides the permutation of the Doshas within us.

The Doshas Have:

- Physical traits that translate into the physical description of a person, for example, height, complexion, eyes, etc.
- Mental and behavioral traits that translate into the kind of people we are, how we sleep, dream and think, how we react to external situations, our emotional strengths and weaknesses and our attitude towards money.
- Intellectual traits that translate into whether we are thinkers and dreamers, designers and planners or silent plodders and solid workers.
- Disease and digestive traits that are affected by different kinds of food, the climate and whether the environment is beneficial or detrimental to us.

All this, and more, Nature decides at the time of conception and during the period we spend in the mother's womb.

Doshas can be managed by the six tastes of Sweet, Sour, Salty, Pungent, Bitter and Astringent. These tastes can aggravate or pacify the different Doshas.

With this knowledge we are able to prevent disease, heal ourselves and understand our interpersonal relationships better.

3.4 Doshas and Their Attributes

VATA	PITTA	KAPHA
Dry	Oily	Oily
Cold	Hot	Cold
Light	Light	Heavy
Irregular	Intense	Stable
Mobile	Fluid	Viscous
Rarefied	Malodorous	Dense
Rough	Liquid	Smooth

In our bodies, these three doshas, also called humors, govern our psychobiological functioning. Vata, Pitta and Kapha are present in every cell, tissue and organ. When in balance, they create health; when out of balance, they are the cause of disease. These three doshas are responsible for the huge variety of individual differences and preferences and they influence all we are and all we do, from our choices of food to our modes of relating to others. They govern the biological and psychological processes of our body, mind and consciousness. They regulate the creation, maintenance and destruction of bodily tissue as well as the elimination of waste products. They even govern our emotions. When in balance, they generate noble qualities such as understanding, compassion and love. When their balance is disturbed by stress, improper diet, and environmental conditions, they can give rise to a disturbed disposition.

In Ayurveda, Vata is the bodily air principle, the energy of movement. Pitta is the principle of fire, the energy of digestion and metabolism and Kapha is the principle of water, the energy of lubrication and structure. While we are made up of all three doshas, one is usually primary, one secondary and the third least prominent. Thus, each person has a particular pattern of energy, an individual combination of physical, mental and emotional characteristics that make up their Prakruti constitution.

Health is order; disease is disorder. The internal environment of the body is ceaselessly reacting to the external environment. Disorder occurs when these two are out of harmony with each other. But since order is inherent within disorder, the wise person learns to be aware of the presence of disorder and sets about to reestablish order.

The three fundamental doshas combine to create ten basic constitutional types. For the moment, let us look a little more deeply into the characteristics of the three basic energies of life.

3.5 Attributes of Vata

Attributes	Manifestations in the Body, Mind and Emotions
Dry	Dry skin, tongue, hair, lips, tongue, tending towards constipation, hoarse voice
Light	Underweight, light bones, muscles, slender skeletal system, scanty sleep
Cold	Poor circulation, cold hands and feet; stiff muscles, dislikes cold
Rough	Cracking joints, skin, hair, nails, teeth, rough hands and feet
Subtle	Emotional anxiety, insecurity, fears, tremors and muscle twitching
Mobile	Restless in body, mind and emotions, moves and walks fast, unstable joints, does numerous things simultaneously, always traveling, scattered mind and moody
Clear	Experiences loneliness, learns quickly but just as quickly forgets, absent minded and spacey
Astringent	Tendency towards constipation, gets hiccups easily and hiccups frequently, craves Sweet, Salty and Sour
Brownish-Black	Coated tongue, dark complexion, hair and eyes

3.6 Attributes of Pitta

Attributes	Manifestations in the Body, Mind and Emotions
Hot	Strong appetite and digestive capacity, high body temperature, soft brownish-red body, facial and skin hair, gray hair and balding
Sharp	Sharp teeth, pointed nose and chin, piercing eyes, sharp complexion, strong digestive assimilation, good memory, grasps information well, intellectual, irritable, sharp vision/eyesight
Light	Bright eyes, fair glossy skin, medium-light skeletal frame, sensitive to sunlight
Liquid	Soft delicate muscles, excess urine, sweat and thirst, diarrhea symptoms
Mobile/ Spreading	Inflammation throughout the body, skin and muscles, a tendency to spread like wide fire
Oily	Oily skin, hair, feces
Body Odor	Strong body odor under armpits, soles of feet and mouth
Red	Red flushed skin, nose, cheeks, eyes appear red, sensitive to heat and sunlight
Yellow	Bright yellow color of eyes, skin, urine and feces, over production of bile, dark yellow is color of Pitta Ama, pale yellow coloring is healthy Pitta
Pungent	Burning sensation, heartburn, emotionally strong feelings of hate and anger
Sour	Acidic pH of body tissues and digestive juices, excess salivation and sensitive mouth and teeth
Bitter	Bitter acid taste in mouth, feelings of nausea and vomiting

3.7 Attributes of Kapha

Attributes	Manifestations in the Body, Mind and Emotions
Heavy	Grounded, overweight, heavy skeletal and muscular systems, heavy voice
Slow/ Dull	Sluggish metabolism and digestion, body gestures, walk and talk slow and lazy
Cold	Reoccurring colds, flues, cough, and nasal congestion, clammy skin, cold and slow digestive system
Liquid	Congestion in the chest, sinuses, throat and head, excess salivation
Smooth	Smoothness of organs and skin, calm, gentle mind and personality
Dense	Firm and solid muscles, condensed, strong tissues, well rounded organs, thick skin, hair and feces
Soft	Gentle pleasant character, compassionate, kind, caring and forgiving
Static	Enjoys lying around and sleeping a lot
Oily	Oily internal organs, joints, skin, hair and feces
Sticky	Cohesive quality, compact and firm joints and organs, viscous, emotionally is very loving, a great friend and loyal in relationships
Hard	Strong muscles and body, lots of strength and vigor
Gross	Obese, may have numerous internal obstructions
Cloudy	Mucousy congestion, mind and emotions are cloudy and foggy
White	Tongue is coated with a white film, pale complexion
Sweet	Abnormal function may cause cravings for sweets, the anabolic action of Sweet taste stimulates sperm formation increasing quality of semen
Salty	Water retention, assists with growth and metabolism, gives strength and stamina, abnormal function may create craving for Salt

3.8 Functions of Vata

PHYSICAL FUNCTIONS	PSYCHOLOGICAL FUNCTIONS
Respiratory Heart Function Circulation Ingestion Peristalsis and enzyme secretion Assimilation and absorption Elimination of urine, feces, sweat Menstruation Orgasm Hearing Touch	Governs the mind, sensory perception, and motor functions (speech and muscular co-ordination) Movement of all thoughts, feelings and nerve impulses Communication Clarity Joy Creativity

3.9 Functions of Pitta

PHYSICAL FUNCTIONS	PSYCHOLOGICAL FUNCTIONS
Maintenance of body temperature Governs bodily metabolism Digestion, absorption, assimilation of food Appetite Thirst Color Luster of eyes, hair, skin, body Visual perception	Intelligence, understanding, comprehension, knowledge Courage Transformation Ambition

3.10 Functions of Kapha

PHYSICAL FUNCTIONS	PSYCHOLOGICAL FUNCTIONS
Water electrolyte balance	Memory perception
Gastric secretions	Compassion
Repair and regeneration	Contentment
Fat regulation	Forgiveness
Groundedness	
Nourishment	
Lubrication	
Growth	
Energy	
Sleep	
Support and stability	
Stamina and Strength	
Taste perception	

VATA

The term Vata stems from a Sanskrit word vyv (vaya) that means "that which moves things". It is commonly translated as wind. Vata is the energy of movement. Although it is the air principle, it is not considered the same as actual air in the external environment, but rather as the subtle energy that governs biological movement. Vata is intimately related to our vital life essence, known as Prana. Prana is the pure essence of Vata. It is the life force, the play of intelligence. That flow of intelligence is necessary for communication between two cells, and it maintains the life function of both. As the principle of mobility, Vata regulates all activity in the body, both mental and physiological. It is responsible for breathing, the blinking of our eyes, the beating of our hearts, and all movement, thoughts, emotions, eating, drinking, elimination and our general functioning. Vata governs all the impulses in the vast networks of our nervous system.

When Vata is in balance, it promotes creativity and flexibility and evokes feelings of freshness, lightness, happiness and joy. Out of balance, Vata produces fear, nervousness, anxiety, even tremors and spasms. Vata is dry, light, cold, subtle, clear, mobile and dispersing. We shall soon see how these qualities are expressed in a person with a Vata constitution.

3.11 Effects of Vata Dosha

Effects of Balanced Vata	Effects of Unbalanced or Excess Vata
A healthy coordination of all body functions	Bodily functions impaired
Healthy regular movements associated with eating	Disturbed movements associated with eating, digestion, and elimination with symptoms of flatulence, bloating and constipation
Stimulation of digestive juices and function	Deficiency or irregularity of the digestive juices
Mental activity controlled and precise	Mental agitation, confusion, impaired memory
Control of organs of action and perception	Dulled and impaired senses, inappropriate perception and action, responses ill-timed
Energy level good	Anxiety, fatigue, worry, cold intolerance, depletion of life-force
Excellent respiratory function	Respiratory symptoms: dry cough, shortness of breath, hiccups
Healthy function of mucous discharge	Unhealthy and constant bodily discharge
Healthy sleeping pattern	Sleep is disturbed and irregular, insomnia
Zest for life, active with vitality, curiosity and natural interest	Loss of enthusiasm, zest, joy and spark for life, loss of energy

PITTA

The term Pitta comes from the Sanskrit word pinj, meaning, "to shine," it can also mean "that which digests." Pitta is translated as fire, but this is not meant literally. Rather, it is the principle of fire, the energy of heating or metabolism. Pitta governs all the biochemical changes in the body, regulating digestion, absorption, assimilation and body temperature. From the standpoint of modern biology, Pitta comprises the enzymes and amino acids that play a major role in metabolism. Pitta regulates body temperature through the chemical transformation of food. It promotes appetite and vitality. We not only metabolize food, but also every impression coming in from the outside is processed, absorbed and made a part of us. Pitta produces heat, providing color to the blood, luster to the skin and clearer vision. When Pitta is in balance it promotes intelligence and understanding and is crucial in learning. When out of balance Pitta may arouse fiery emotions such as frustration, anger, hatred, criticism and jealousy.

Pitta is the energy stored in the chemical bonds, the organic substances that make us up: it is encoded in our hormones, enzymes, organic acids and neurotransmitters. Pitta is hot, sharp, light, oily, liquid, pungent, sour and dispersing. These qualities occur in various ways in people of Pitta constitution.

3.12 Effects of Pitta Dosha

Effects of Balanced Pitta	Effects of Unbalanced or Excess Pitta
Complete and strong digestion	Incomplete digestion with numerous symptoms
Efficient absorption of foods	Digestive symptoms: diarrhea, hemorrhoids, heartburn, peptic ulcer, irritable bowels
Vision is perfect and sharp	Vision is poor and impaired
Complexion healthy with good facial tone	Unhealthy skin tone and may be inflamed
Healthy body temperature	Irregular body temperature and perspiration
Lustrous healthy hair	Unhealthy dry hair, graying or balding
Spiritually focused, disciplined, responsible, truthful	Spiritually lost, constantly seeking
Character is joyful, cheerful, brave, open, imaginative and intellectual	Character is anxious, angry, irritable, obsessed, dull and uninterested

KAPHA

The term Kapha comes from the Sanskrit word "shlish", meaning, "that which holds things together, to embrace, coherent." Kapha combines Water and Earth. It is the energy that forms the body's structure, the glue that holds the cells together. Kapha also supplies the liquid needed for the life of our cells and bodily systems. It lubricates our joints, moisturizes the skin, helps to heal wounds, and maintains immunity. Kapha imparts stability and resilience to the body-mind emotions. It is the anabolic force in the body that governs the formation of neuropeptides, stomach linings and all new cells and tissues of the body that are constantly being destroyed and re-created. Kapha provides strength, vigor and stability. Psychologically, excess Kapha is responsible for the emotions of attachment, greed, lust and envy. When Kapha is in balance, it expresses itself in tendencies toward love, calmness and forgiveness. When Kapha is out of balance the qualities are displayed as heavy, slow, cool, oily, damp, smooth, soft, static and viscous. Kapha individuals display these qualities in various ways.

3.13 Effects of Kapha Dosha

Effects of Balanced Kapha	Effects of Unbalanced or Excess Kapha
Appetite and digestion: regular and strong	Appetite and digestion: sluggish and unregulated
Nutritionally and minerally nourished tissues, muscles and bones	Nutritionally and minerally depleted, fatigued and flabby
Respiratory system well lubricated and moist	Respiratory system excess amounts of mucous
Bodily fluids good and moist, lubricated through all body systems	Bodily fluids depleted, dry in all tissues and organs
Character traits: patient, forgiving, calm, steady and compassionate	Character traits: insecure, jealous and intolerant
Physical physique: strong and well-built	Physical physique: weak and obese
Sexual potency and immunity: healthy and strong	Sexual potency and immunity: low, weak and diminished

Together, these three doshas govern all the body's metabolic activities.

- Kapha promotes anabolism, the process of building up the body, the growth and creation of new cells as well as cell repair.
- Pitta regulates metabolism, digestion and absorption.
- Vata triggers catabolism, the necessary deterioration process in which larger molecules are broken down into smaller ones.

Vata, the principle of movement, moves both Pitta and Kapha, which are immobile. Thus, when Vata is out of balance, it influences and disturbs the other doshas. The majority of illnesses have aggravated Vata at their source.

The whole of life's journey is divided into three major milestones. From birth to age 20 is the Kapha age, from 21 to 55 is the age of Pitta, and from 55 to 100 the age of Vata. In childhood, Kapha and the process of anabolism are predominant; this is the time of greatest physical growth and the structuring of the body. Kapha disorders, such as lung congestion, cough, colds and mucus secretions, are common at this time. In adulthood, at times of activity and vitality, Pitta is most apparent. Vata and the catabolic processes of deterioration take over in old age bringing Vata disorders such as tremors, emaciation, breathlessness, arthritis and loss of memory.

3.14 Characteristics of Vata Types

Here are some of the common characteristics of people who have a predominantly Vata constitution.

Physical Traits

- Variable appetite and digestive efficiency
- Generally have dry skin and dry hair and don't perspire much
- Irregular daily routine
- Sexually easily excited but quickly satiated
- Slender, lightest of the three body types
- Talk and walk quickly
- Tendency toward cold hands and feet, discomfort in cold climates

Psychological Traits

- High energy in short bursts, tendency to tire easily and to overexert
- Creative, mental quickness
- Highly imaginative
- Changeable moods
- Full of joy and enthusiasm when in balance
- Quick to learn and grasp new knowledge, but also quick to forget
- Respond to stress with fear, worry and anxiety, especially when out of balance
- Tendency to act on impulse
- Often have racing, disjointed thoughts
- Excitable, lively, fun personality

Typical Health Problems

Headaches, hypertension, dry coughs, sore throats, earaches, anxiety, irregular heart rhythms, muscle spasms, lower back pain, constipation, abdominal gas, diarrhea, nervous stomach, menstrual cramps, premature ejaculation and other sexual dysfunctions, arthritis. Most neurological disorders are related to Vata imbalance.

Physical Features

People of Vata constitution are generally physically underdeveloped. Their chests are flat and their veins and muscle tendons are visible. The complexion is brown; the skin is cold, rough, dry and cracked.

Vata people generally are either tall or short, with thin frames, revealing prominent joints and bone-ends because of poor muscle development. The hair is curly and scanty, the eyelashes are thin and the eyes lusterless. The eyes may be sunken, small, dry and active. The nails are rough and brittle. The shape of the nose is bent and turned-up.

Appetite and digestion are variable. Vata people love Sweet, Sour and Salty tastes and like hot drinks to balance their excess Air quality. The production of urine is scanty and the feces are dry, hard and small in quantity. They have a tendency to perspire less than other constitutional types. Their sleep may be disturbed and they will sleep less than the other types. Their hands and feet are often cold.

Psychologically, they have a short memory but quick mental understanding. They will understand something immediately, but will soon forget it. They have little willpower, tend toward mental instability and possess little tolerance, confidence or boldness. Their reasoning power is weak and these people are nervous, fearful and afflicted by much anxiety.

Vata people tend to earn money quickly and also to spend it quickly. Thus, they tend to remain poor.

3.15 Characteristics of Pitta Types

Here are some of the common characteristics of people who have a predominantly Pitta body type.

Physical Traits

- Medium physique, strong, well-built
- Perspire a lot
- Skin fair or reddish, often with freckles, sunburns easily
- Hair usually fine and straight, tending toward blond or red, typically turns gray early; tendency toward baldness or thinning hair
- Strong digestion, strong appetite, get irritated if they have to miss or wait for a meal
- Uncomfortable in sun or hot weather; heat makes them very tired

Psychological Traits

- Orderly, focused
- Competitive, enjoy challenges
- Sharp mind, good concentration powers
- Assertive, self-confident and entrepreneurial at their best; aggressive, demanding and pushy when out of balance
- Others may find them stubborn, pushy, opinionated
- Passionate and romantic, sexually have more vigor and endurance than Vata individuals but less than Kapha individuals

- Good public speakers; also capable of sharp, sarcastic, cutting speech
- Generally good management and leadership ability, but can become authoritarian
- Like to be in command
- Like to spend money, surround themselves with beautiful objects
- When under stress, Pitta individuals become irritated and angry
- Subject to temper tantrums, impatience and anger

Typical Health Problems

Rashes or inflammations of the skin, acne, boils, skin cancer, ulcers, heartburn, acid stomach, hot sensations in the stomach or intestines, insomnia, bloodshot or burning eyes and other vision problems, anemia, jaundice.

Physical Features

These people are of medium height, are slender and their body frame may be delicate. Their chests are not as flat as those of Vata people and they show a medium prominence of veins and muscle tendons. The bones are not as prominent as in the Vata individual. Muscle development is moderate.

The Pitta complexion may be coppery, yellowish, reddish or fair. The skin is soft, warm and less wrinkled than Vata skin. The hair is thin, silky, red or brownish and there is a tendency toward premature graying of hair and hair loss. The eyes may be gray, green or cooper-brown and sharp; the eyeballs will be of medium prominence. The nails are soft. The shape of the nose is sharp and the tip tends to be reddish.

These people have a strong metabolism, good digestion and resulting strong appetites. The person of Pitta constitution usually takes large quantities of food and liquid. Pitta types have a natural craving for Sweet, Bitter and Astringent tastes and enjoy cold drinks to balance their excess Fire quality. Their sleep is of medium duration but uninterrupted. They produce a large volume of urine and the feces are yellowish, liquid, soft and plentiful. There is a tendency toward excessive perspiring. The body temperature may run slightly high and hands and feet will tend to be warm. Pitta people do not tolerate sunlight, heat and enjoy hard work.

Psychologically, Pitta people have a good power of comprehension; they are very intelligent and sharp and tend to be good orators; they have emotional tendencies toward hate, anger and jealousy.

They are ambitious people who generally like to be leaders. Pitta people appreciate material prosperity and they tend to be moderately well off financially. They enjoy exhibiting their wealth and luxurious possessions.

3.16 Characteristics of Kapha Types

Here are some of the common characteristics of people who have a predominantly Kapha constitution.

Physical Traits

- Excellent health, strong resistance to disease
- Tend toward being overweight; may also suffer from sluggish digestion
- Tend to be possessive and hold on to things, such as people and money
- Dislike cold, damp weather
- Soft hair and skin, tendency to have large "soft" eyes and a low, soft voice
- Physically strong with a sturdy, heavy build
- Have the most energy of all constitutions, but it is steady and enduring, not explosive
- Slow moving and graceful
- Slow speech, reflecting a deliberate thought process
- More self-sufficient, need less outward stimulation than do the other types
- A mild, gentle and essentially undemanding approach to life
- Sexually, Kapha individuals are the slowest to be aroused, but they also have the most endurance

Psychological Traits

- Affectionate and loving

- Easygoing, relaxed, slow-paced
- Slower to learn, but never forgets; outstanding long-term memory
- Forgiving, compassionate, nonjudgmental nature, stable and reliable, faithful
- Slow to anger; strive to maintain harmony and peace in their surroundings
- Not easily upset
- Can be a point of stability for others
- Prone to heavy, oppressive depressions

Physical Health Problems

Colds and congestion, sinus headaches, respiratory problems including asthma and wheezing, hay fever, allergies and arteriosclerosis (hardening of the arteries).

Physical Features

People of Kapha constitution have well-developed bodies. There is, however, a strong tendency for these individuals to carry excess weight. Their chests are expanded and broad; their veins and tendons are not obvious because of their thick skin and their good muscle development, and their bones are not prominent.

Their complexions are fair and bright. The skin is soft, lustrous and oily; it is also cold and pale. The hair is thick, dark, soft and wavy. The eyes are dense and black or blue: the white of the eye is generally very white, large and attractive.

Physiologically, Kapha people have regular appetites but due to slow digestion, they enjoy larger servings at one setting, they are usually not nibblers . They crave Pungent, Bitter and Astringent foods to balance their excess Water qualities. Their stools are soft and may be pale in color; evacuation is slow. Their perspiration is moderate. Sleep is sound and prolonged. There is a strong vital capacity evidenced by good stamina and Kapha people are generally healthy, happy and peaceful.

Psychologically, they tend to be tolerant, calm, forgiving and loving; however, they also exhibit traits of greed, attachment, envy and possessiveness. Their comprehension is slow but definite; once they understand something, that knowledge is retained.

Kapha people tend to be wealthy. They earn money and are good at holding on to it.

3.17 Signs of Vata Imbalance

There are a number of signs of dosha imbalance. Some people will get very angry, some will get depressed, etc. Here is a summary of the signs of Vata imbalance:

Physical Traits

- Rough, flaky skin, chapped lips
- Tired, yet can't relax, fatigue, poor stamina
- Very sensitive to cold
- Nail biting
- Nervous, can't concentrate
- Insomnia, wake up at night and can't go back to sleep
- Heart palpitations
- Constipation, intestinal bloating, gas, belching, hiccups
- Dry, sore throat, dry eyes

Psychological Traits

- Worried
- Anxious, fearful
- Nervous, can't concentrate
- Agitated movement
- Cannot make decisions
- Shy, insecure, restless
- Self-defeating
- Fainting spells
- Agitated mind
- Impatient, antsy, hyperactive
- Spaced out

Symptoms of Increased Vata

- Eye dilation

- Cutting pain
- Loss of sensation
- Weakness
- Continuous pain
- Pricking pain
- Splitting pain
- Crushing pain
- Contraction (constriction)
- Twisting
- Tingling
- Thirst
- Tremors
- Dryness
- Pulsations (throbbing
- Stiffness (rigidity, withholding, loss of movement)
- Black color of skin
- Desire for hot things
- Distension of the abdomen
- Constipation
- Loss of strength, sleep and sensory functions, irrelevant speech
- Giddiness and timidity (peevishness)

Symptoms of Decreased Vata

- Debility of the body
- The person speaks very little and is not very active
- Loss of sensation (awareness) and consciousness
- Unctuousness
- Hardness, coldness and heaviness of the body's organs
- Indigestion
- Sweet and salty tastes in the mouth
- Delay in all activities

Indications of balanced Vata influences are mental alertness and abundance of creative energy, good elimination of waste matters from the body, sound sleep, a strong immune system, enthusiasm, emotional balance and orderly functioning of the body's systems.

3.18 Signs of Pitta Imbalance

Physical Traits

- Skin rashes
- Very sensitive to heat, hot flashes
- Boils
- Bloodshot eyes
- Acne
- Weakness due to low blood sugar
- Fevers, night sweats
- Acidity, heartburn, stomach ulcer
- Fitful sleep, disturbing dreams
- Diarrhea, food allergies
- Bad breath, sour body odor

Psychological Traits

- Angry, irritable
- Impatient
- Hostile, enraged, destructive
- Critical of self and others
- Argumentative, aggressive
- Bossy, controlling
- Frustrated, willful, reckless

Symptoms of Increased Pitta

- Burning sensation
- Reddish discoloration
- Increased digestion
- Formation of pus, ulcers, etc
- Perspiration
- Debility
- Fainting

- Bitter and sour taste in the mouth
- Yellow color of the feces, urine, eyes and skin
- Excess of hunger and thirst
- Burning sensation throughout the bod
- Very little sleep

Symptoms of Decreased Pitta

- Weakness in digestion
- Coldness of body organs
- Loss of luster (complexion)

Indications of balanced Pitta influences are strong powers of digestion, vitality, goal-setting inclinations, good problem-solving skills, keen powers of intelligence, decisiveness, boldness and courage and a bright complexion.

3.19 Signs of Kapha Imbalance

Physical Traits

- Nausea
- Diabetes
- Aching joints or heavy limbs
- Hay fever
- Pale, cool, clammy skin
- Edema, water retention, bloated feeling
- Sluggish digestion, food "just sits" in the stomach
- High cholesterol
- Sleeping too much
- Very tired in the morning, hard to get out of bed
- Weight gain, obesity
- Mucus and congestion in the chest or throat
- Mucus and congestion in the nose or sinuses

Psychological Traits

- Sluggish and dull thinking
- Apathetic, no desire

- Depressed, sad, sentimental
- Slow to comprehend, slow to react
- Procrastinating, lethargy
- Clingy, hanging on to people and ideas
- Drowsy or groggy during the day
- Greedy, possessive, materialistic

Symptoms of Increased Kapha

- Unctuousness
- Itching (irritation)
- Coldness
- Heaviness
- Obstruction and coating of channels
- Loss of movement
- Swelling
- Indigestion
- Excess sleep
- White color of feces
- Sweet and salty taste in mouth
- Delay in all activities
- Debility of digestive activity
- Excess saliva
- Looseness of the body parts
- Cough

Symptoms of Decreased Kapha

- Dizziness
- Emptiness of the organs of Kapha
- Palpitation
- Looseness of the joints

Indications of balanced Kapha influences are physical strength, a strong immune system, serenity, mental resolve, rational thinking, and the ability to conserve and use personal resources, endurance and adaptability.

3.20 DAILY COURSE OF THE DOSHAS AND ORGANS

Time	Dosha	Internal Organ
11:00 am-1:00 pm	Pitta	Heart
1:00 pm -3:00 pm	Pitta	Small Intestine
3:00 pm -5:00 pm	Vata	Bladder
5:00 pm -7:00 pm	Vata/Kapha	Kidney
7:00 pm -9:00 pm	Kapha	Pericardium
9:00 pm -11:00 pm	Kapha/Pitta	Body Cavities-Triple Warmer
11:00 pm -1:00 am	Pitta	Gall Bladder
1:00 am -3:00 am	Pitta	Liver
3:00 am -5:00 am	Vata	Lungs
5:00 am -7:00 am	Vata	Colon
7:00 am -9:00 am	Kapha	Stomach-Pancreas
9:00 am-11:00 am	Kapha/ Pitta	Spleen

The Ten Constitutional Types

According to Ayurveda, in addition to the basic three constitutions of Vata, Pitta and Kapha, there are the mixed types. An important note to make here is that the first three types in pure form are rare; seldom is anyone influenced by one dosha alone. The primary difference is the degree to which the three doshas interact within each type. In most cases, a mixed type will have one dominant dosha with a second dosha being a close second. For example, a Vata - Pitta individual will have stronger Vata tendencies than Pitta compared to a Pitta - Vata individual will have more Pitta attributes. A Vata - Pitta type contains more Air energy, whereas a Pitta-Vata type contains more Fire energy. These are called dual types and are also referred to as dual Prakruti. There is also another category and this one is a balanced tridosha called Vata – Pitta – Kapha (VPK). This is where one type is not predominant. In total, there are ten constitutional categories. They are:

Four Classic Types

Vata
Pitta
Kapha
Sama (Tridosha - equal proportion of all three doshas)

Three Classic Dual Types

Vata - Pitta
Vata - Kapha
Pitta - Vata

Three Additional Dual Types

Pitta - Kapha
Kapha - Vata
Kapha - Pitta

Sites of the Doshas

3.21 Sites of the Doshas

Sites of Vata

- Large intestines
- Pelvic cavity, waist
- Thighs
- Head
- Bones
- Ears (organs of hearing)
- Skin (organ of touch)

Sites of Pitta

- Small intestines
- Liver, spleen and gallbladder
- Belly button
- Blood

- Skin
- Sweat
- Sebaceous secretions
- Subcutaneous fat
- Heart
- Gray matter of the brain
- Eyes (organ of sight)

Sites of Kapha

- Stomach
- Pancreas
- Lungs
- Sinuses
- Plasma
- Joints
- White matter of the brain
- Cerebrospinal fluid
- Nose (organ of smell)
- Tongue (organ of taste)

The Fivefold Division

The Five Functions of Vata

The normal function of Vata is to sustain the body, making it the originator of every kind of action in the body. Vata occupies the space and movement among the three doshas. As the wind controls the direction of the clouds, so Vata controls the functioning of Pitta and Kapha.

There are five functions of Vata or vayu: Prana, udana, vyana, samana and apana. Prana vayu is responsible for breathing and the swallowing of food. It is also responsible for the functioning of the heart and the parts of the body directly connected with the heart. Not only does it maintain the functioning of the heart, it also sustains the mind, the senses, the intellect, the arteries, the veins and the nerves. Udana vayu is responsible for the production of various sounds and speech as well as the action and the effort to keep up the strength of the body, mind, memory, and intellect. Samana vayu helps in the action of the digestive enzymes. It separates the essences vital for the nourishment of the body and sends the wastes to the large intestines. Apana vayu is situated in the lower part of the digestive tract, the urinary system and the reproductive organs. Its function is to hold the feces, urine, menses and semen for a normal period of time and then expel them through the various orifices of the body. This vayu is one of the most important factors in the body since its proper functioning keeps a person healthy. In an abnormal state, it moves upwards and depresses the diaphragm giving rise to a sense of acute discomfort. Vyana vayu flows through the whole body carrying the nutrients with it. It also helps with the excretion of perspiration and controls the opening and closing of the eye lids and other movements of the body.

3.22 The Fivefold Division of Vata

Subtype	Governing Element	Primary Sites	Functions	Direction
Prana	Ether	Head, Brain	To fill the space	Downward, Inward
Udana	Air	Diaphragm, Throat	Moves upward	Upward
Samana	Fire	Small Intestine, Navel	Isolation, separation, splitting	Linear
Apana	Earth	Colon, Pelvic Cavity	Holding	Downward, Outward
Vyana	Water	Heart, Whole Body	Pulsation, throbbing	Circular Circulation

The Five Subtypes of Pitta

Like the vayus, Pittas are also of five subtypes: pachak, ranjaka, sadhaka, alochaka, and bhrajaka. Pachaka Pitta is mainly responsible for the digestion of food. It divides the food juice into the useful and waste parts, and helps the other four types of Pittas to function normally in the body. Ranjaka Pitta, as the very name indicates, adds colour to the food juices when they travel from the stomach to the liver. Sadhaka Pitta has its seat in the heart and is the finest of all the Pittas. It helps in the normal functioning of the intellect and memory. Alochaka Pitta is responsible for the maintenance of normal vision in the eyes. Bhrajaka Pitta is situated in the skin of the body and is responsible for the normal pigmentation of the skin.

3.23 The Fivefold Division of Pitta

Subtype	Governing Element	Primary Sites	Functions
Pachaka	Fire	Small Intestine, Stomach	Digestion, absorption and assimilation of food
Ranjaka	Water	Liver, Spleen, Intrinsic Factor in Stomach	Produces bile, liver enzymes; gives color to blood
Sadhaka	Ether	Brain (gray matter), Heart	Conscious thinking
Alochaka	Air	Eyes	Maintains iris color; visual perception
Bhrajaka	Earth	Skin	Maintains skin color, texture and temperature; stereognosis

The Five Subtypes of Kapha

Like the Vatas and the Pittas, the Kaphas are also of five subtypes. The first of these is Kledaka, which, as its name indicates, is responsible for moistening the food in the stomach. It nourishes the other Kaphas by its special humid properties. The second Kapha, the Avalambaka, has its seat in the thorax and protects the heart from excessive heat by its cooling influence and gives a special power to the heart. The Bodhaka Kapha moistens any substance that comes in contact with the tongue and helps the individual to recognize the taste of substances ingested. Its seat extends from the root of the tongue to the throat and it plays a part in increasing appetite. The fourth Kapha, the Tarpaka, cools the sight and hearing sense organs. The Shleshaka Kapha is situated in the joints of the body and maintains them in good order so that the various parts of the body not only remain firm, but also have the flexibility to move.

3.24 The Fivefold Division of Kapha

Subtype	Governing Element	Primary Sites	Functions
Kledaka	Fire	Stomach, Gastrointestinal Tract	Gastric secretions, digestion and absorption, nourishes rasa
Avalambaka	Air	Lungs, Pleural Cavity; Heart, Respiratory Tract, Spine	Support, holds emotions, supports all Kapha Systems
Bodhaka	Water	Oral Cavity	Salivary secretions, taste, swallowing, speech
Tarpaka	Ether	Brain (white matter), Myelin Sheath, Cerebrospinal Fluid	Subconscious thinking and emotions, memory
Shleshaka	Earth	Joints	Lubricates joints (synovial fluid) nourishes bones

Causes of Constitutional Imbalance

General Causes of Disease

All diseases or sicknesses are caused by an imbalance in the tridosha. The imbalance may be an increase or decrease in one, two or all three of the doshas. Once the doshas are imbalanced, symptoms of disease manifest. For example, excess Vata can cause arthritis and excess Pitta can cause acidity, ulcer and liver disorders.

Factors that cause an imbalance of doshas include diet, our thoughts, emotions, activity, exercise and overall lifestyle. If you want to maintain health, you must know which factors create an imbalance of doshas.

Factors That Increase Vata

Eating large quantities of foods that contain the Vata elements of Air and Ether will increase Vata. These foods are light, dry, airy, cold or gas forming. This food group includes the cabbage family, (such as cauliflower and broccoli), beans, sprouts, dried fruits, mushrooms, and junk foods or frozen foods. Other factors are: too much traveling by any means of transportation, staying awake, late nights or not sleeping adequately, an excessive exposure to loud or high-pitched sounds, watching too much television and over-exposure to computers or any other kind of electrical appliance, indulging in excessive sexual activity, excessive imagination, overwork or sporting activity, taking medicinal, recreational or stimulating drugs.

Factors That Increase Pitta

Eating large quantities of foods that contain the Pitta element of Fire will increase Pitta. These foods are Pungent, Hot, Spicy, Sour and Acidic. This group includes tomatoes, pineapples, citrus fruits, all sour fruits, chilies, eggplant, onion and garlic. The extremes that increase Pitta even more than fried foods are pickled foods, mustard and vinegar. Actions that increase Pitta are: eating while angry, experiencing anger frequently, exposure to heat and sun, drinking tea, coffee or alcohol, smoking and engaging in competitive activities.

Some of the symptoms caused by excess Pitta are: hyperacidity, skin diseases, burning sensations, fever, infections, ulcers and liver disorders.

Factors That Increase Kapha

Eating large quantities of food that contain the Kapha elements of Water and Earth will increase Kapha. These foods are heavy, dense, sweet, oily and moist. Foods in this group include nuts, seeds, avocado, banana and melons. These are the extremes that increase Kapha. Even higher on the scale are meats and dairy products, pasta, rice, cakes, breads, custards and puddings, overeating, eating while experiencing grief or sadness, sedentary lifestyle or minimal activity, sleeping too much or sleeping during the day.

3.25 Qualities Comparing Vata Prakruti to Vata Vikruti

Vata Prakruti	Becomes	Vata Vikruti
Gets fatigued easily	>	Constantly fatigued
Active and motivated	>	Hyperactive
Moderate body weight	>	Loses weight & structure
Fast metabolism & elimination	>	Irregular digestion & elimination
Dry skin	>	Extremely dry skin
Cracking in joints	>	Cold & stiff extremities
Temperament Initiates action quickly Thoughts & decisions are quick Not easily satisfied Motivator and precise	>>>>	*Temperament* Initiates action slower Thoughts & decisions are confused Unsatisfied Prone to psychological problems

3.26 Qualities Comparing Pitta Prakruti to Pitta Vikruti

Pitta Prakruti	Becomes	Pitta Vikruti
Strong metabolism & elimination	>	Sluggish metabolism & elimination
Appetite is strong	>	Appetite is poor
Skin is soft & radiant	>	Skin is red, spotty with rashes
Temperament Warm, intelligent, witty, clever, Thoughts are clear Sharp & quick natured Reactive	>>>>	*Temperament* Hot, irritated, angry, Thoughts are confused, Sensitive & impatient in nature Overly reactive

3.27 Qualities Comparing Kapha Prakruti to Kapha Vikruti

Kapha Prakruti	Becomes	Kapha Vikruti
Slower metabolism & elimination	>	Sluggish metabolism
Tissues are bulky	>	Tissues carry an excess of bulk & fat
<u>Temperament</u> Friendly, easy-going Pleasant character Less expressive	>>>>	<u>Temperament</u> Introverted, hard to get going Variable in character Non-expressive

3.28 Dosha Correspondences

Dosha	**Vata**	**Pitta**	**Kapha**
Element	Air	Fire	Water
Cosmos	Preserver	Creator	Destroyer
Metabolic Energy	Nerve	Catabolic Fire	Anabolic Nutritive
Physics	Neutron	Electron	Proton
Time	Afternoon, early morning	Noon, midnight	Morning, late evening
Season	Autumn	Spring/ Summer	Winter/Spring
Age (Stage of Life)	61 to end of life (Maturation)	31 to 60 (Ripening)	1 to 30 (Growing)
Color	Blue	Red	White
Tastes	Bitter, Astringent, Pungent	Sour, Bitter, Pungent	Sweet, Sour, Some Pungent

Prana, Tejas, Ojas

The Tridoshas (Vata, Pitta, and Kapha) play a very important role in the maintenance of cellular health and longevity. Each dosha plays a vital part in upholding the functioning of the billions of cells that constitute the human body. Kapha maintains longevity on the cellular level. Pitta governs digestion and nutrition. Vata, which is closely related to Pranic life energy, governs all life functions.

Vata, Pitta and Kapha display a subtle correspondence at the level of vital energy. This complement is represented by the concepts of Prana, Tejas and Ojas, also known as the "Three Vital Essences." Prana, Tejas and Ojas are the masterful forms of Vata, Pitta and Kapha. They control the common functions of body and mind, maintaining health.

From the time of physical birth until physical death, the body is engaged in a continuous transformational journey against the aging process. Because continuous breakdown of the bodily tissues and organs at the cellular level causes deterioration and degeneration, it is therefore at the cellular level that rejuvenation must take place. The functioning of Prana, Ojas and Tejas corresponds at a subtler level of creation to the functioning of Vata, Kapha and Pitta respectively. Proper diet, exercise and lifestyle can create a balance among these three essences, thus ensuring a long, healthy life.

Prana, as the cosmic life force, corresponds to air and ether; Tejas, as the power of will and vigor, is the primal fire, and Ojas, as stamina and determination, is the essence of Water.

The subtle form of Vata is called Prana
The subtle form of Pitta is called Tejas
The subtle form of Kapha is called Ojas

PRANA (Original Force of Life)

Prana is the subtle energy of the Air-like masterful force behind all the functions of the body and the mind. It is responsible for the coordination of breathing, the senses and the mind. At a deeper level it governs the development of elevated states of conscience.

TEJAS (Inner Radiance)

Tejas is the subtle energy of the Fire through which we take in impressions and feelings. At a deep level it regulations the expansion of the elevated perceptual capacities.

OJAS (Original Vigor)

Ojas is the subtle energy of Water like our reserve of vital energy, the essence of the digestion of the meals, the impressions and the feelings. At a deep level it supports and nourishes all the elevated states to of conscience.

Vitality, luster and splendor are essences of Kapha. Kapha prevents decay and degeneration of the body and supports the body providing strength against dis-ease. Ojas is a biological substance and the biological strength of the tissues depends upon it. Ojas is a protoplasmic biological substance called albumin and globulin that is formed during the biosynthesis of bodily tissue. This protoplasmic biological substance is the pure essence of biological tissue. The final product of digested food plus Agni creates the nutritional precursor called Rasa. In that transformation, dhatu waste products, dhatu by-products and Ojas is created. It is the Tejas of Rasa Agni that separates out the pure essence of Rasa and that pure essence is called Ojas. The same process occurs with all bodily tissues. Every tissue has its own Ojas. The same process occurs with all bodily tissues, so Ojas is the pure essence of all tissues. In a way every tissue has its own Ojas.

PRANA: The Life Force

A key concept in Ayurveda is the life force that enters the body at birth. It imbues our whole body and leaves at the moment of death. This life force is called Prana. Prana strings body, mind and spirit together like beads on a strand. Prana is the force necessary to keep all living beings alive; it is found in all life.

Prana gets its nutrition through:

- the lungs that absorb the essence found in the air;
- the colon that absorbs the Prana found in well digested food.

TEJAS: The Essence of Internal Fire

Tejas is the essence of the light and heat we take into the body from the sun. This is especially true from our sensory impressions of sight and skin. Tejas is the heat that is produced by our breath. It dominates in the eyes and allows us the ability to assimilate sensory impressions. This quality allows us to communicate and articulate ourselves through our spoken word; it permits us to discriminate things with our intellect.

To develop Tejas, the regular practices of fasting or staying awake at night are helpful due to their ability to increase our inner fire of determination.

Tejas gives vigor, bravery and courage allowing us to achieve astonishing actions. It governs both physical and mental digestion and assimilation, without which we lack precision and willpower. In addition, Tejas predominates in functions of the thyroid, pancreas and the immune system, providing the ability to burn and eliminate toxins. It gives us the capability to mobilize our immune system's forces. When pathogens enter the body, it is the Tejas that generates the fever that eliminate them. Without Tejas we would be unable to overcome acute diseases that are usually infectious. When Tejas are deranged, they will cause a burn out of the nervous system and scarring and inflammations of the nerve tissue.

Tejas is the activated state of the reproductive fluid when it is transformed into heat, passion and will power. This takes place whenever we are challenged or need to exert ourselves. Excess Tejas will cause burning sensations in the eyes and head area. Nothing seems to satisfy the senses when Tejas are over stimulated. When Tejas are in excess we experience annoyance, bad temper, as well as doubt. However, when Tejas are deficient we become easily submissive and vulnerable and fall under control or manipulation of others.

OJAS: The SubstanceThat Sustains Life

Ojas is the by-product of a healthy, efficient, contented physiology. It is the "sap" or "juice" that remains after food has been properly digested and absorbed. When you are generating Ojas, it means all your organs have incorporated vitality and you are receiving the sustenance your mind and body needs. Your whole being hums with high-quality vibration since you are producing and feeling delight and enchantment. However, when your Agni (fire) isn't functioning correctly, you don't create Ojas; causing food, thoughts and feelings to turn into Ama (toxins).

Ojas is the subtle adhesive that fortifies the body, mind and spirit as one, integrating them into a functioning human being.

A person's capacity to live, to enjoy life and good health, to do day-to-day routine work, etc., are manipulated by many factors. On the one hand, out of the three doshas, Kapha is held responsible for conferring the strength required to perform vigorous physical work, and on the other, the power to resist and overcome forces or factors that bring about disease and decay.

Ojas is described as an unseen source of energy and vigor in the body. Ojas is a foundation of physical and mental potency and it must be conserved by all living beings. According to Ayurveda, the substance situated in the heart is Ojas and with the increase of this substance the individual cultivates, expands and grows. With its reduction, these things decrease. Ayurveda emphasizes that sweet, unctuous, warm and light substances are beneficial and are said to increase the Ojas, and therefore children should be given these.

Ojas is the resistance to decay and degeneration of the body and provides natural immunity against disease. It is the essence of all tissues and it represents the signs of growth and formation.

1. It is antagonistic to the strength and virulence of disease.
2. It has the capacity to restrain or bind the causes or factors of disease.

Ojas is the essence of the seven Dhatu or bodily tissues. It is the vital energy that governs the hormonal balance. Ojas is the energy that controls the life-functions with the help of Prana. Ojas contains all of the five basic elements and all the vital substances of the bodily tissues. It is responsible for the autoimmune system and for mental intelligence.

Because Ojas is related to Kapha, aggravation of Kapha displaces Ojas and vice-versa. Displaced Ojas creates the Kapha related disorders of diabetes, looseness of the bones and joints and numbness of the limbs. Decreased Ojas will create Vata related reactions such as fear, general weakness, inability of the senses to perceive, loss of consciousness and death. Balanced Ojas is necessary for optimal biological functions and immunity.

High quality organic fresh nuts and seeds help to enhance Ojas. Mother's milk promotes Ojas in the body of the child, so it is important that the child receives mother's milk in order to develop biological strength. During the eight months of pregnancy, Ojas travels into the fetus from the body of the mother. Thus, if birth takes place prematurely, before the transference of Ojas, the baby will have difficulty surviving. This phenomenon demonstrates the importance of Ojas in the maintenance of life functions. Just as Ojas is necessary at the beginning of life, it is also necessary for longevity.

On the psychological level, Ojas is responsible for compassion, love, peace and creativity. Through spiritual practices, breathwork and Tantric techniques, a person can transform the Ojas into spiritual strength. This powerful spiritual energy creates a dynamic radiant individual. A person with strong Ojas is attractive, with lustrous eyes and a spontaneous and calming smile. Such an individual is full of spiritual energy and power. Spiritual practices enhance these qualities in the individual. Those who indulge excessively in losing their Ojas will directly affect their immune system. Such an individual becomes susceptible to psychosomatic ailments.

Types of Ojas

Para Ojas

- Situated in the heart.
- Eight drops in quantity.

Ojas is sweet in taste and smells like parched paddy. In the body, the color of Ojas is red or slightly yellowish and it is unctuous, slightly cooling, stable, pure and clean, soft and minute.

Apara Ojas

- Present all over the body
- Half a handful (when both the hands are joined) in quantity.

Qualities of Ojas

- Slightly cooling, watery, viscous clear, white
- High endurance potential
- Responsible for promoting the stability and strength of the organs of the body

- Capable of flowing and permeating through the body
- Nutritional substance of life

The entire body is permeated with Ojas and the loss of it leads to wasting, decay and destruction. Disturbance in its physiology may lead to three conditions:

1. Displacement of Ojas

This is the impairment of the circulation of the Ojas due to its leakage. This may cause:

- Looseness of the joints
- Inert extremities
- Displacement of dosha from their locations
- Impairment of the functions of the body including speech and/or mind

2. Disorder of Ojas

This condition is due to the change or modification in the natural properties of Ojas, under the influence of vitiated dosha. It may be present with symptoms like:

- Inertness and heaviness of the extremities
- Swelling all over the body
- Discoloration of the skin or change of complexion
- Drowsiness
- Excessive sleepiness

3. Decline of Ojas

This condition is due to the excessive loss and wasting of Ojas. It is manifested as:

1 Loss of consciousness
2 Wasting of muscles
3 Wasting of bones
4 Loss of memory
5 Death

Many scholars have correlated the condition of lose of Ojas with AIDS.

Ojas is present in the organism from the time of fertilization. Disturbance may be due to the production of quantitatively and qualitatively deficient Ojas or loss of Ojas from its channels of distribution.

Ojas is produced in the body after assimilation of the food. If one consumes food of rajasic and tamasic nature, the Ojas will be depleted from the body. By taking Sattvic food, Ojas will increase in our body and one will become strong, stout, good in appearance and pleasant. Proper and efficient functioning at all levels, be it cellular, tissue, organs or of a system, depends on Ojas. Ojas is a material and can be stored and used successfully

The Sattvic Diet

At the breast, a young infant naturally turns the mother's milk into Ojas, but it would take a most remarkable digestive system to produce Ojas from day old cold, cooked leftovers. Whole, organic, fresh foods are the highest in Prana, Tejas and Ojas. Sattvic foods are high in essential lifeforce; they haven't been tampered with. Sattvic foods are those foods that purify and uplift the body and calm the mind.

According to Ayurveda this is the healthiest way to eat and live. A Sattvic way of eating and living is the best way to build up strength, a good mind, good health and longevity. It is the most conducive way to create joy, happiness and radiant loving emotions because it is in tune with nature as a whole. We cannot separate ourselves from nature and expect to stay healthy.

If we return to a peaceful state of living, in accordance to nature's laws, it will bring health within ourselves and all life on this planet.

A Sattvic Diet Contains:

Foods that are high in Prana, Tejas and Ojas are:

- Balance of all Six Tastes
- Emphasis on Nutrient-Rich Mineral Foods
- Fresh Produce
- Spring Water

- Light, Soothing and Sweet Foods
- Easily Digested Food
- Moderate Portions

Sattvic Foods:

- Fresh, sweet fruits and juices
- Ripe pleasant-tasting nuts and seeds
- Oily fruits
- Sprouted whole grains
- Naturally sweet tasting foods in general

Prana "life-force" means "the energy that is able to create life." The sprouting ability of a seed demonstrates the presence of the life force within them. All whole grains, nuts, seeds, legumes, beans and nuts in the shell sprout. Apple seeds create apple trees; avocado pits and mango pits sprout. This is due to the life force of Prana, Tejas and Ojas present in the seed.

If you take the same seed and process or alter it in some way, then put it into soil, you will see that a plant will not grow from it. A food that has lost its life force begins to decay and rot and a new plant does not come forth. Through observation, you can easily demonstrate for yourself what you are losing by consuming foods that have been aged, cooked at excessively high temperatures, processed or been genetically altered. A food that has had its life force damaged (oxygen quality, enzymes destroyed and water molecules rearranged) cannot create life and cannot maintain the life-force energy in our bodies. Only life gives life.

> *"From the earth came herbs and from herbs came the seed that gave life to humans."*
>
> — Taittiriya Upanishad (11.1)

Prana, Tejas and Ojas are the essence of the nutrients that we take into our bodies. The importance of understanding these vital essences is a way of comprehending the deeper meaning of Vata, Pitta and Kapha. In addition, it will assist in knowing the dynamic interplay of the five elements.

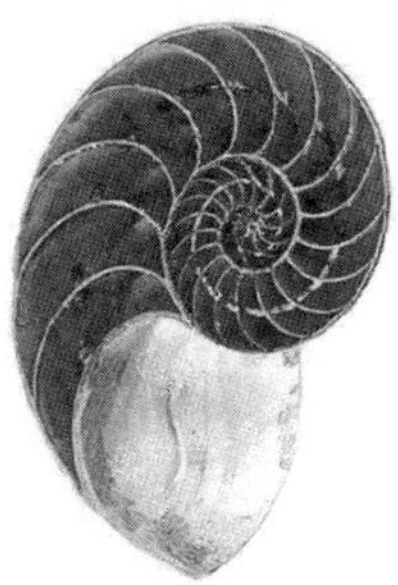

PART THREE

The Terrain

"In reality, it is not the bacteria themselves that produce the disease, but we believe it is the chemical constituents of these micro-organisms enacting upon the unbalanced cell metabolism of the human body that actually produces the disease. We also believe that if the metabolism of the human body is perfectly balanced or poised, it is susceptible to no disease."
— Royal Rife

For a seed to grow strong and vibrant, the terrain has to be fertile, healthy and balanced. The terrain is just as important as the seed. The terrain is the nourishment to feed the seed (the constitution).

In beginning to understand tongue diagnosis we need to understand that for health to exist there needs to a balance of health and vitality both in the seed and in the terrain. We can see both in the tongue and interpret the constitution and the terrain. The tongue is an essential and direct link to our whole organism. The seed is the Prakruti constitution and the terrain is the Vikruti constitution or the present state of the elements. This means the flow, stagnation and proportions of the elements. We are made of the elements. All that we take in either supports our constitution for growth or creates imbalance.

"The basic constitution of the individual remains unaltered during the lifetime, as it is genetically determined. The combination of the elements that governs the continuous physio-pathological changes in the body alters in response to changes in the environment.
— Dr. Vasant Lad, "Ayurveda: The Science of Self-Healing"

Just as each of us is born with a particular ratio of elements that make up our constitution, it is the internal presence of the elements that make up our present terrain. Knowing our present terrain or Vikruti helps us to know the immediate steps we need to take to return to balance. A healthy terrain balances Prakruti and Vikruti

Every cell, organ, system and body function is made up of the basic building blocks of Air, Fire, Water, Earth and Ether. Through touch, sight, taste, smell and hearing we absorb the elements to create our inner landscape. The beautiful thing is that we all crave the elements, each one in their own way. As has been written, 'we are the breath of life', 'we are pure sunlight', 'within us are the rivers of life', 'we are the dust of the earth', 'within us is all knowing'.

A person's tongue reveals their inner terrain. This is made known through the tongue coating, cracks, shape and moisture. The tongue is one of the best tools we have to see the activity of the internal digestive organs. We can even determine the energetic activity of the elements.

There are numerous substances that disrupt the quality of nourishment we receive from the elements. There are thousands of substances in the market now that were not around 100 years ago. The following list of items creates an unhealthy terrain and diminishes blood quality. These are foods that are high in sugar content, animal fats, commercial salt, saturated vegetable oils, pasteurized foods, dairy products, pastries, creams; commercial irradiated and genetically engineered foods, microwaved and fast foods. The number one substance that deranges the biological terrain is food high in processed sugars.

Each constitutional type requires different fuel proportions in order to create the right conditions for maximum cellular energy and expression of health. When we give our body the correct balance of proteins, fats, carbohydrates, vitamins and minerals, and include healthy lifestyle habits, we will reach our optimal level of health.

For true healing to occur, the imbalance in the terrain must be considered and addressed. Another way of stating this is that bacteria, virus, and yeasts are pleomorphic, and do not cause disease, but are the affect of disease. Attacking these "disease agents" may help to clear disease symptoms, but does address the underlying cause.

4 The Elements

The Terrain: An Introduction

We have been exploring the importance of the constitution or the seed of the individual. This is the first step. As mentioned, how can you grow a plant from seed if you don't know what kind of seed you have? Once we know what kind of seed it is, the next step is determining what kind of soil or terrain you are working with. Terrain is composed of: the soil (quality and pH), the nutrients in the soil, climate and weather conditions, amount of sunshine and water that is available for the plant to grow in. The healthier and more fertile the soil; the healthier and more vibrant the plant.

The terrain of our environment has shaped and molded us to what we are today. By testing and checking our terrain on a regular basis we can determine if the conditions of our environment continue to support our maximum growth or not.

The terrain of our inner landscape is created by the elements of nature - Air, Fire, Water Earth and Ether or Space. From the elements come the tissues. In Ayurveda, there are seven tissues that are called dhatus. These seven dhatus we can see reflected in the tongue. They are seen by the markings, shape and coating of the tongue. A person's terrain also has the srotas or energy channels that tell us of the flow of energy through the body. The last part of understanding the terrain is the Malas, or wastes, of the body. They are sweat, urine and feces. A comprehensive understanding of the terrain allows us a clear understanding of one's inner environment, needs and possibilities. With this knowledge, we can use the art of Tongue Diagnosis as a guide to help others and ourselves in treating illness or maintaining existing health.

The Elements

The Five Great Elements

Everything in the universe is composed of the five element- Air, Fire, Water, Earth and Ether. They represent the five states or qualities of energy or matter. We know these elements because we live in them and we experience their action in our physical, mental, and emotional bodies. They exist in all things, in an infinite variety of proportions. This variety of proportions and attributes allows for the enormous diversity of life. These elements are always in motion and are constantly changing and interacting with each other. While each element has its own unique nature, it cannot assume form without being absorbed by each other. This is to say, a change in one element affects the others; this is the dynamic dance of creation that we are a part of. The bonding of the elements is what makes the universe emerge and exist.

The Five Elements and Man: Creation Originating in Cosmic Consciousness

Ayurveda evolved in the meditative minds of seers. Originating in Cosmic Consciousness, this wisdom was intuitively received in the hearts of the Rishis Masters. They perceived that consciousness was energy manifested into the five basic principles, or elements: Ether (space), Air, Fire, Water and Earth.

In the beginning, the world existed in an unmanifested state of consciousness. From that state of unified consciousness, the subtle vibrations of the cosmic soundless sound "aum" manifested. From that vibration, the Ether element appeared. This ethereal element then began to move, its subtle movements created the Air, which is Ether in action. The movement of Ether produced friction, and through that friction heat was generated. Particles of heat-energy combined to form intense light and from this light the Fire element manifested.

Thus, Ether manifested into Air, and it was the same Ether that further manifested into Fire. Through the heat of the Fire, certain ethereal elements dissolved and liquefied, manifesting the Water element, and then solidified to form the molecules of Earth. In this way, Ether manifested into the four elements of Air, Fire, Water and Earth.

All organic living bodies, including those in the vegetable kingdom such as herbs and grains, and those in the animal kingdom, including man, are created from Earth. Earth also contains the inorganic substances that comprise the mineral kingdom. Thus, out of the womb of the Five Elements all matter is born.

Origination of the Elements

Ether is the original element. Through movement it becomes air, which manifests the idea of motion inherent in the idea of space.

Air through repeated movement creates friction that becomes fire, which manifests the idea of illumination inherent in the idea of movement.

Fire through densification becomes water, which manifests the idea of life inherent in the idea of illumination. Water as it coagulates becomes earth, which manifests the idea of form inherent in the idea of life.

Hence, all the five elements are different densifications of one great element, Ether, and one great idea, space, or location.

The element Ether is set in motion and condenses to become Air.

The element Air, by its constant movement and density, leads to friction to become Fire.

The element Fire, when heated, condenses to become Water.

The element Water, when cooled, becomes a solid mass, Earth.

4.1 Process of Materialization

VATA	PITTA	KAPHA
Ether and Air	Fire and Water	Water and Earth
Bodily air	Digestion acids, enzymes and fats	Bodily mass, structure and fluids

4.2 The Five Elements

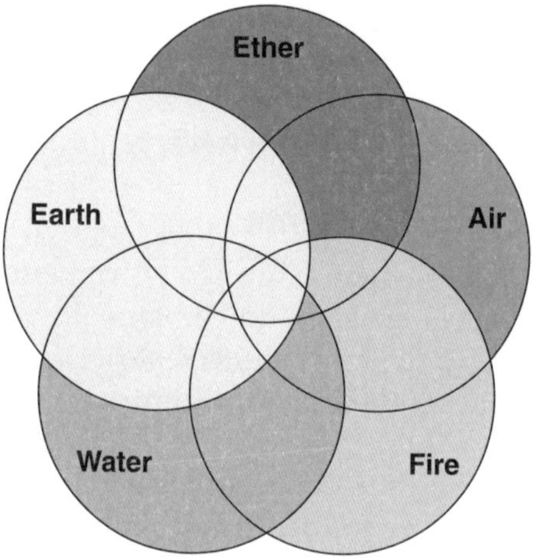

All the elements are derivations from the same basic etheric substance.

One-tenth of ether becomes air.
One-tenth of air becomes fire.
One-tenth of fire becomes water.
One-tenth of water becomes earth.

In this way earth contains all five elements;
Water contains four elements (all but earth);
Fire contains three (including air and ether);
and Air two (with ether).

Each element is distinguished according to the general rule that an item is named according to a quality or component which is in excess. These Five Elements are thus neither discrete nor individually objectifiable.

Each element has the quality of the one that preceded it, which means that:

Ether has just one quality- sound.
Air has sound and density.
Fire consists of sound, density, shape and color.
Water has sound, density, shape, color and taste.
Earth has sound, density, shape, color, taste and its own unique quality of smell.

4.3 The Five States of Material Existence

Five Elements	Manifestation	Nature	Action		Humor (Dosha)
Ether	Space	Etheric	Field	>	= V = Dry, Propulsion
Air	Motion	Gaseous	Propulsion		
Fire	Energy	Heat	Conversion	> >	= P = Hot, Conversion
Water	Cohesion	Fluid	Liquidity		
Earth	Mass	Solid	Density		= K = Cool, Cohesion

Ayurveda & The Five Elements

Ayurveda believes that everything in this universe is made up of combinations of the Five Great Elements or building blocks. This includes human beings who also acquire a soul or spirit. It should be understood; we derive from and are expressions of an un-manifest and undifferentiated Creative Principle, which is One. These Five Elements are to be understood in a material sense as well as a subtle sense.

Earth represents the solid state of matter. It manifests stability, permanence and rigidity. In our body, the parts such as bones, teeth, cells and tissue are manifestations of the Earth. Earth is considered a stable substance. By Earth we are to understand not only the terrain of our planet or the iron in our red blood cells and spleen, but also the quality of steadfastness of mind, the strength of one's moral fiber, one's slow and quiet undeterred advancement towards a goal, and the resistance to the manifestations of others.

Water characterizes change and represents the liquid state. Water is necessary for the survival of all living things. A large part of the human body is made up of water. Our blood, lymph, and other fluids move between our cells and through our vessels, bringing energy, carrying away wastes, regulating temperature, bringing disease fighters and carrying hormonal information from one area to another. By Water we mean to imply the cohesive aspects of reality that flows into and holds things together perfectly and simply witnessed in the ubiquitous H_2O molecule.

Fire is the power to transform solids into liquids, to gas, and then back again. In other words, it possesses power to transform the state of any substance. Within our bodies, the fire or energy binds the atoms together. It also converts food to fat (stored energy) and muscle. Fire transforms food into energy. It creates the impulses of nervous reactions, our feelings and even our thought processes. Fire is considered a form without substance. By Fire we mean the universal force in nature that produces heat and radiates light; it is our passion to pursue despite obstacles and delays; it is what burns away the cloak of ignorance and allows the Truth to shine with brilliance. Fire removes doubt from the mother-substance of human heart and replaces it with joy.

Air is the gaseous form of matter, which is mobile and dynamic. Within the body, air (oxygen) is the basis for all energy transfer reactions. It is a key Element required for Fire to burn. Air is existence without form. By Air we mean the transparent, rarefied, kinetic force that sets the universe in motion; it moves the blood through the vessels; removes wastes from the body; thoughts through the mind; it moves the birds to warmer climates in winter and the planets around their suns.

Ether is the space in which everything happens. It is the field that is simultaneously the source of all matter and the space in which it exists. Ether is the distance that separates matter. The chief characteristic of Ether is sound. Here sound represents the entire spectrum of vibration. By Ether we mean the subtlest of all Elements that are everywhere and touch everything; in the mind it is the vessel that receives all impressions; in the heart the space that accepts love. Space is receptivity and non-resistance to what is true.

Every substance in our world is made up of these five substances. All substances can be classified according to their predominant element. For example, a mountain is predominantly made up of the Earth Element but also contains Air, Fire, Water and Ether; however, these Elements are very small compared to the Earth Element. Ayurveda defines a human as the assemblage of the five great Elements plus the "immaterial self".

These Five Subtle Elements form the basis for all things found in the material creation; from a grain of sand to the complex physiology of every human being. Balancing these Elements in just the right way for each unique individual is the key to maintaining health and treating disease, should it arise, whether it is physical, mental, or spiritual.

4.4 Attributes of Ether

Qualities	Clear, light, subtle, soft, immeasurable
Actions	Vibration, expansion, non-resistance, freedom, love
Object of Perception	Sound
Type of Energy	Nuclear energy

4.5 Attribute of Air

Qualities	Mobile, dry, light, cold, rough, subtle
Actions	Movement in a particular direction
Object of Perception	Sound and touch
Type of Energy	Electrical energy

4.6 Attributes of Fire

Qualities	Hot, sharp, light, dry, subtle
Actions	Brilliance, luminosity, penetration
Object of Perception	Sound, touch, form
Type of Energy	Radiant energy

4.7 Attributes of Water

Qualities	Cool, liquid, dull, soft, oily, slimy
Actions	Downward movement, cleansing, adhesiveness, percolation, cohesiveness
Object of Perception	Sound, touch, form, taste
Type of Energy	Chemical energy

4.8 Attributes of Earth

Qualities	Heavy, dull, dense, hard, gross, static
Actions	Gravitation, downward attraction
Object of Perception	Sound, touch, form, taste, odor
Type of Energy	Physical, mechanical energy

Memory and the Five Elements

When we experience the elements through our senses, we are activating ancient cognitive memory. This memory is carried in the impulse and life force of everything that existed from the beginning of time. The smell of Earth stirs fresh memory and is also our most essential link to cognitive remembrance. Everything that we take into ourselves from nourishing food, physical movement or dream is a memory of past and future. All vital memory is contained and congealed within these three aspects of the whole. To consciously become aware that we are the inherent knower of the elements is to remember from the beginning of time to the present. We discover our true self when we observe ourselves within the primacy of the elements of nature.

The memory of the five elements is stored in our being. We hold the memory of the elements in the following organs:

Earth memory is stored in the heart.
Water memory is stored in the kidneys.
Fire memory is stored in the intestines.
Air memory is stored in the lungs.
Ether memory is stored in the brain.

The Elements in Life

The five elements are continuously transmuting into each other to create atoms, molecules, minerals, food and life forms. Each of us contains a unique configuration of Earth, Water, Air, and Ether within ourselves.

Earth - is substantial, with the qualities of heaviness, hardness and some downward movement

Water - is liquid, cool and flows downward.

Fire - is the power of change and transformation; its qualities are heat, dryness and upward movement.

Air - is gaseousness and has airy qualities; its light, clear, dry and dispersing.

Ether - is subtle; it's equated to size or space.

Earth - predominates in the cell membrane giving structure to the cell.

Water - predominates in the cytoplasm, the liquid in the cell.

Fire - predominates in the metabolic processes regulating the cell.

Air - predominates in the gases in the cell.

Ether - predominates in the empty space occupied by the cell

Locations of the Five Elements in the Body

Earth is our physical body and is found in the lower part of the body from the region of the knees to the feet and governs stability and the ability to stand.

Water is our body's fluid and is found in the urino-genital system, lower abdomen, hips and buttocks.

Fire is the acids and enzymes of the body and is found in the digestive system and relates to the mid-abdomen from its center in the navel.

Air is the Prana and breath and is found in the heart and chest. It is the center of the circulatory and respiratory systems and arms.

Ether is the vibration of all vital systems together and is found in the head governing the mind and senses and the nervous system.

4.9 The Five Elements in Relation to the Body

Earth	Relates to the bones and solid bodily tissues, skull, muscles, intestines, skin, hair and nails.
Water	Relates to the liquid bodily tissues, plasma, blood, urine, sweat, saliva and mucus.
Fire	Relates to digestive and reproductive systems and urges such as hunger, thirst, delirium and sexuality.
Air	Relates to the respiratory system, movement of all types, effort and breath.
Ether	Relates to our mental space or environment and well as emotions such as desire, anger, fear and delusion.

External increase of an Element increases its internal twin; likewise, an external decrease decreases the internal twin.

4.10 Actions of the Five Elements

Earth	Is our memory and referent of our being.
Water	Allows us to taste and discern life.
Fire	Allows us the power to digest the world around us.
Air	Allows us to feel, to touch and to know.
Ether	Gives us the power to resonate within our observation and cognition.

4.11 The Connection of the Elements and Foods

EARTH	WATER	FIRE	AIR	ETHER
Sprouted whole grains Root Vegetables Dried Fruits Beans and Legumes Seeds & Nuts Sea Salts Trace Minerals	Coconut Water Juicy Fruits Juicy Vegetables Nut & Seed Milks	Sour Fruits Tart Berries Culinary Seeds Heating Spices Warming Herbs Fermented Foods Alcohol	Dried Fruits Cabbage Family Nightshades Leafy Greens Sprouts Rough Vegetables Beans and Legumes	Hypnotics Narcotics Drugs L.S.D. Cocaine Tobacco Marijuana

4.12 Nourishing Elements

Element	Found Within	Nourishes
Earth	Solid food	Internal organs, muscles, skin, bones and all other Earth predominant tissues
Water	Liquid food	Mucous membranes, secretions, lymph, plasma, fat, nerves, reproductive system and all other watery predominant tissues
Fire	Sunlight, heat and the heating element as found in food	Digestion and metabolism, blood and all Fire predominant digestive secre-tions and enzymes, also tissue enzymes
Air	Breath and the Air Element	Vitalizes nervous system, promotes discharge of impulses and secretions
Ether	Space in breath and in food	Nourishes and clears the mind and the five sense organs

4.13 Elements and the Six Tastes

EARTH	WATER	FIRE	AIR	ETHER
Sour Sweet	Sweet Salty	Pungent Salty	Bitter Astringent	Astringent Pungent

The Three Principles (Air, Fire, and Water)

Air, fire and water are the three principles most fundamental to life.

Air and Ether are both ethereal and together constitute Vata. Air can exert its effects only when there is empty space available.

Fire and Water together constitutes Pitta. Fire cannot exist within the body except in association with water, such as in the stomach where water protects it from stomach acid. A burn from stomach acid has the same amount of burning effect as an open flame or a lightning burn.

Water and Earth combine to make up Kapha. Pure Earth in the body obstructs its functions and pure solidity in the body means a disease condition. Earth is only beneficial to the body when it is in a solution of Water.

The Five Elements and the Gunas

The Subtle Aspects of the Elements

The five elements originate in the energy issuing from cosmic consciousness. They are present in all matter of the universe, meaning that energy and matter are one. From the three Gunas stem the five elements:

4.14 The Five Elements and the Three Gunas

GUNA:	SATTVA	RAJAS	TAMAS
ELEMENT:	Ether / Air	Fire / Water	Earth

Discovering Your Elemental Constitution

Each of the three living, moving elements can be easily transformed by changing the proportion of elements ingested from the world around you.

If you are experiencing too much scattered energy and your mind is racing here there and everywhere (excessive Air Element), seek out stability of the Earth and Water Element. Find a gentle stream, lean yourself against a tree, or simply be still and feel the balance come back to your mind and body.

If you are over heating (excessive Fire Element), seek out the cooling influence of the Water Element or expand your perspective through the Element of Ether/Space through meditation;

where there is less oxygen, there is less fuel to feed the flames.

If you are feeling dull and lethargic (excessive Water Element), seek out more movement and expansion through the Elements of Air and Ether and you will find yourself feeling lighter and freer.

We are surrounded by nature's medicine in the form of the five elements and we can access and take in the nourishment through our senses. Our senses are our way to ingest the revitalizing energy from the healing Earth and her Elements.

Elemental Questionnaire

The following questionnaire has been designed to help you determine your true Elemental body-mind nature. Don't spend more than a few moments considering your response. There is no right or wrong response, so simply answer the questions as truthfully as you can. Answer with one or two of the letters indicating which element describes you the best.

Code to Answers

A - Air/ Wind

F - Fire/ Sun

W - Water/ Rain

E - Earth/ Soil

S - Space/Ether

- Which element(s) were present when you felt the healthiest?
- Which elements(s) are present during your favorite season?
- Which environment and element(s) nourished you growing up?
- Which element(s) do you crave when you feel under the weather?
- Which of the element(s) are you aware of that you enjoy at your work place?
- Which of the elements(s) do you appreciate in your own home?
- Which is your favorite season - which element(s) are present?
- If you could live anywhere in the world which element(s) would you want to be present?

- Which element(s) best describes your body?
- Which element(s) best describes your personality and emotional realm?
- Which of element(s) best describes your mental state of mind?
- Which element(s) could you say you feel that you know most intimately?
- Which element(s) were you aware of today as expressing a prominent quality?
- In a stressful and irritating situation, which of your element(s) would reveal themselves?
- If people were going to describe you using the element(s), which would they be?
- Which element(s) do like to play with/in?
- Which element(s) comfort you?
- Which element(s) give you the most strength and vitality?
- How fast do you move, describe your speed?
- How light or heavy do you feel most of the time, according to the element(s)?

> *"The real voyage of discovery consists not in seeking new landscapes, but having new eyes."*
> — Marcel Proust

The Return of the Elements

As death approaches the Earth element, the feeling of the solidity and hardness of the body begins to melt. The body seems very heavy. The boundaries of the body, its edge, are less solid. There is not so much a feeling of being "in" the body. One is less sensitive to impressions and feelings. One can no longer move the limbs at will. Peristalsis slows, the bowels no longer move without aid. The organs begin to shut down. As the Earth element continues to dissolve into the Water element, there is a feeling of flowingness, a liquidity as the solidity that has always intensified identification with the body begins to melt, a feeling of fluidity.

As the Water element begins to dissolve into the Fire element, the feeling of fluidity becomes more like a warm mist. The bodily fluids begin to slow, the mouth and eyes become dry, circulation slows, blood pressure drops. As the circulation begins to thicken and stop, blood settles in the lowest extremities. A feeling of lightness ensues.

As the Fire element dissolves into the Air element, feelings of warmth and cold dissipate; physical comfort and discomfort no longer have meaning. The body temperature drops until it reaches a stage where the body begins to cool and becomes pale. Digestion stops. A feeling of lightness, as of heat rising, becomes predominant. A feeling of dissolving into yet subtler and subtler boundarylessness.

As the Air element dissolves into Consciousness itself there is a feeling of edgelessness. The out breath having become longer than the in breath has dissolved into Space and there is no longer the experience of bodily form or function but just a sense of vast expanding airiness, a dissolving into pure being.

So the human nervous system returns to the Source of its being. Yet the ending of that cycle,... marks the beginning of the journey for you.

— Dr. Vasant Lad, Ayurveda, Science of Healing

The Elements and the Six Tastes

While the elements give us a foundation from which to understand constitution, the six tastes provide us with a practical method of determining the elemental aspects present in what nourishes us. The science of the six tastes will be covered in greater depth later in the book; however, it is valuable to touch on them at this point.

4.15 Classification According to the Fundamental Elements

Element	Taste	Properties	Effects
Earth	Sweet, Slightly astringent	Heavy, rough, hard, inert, stable, clear, dense, coarse	Promotes growth, weight, compactness, stability, strength, downward movements, aperients
Water	Sweet, slightly Astringent, Sour, and Salty	Cold, oily, inert, mobile, fluid, soft, gelatinous	Moistening, binding, lubricating, cooling, solvent
Fire	Pungent, slightly sour and salty	Hot, dry, fine, light, rough, clear	Burning, digestive, heating, energy-giving, radiant, purifying, upward, movement, emetic
Air	Astringent & Bitter	Cold, light, clear, fine, rough	Purifying, drying, loosening, tiring, alleviating, promoting movement
Ether	Unmanifest	Smooth, subtle, soft	Softening, unblocking

5 The Seven Dhatus

- Dhatus Signs of Deficiency and Excess
- Physical Properties and Functions of the Dhatus
- Causes, Signs and Symptoms
- Malas: Waste Products
- The Energy Channels: Srotas

The elements are the building blocks of the dhatus. The dhatus are constituents that comprise the basic structure of the body. They are seven tissues in the body: blood, muscle tissue, fat tissue, bones, bone marrow, sperm in males and ova in females.

The term "dhatu" reflects its literal meaning, "to support and to nourish." Dhatu, the constructing element is involved in the body's basic physical formation. The dhatus are represented by a specific series of body tissues that function in the development and nourishment of the whole body as well as maintain the natural immunity. The following seven dhatus make and maintain the architecture of the body.

The Seven Dhatus Body Tissue Layers

Each Dhatus is developed or transformed out of the previous tissue layer, starting with Rasa (plasma). Each of the seven tissue layers has a special membrane that allows for the absorption and diffusion of nutrients. If plasma is not healthy, then all the other layers will also be affected.

The seven layers are:

- Plasma (Rasa), which feeds and nourishes the blood. Tissue fluids like chyle, blood plasma, intracellular and tran cellular fluid lymph etc. Its function is nourishment.
- Blood (Rakta); when your body is able to obtain sufficient Rasa, nourishment begins to take place. Blood produces invigoration.

- Muscle (Mamsa); when your blood is healthy and well formed it nourishes the muscles and tissues; function is "plastering." It holds together the skeleton.
- Fat (Meda); well nourished muscle and tissue feeds fat; function is "unctuousness."
- Bone (Asthi); healthy fat makes for healthy bone tissue; function is "support."
- Nerves- Fluid & Marrow (Majja); bone produces marrow; marrow is anything that is entirely encased in bone, includes all body marrows and the brain and spinal cord; function is "filling." Its function is to fill the bones.
- Reproductive tissues (Majja & Shukra); properly nourished marrow goes to nourish all bodily secretions involved in reproduction; function is "creativity." Reproductive elements (male and female sexual fluids). Its function is reproduction and production of ojas, the fluid that produces the strength, aura and controls immunity.

These dhatu are being constantly formed, destroyed and reformed with appropriate materials derived from nutrient substances, from the time of conception till death.

5.1 Dhatus of Deficiency and Excess

Dhatu	Elements	Signs of Decrease	Signs of Increase
Plasma & Lymph (Rasa)	Water	Fatigue, dryness, empty feel, loud noises irritating	Loss of appetite, mouth watering, nausea, obstructed bodily channels
Blood (Rakta)	Fire & Water	Loss of stamina, dry skin and collapsed vessels	Skin diseases, jaundice, redness of eyes and body
Muscle Tissues (Mamsa)	Primarily Earth also Water & Fire	Fatigue, emaciation, looseness of joints	Swollen glands, heavy muscles
Fat (Media)	Water	Dry, rough, lean body structure; cravings for fatty foods	Obesity, pendulousness of breasts, abdomen and buttocks

Dhatu	Elements	Signs of Decrease	Signs of Increase
Bone (Asthi)	Earth & Air	Pain in bones and joints, dryness of teeth, nails or hair	Heavy deposits of minerals and calcification in tissues
Bone Marrow & Nervous System (Majja)	Water & Earth	Dizziness and weak bones	Enlarged and heavy joints
Reproductive Tissues (Shukra & Artava)	Water	Pain in reproductive organs, loss of virility, darkness around the eyes aversion to sex	Excessive lust

5.2 Physical Properties and Functions of the Dhatus

Panchabhautik constitution and physical properties	Special properties	Functions

Plasma & Lymph (Rasa) Dhatu

Liquidity	Liquefying	Oleating
Fluidity	Oleating	Nourishing the blood.
Opacity	Preserving	Preserving
Viscosity	Main gaining, Preserving, bearing Protecting.	Satiating, Refreshing
Unctuous	Soothing	Satiating Refreshing

Blood (Rakta) Dhatu

Liquid	Smell	Imparts colour
Fluid	Fleshy	Nourishes the blood
Opaque	Colored	Nourishes the mamsa
Unctuous	Movement	Enlivening
Soft	Softness	Softness to body parts
Viscous	Neither hot nor cold, warm Sweet Salt	Responsible for tactile sensation, Produces growth or wasting of other dhatu

Muscle (Mamsa) Dhatu

Gross in form	Strengthens the body
Static	Nourishes meda
Heavy	Covers the body
Rough	Nourishes mala.
Hard	Strengthens the body

Fat Tissue (Meda) Dhatu

Liquid	Oleating and produces sweat
Smooth	Nourishes the asthi and secures sturdiness.

Bones & Cartilage (Asthi) Dhatu

Heavy	Bearing, supporting.
Rough	Nourishes the maija.
Hard	Provides support to mamsa.
Gross	Provides strength.
Static	Supports the mamsa and other bodily parts.
Gives form	Supports the mamsa and other bodily parts.

Marrow, Nerve & Connective Tissue (Majja) Dhatu

Unctuous	Oleates.
Soft	Fills the asthi and nourishes the shukra.

Male Reproductive Tissue (Shukra) Dhatu

Crystalline and white Liquid	Produces (Conception).
Viscous	Sensation of ejaculation.
Sweetish	Satisfaction.
Smelling like honey	Fondness.
Heavy	Strengthens the body.
Thick	Strengthens the body.

The dhatus are produced in a kind of progressive pattern beginning with rasa and ending with shukra dhatu.

Decrease in Dhatu

A decrease in Rasa dhatu would lead to a sense of oppression of the heart or chest region, tremors in the extremities, feeling of emptiness in the stomach or in the body as a whole and thirst.

A decrease in Rakta dhatu would lead to roughness of skin, desire for sour and cold things with and flaccidity in the veins.

A decrease in Mamsa dhatu would lead to emaciation of the buttocks, cheeks, hips, loins, chest, thighs, axillac, penis, belly and neck.

A decrease in Meda dhatu would lead to enlargement of the spleen, feeling of emptiness in the joints, general roughness, and desire for oily food.

A decrease in Asthi dhatu would lead to pain in the bones, brittle nails and teeth.

A decrease in Majja dhatu would lead to reduced generation of semen, cracking of knuckles at the joints, pricking pain in the bones.

A decrease in Skukra dhatu would lead to pain in penis and testicles, inability to engage in coitus, ejaculation only after long time, or it contains blood and whiteness in ejaculate.

Dhatu also contribute to the formation, or update, of accessory or supplementary supports. The former pass through tranformative changes, the latter are not subjected to any such changes i.e. they represent the final formed products.

Dhatu	Upadhatu
Rasa	Stanya (Breast milk) and Asrik (Menstrual blood).
Rakta	Kandra (Tendon like structures) and Sira (Blood vessels, especially veins)
Mamsa	Vasa (muscle fat) Twacha (seven layers of the skin)
Meda	Snayu (ligaments, sheaths etc.)

Like the dhatu, updhatu are structural elements that support the body but do not nourish it, and are not subjected to any transformation. Upadhatu appear to arise either as by products of the nutrition dhatu during the course of dhatvagni transactions or are produced from the breakdown products of stable dhatu. They provide supplementary support to the body.

Stanya (Breast milk) - Excellent food for the infant. It nourishes and supports the child.

Rajah (menstrual blood) - It has close relationship to a female's biological functions and is an index of her well being. Also, it closely resembles the circulating rasadhatu and that is why it is considered an upadhatu.

Kandara (Tendon like) - Resemble bones in grossness. They help in various motions such as extension, contraction, flexion etc.

Sira (Blood Vessel or Channel) - According to Sushruta there are seven hundred siras in the human body as veins, nerves and lymphatics.

Vasa (Muscle Fat) - It fills muscle spaces and supports various structures such as blood vessels and nerves. It belongs to the adipose tissue system of the body.

Twacha (Skin) - Belongs to the epithelial group of tissues for support (epidermis and dermis). The seven layered twacha is the largest vital organ with numerous complex function providing protection to the under lying viscera against the physical trauma, chemical trauma and other infections. It is richly supplied with nerves and serves as a sense organ for the perception of local sensation. It activates various system of body in, response to certain environmental changes.

Snayu (ligament like) - Vayu conducts the fat of the adipose tissue and makes the sira, snayu. Snayu binds the muscles, bones, fat tissues and strengthens the joints. Acharya Sushruta says vayu in its normal state, while coursing through its specific siras, helps in the unobstructed performance of its specific functions namely extension, flexion, speech etc. and produces clearness and non illusiveness of the intellect and the sense organs. Snayu are nine hundred in number and may be grouped under four types, namely:

- Pratanvati (Branching and ramifying)
- Vrit (Ring shaped; as in stomach and small intestine)
- Prithu (Thick or broad)
- Sushir (Perforated /hollow as in urinary bladder)

5.3 The Seven Dhatus

Dhatu	**Elements**	**Bodily Tissue(s)**
Plasma & Lymph (Rasa)	Water	Plasma (serum, white blood cells, lymphatic system)
Blood (Rakta)	Fire & Water	Red blood cells
Muscle Tissues (Mamsa)	Primarily Earth also Water & Fire	Muscle
Fat (Media)	Water	Adipose tissue/ fat
Bone (Asthi)	Earth & Air	Bones & cartilage
Bone Marrow & Nervous System (Majja)	Water & Earth	Marrow, Nerve tissue, connective tissue
Reproductive Tissues (Shukra & Artava)	Water	Male & Female reproductive tissue

5.4a Causes of Plasma and Lymph (Rasa) Disorders

- Heavy food
- Overeating
- Cold beverages & food
- Fried, oily, processed, leftover foods
- Unhealthy food combining
- Excess sugar or salt
- Hydrophilous substances: cheese and yogurt
- Bacteria
- Excess bodily Ama
- Excessive or insufficient physical exercise (beyond one's constitutional capacity)
- Emotionally: worry, anxiety & lack of trust.

5.4b Signs and Symptoms of Plasma and Lymph (Rasa) Disorders

Increased Tissue	Decreased Tissue	Disturbed Tissue
• Lymphatic & venous congestion • Reoccurring colds, bronchial & sinus congestion • Excess salivation • Edema & swelling • Pallor • Feeling of heaviness in heart	• Anemia • Dehydration • Dizziness • Dry skin • Emaciation • Excess thirst • Fatigue • Hypersensitive • Palpitations • Shock	• Dizziness & Nausea • Fatigue • Fever • Lack of taste • Lack of faith • Lack of perception • General bodily aches & pains

5.5a Causes of Blood (Rakta) Disorders

- Bacteria
- Deficiency of iron &/or vitamin B12
- Excess sugar & salt
- Excessive exposure to the sun
- Exposure to radiation
- Heated oils & fried foods
- Unhealthy food combinations
- Liver & spleen disorders
- Sour fermented foods: cheese, yogurt & pickles
- Working in a hot environment
- Excessive or insufficient physical exercise (beyond one's constitutional capacity)
- Emotionally: repressed aggression, anger, envy, & hate

5.5b Signs and Symptoms of Blood (Rakta) Disorders

Increased Tissue	Decreased Tissue
• Bleeding tendencies • Enlarged liver or spleen • Fullness of blood vessels • Hypertension • Red eyes • Skin conditions such as: Acne, eczema, dermatitis, rash	• Anemia • Breathlessness on exertion • Craving for hot spicy foods, sour, citrus fruit & iron rich-food • Cracked, dry & rough skin • Lack of energy, vitally & enthusiasm • Loss of luster • Poor circulation

5.6a Causes of Muscle (Mamsa) Disorders

- Emotional stress
- Daytime sleeping
- Unhealthy food combinations
- Lack of sleep or rest
- Insufficient or excess protein intake
- Heavy acid foods such as meats & dairy products
- Over or undereating
- Excessive or insufficient physical exercise (beyond one's constitutional capacity)
- Physical trauma
- Liver imbalances & diseases
- Typhoid
- Tuberculosis
- Sleeping during day
- Hydrophilous substances: cheese and yogurt
- Emotionally: stressed & uneasy

5.6b Signs and Symptoms of Muscle (Mamsa) Disorders

Increased Tissue	Decreased Tissue
• Fibrocystic changes in the breasts • Enlarged lips, cheeks, tongue • Uterine fibroids • Muscle flaccidity & hypertrophy • Undue growth of muscle, fibromas & myomas	• Cravings for protein • Emaciation • Dislocation of joints • Fatigue • Loss of muscle power • TMJ disorders • Muscle rigidity, atrophy & wasting away

5.7a Causes of Fat (Meda) Disorders

- Excess sugar & sweets
- Excess salt or dairy products
- Cold beverages & foods
- Consumption of meat
- Heated oils & fried foods
- Lack of high-quality fats in the diet
- Unhealthy food combinations
- Excess water
- Sleeping during the day
- Excessive or insufficient physical exercise (beyond one's constitutional capacity)
- Typhoid
- Artificial drugs & substances: alcohol, tobacco, marijuana, steroids & other medication
- Emotionally: stress & unresolved emotions
- Frequent emotional eating

5.7b Signs and Symptoms of Fat (Meda) Disorders

Increased Tissue	Decreased Tissue
• Diabetes	• Dry skin
• Gallstones	• Cracking joints
• Lethargy	• Emaciation
• Pains in the joints	• Osteoarthritis
• Breathlessness	• Lumbago
• Sluggish metabolism	• Overactive thyroid
• Underactive thyroid	• Osteoporosis
• Excess sweating	• Enlarged spleen
• Lipomas-fatty tumors	
• Hypertension	
• Gallstones	
• Low libido	
• Excess thirst & sweet taste in mouth	

5.8a Causes of Bone (Asthi) Disorders

- Excess or low consumption of protein
- Lack of minerals
- Menopause & hormone replacement therapy
- Poor posture
- Physical trauma, such as an accident
- Thyroid & Parathyroid disorders
- Excessive or insufficient physical exercise (beyond one's constitutional capacity) & irregular intense exercise which can provoke Vata, such as running & mountain climbing
- Unbalanced diet- particularly excessive Vata promoting foods: dry foods & beans, stale food & leftovers
- Emotionally: loneliness, insecurity, lack of support, trauma

5.8b Signs and Symptoms of Bone (Asthi) Disorders

Increased Tissue	Decreased Tissue
• Bony protuberances, spurs	• Hair loss
• Bone fusion & /or tumors	• Joint pain
• Calcification	• Osteoporosis
• Extra teeth	• Osteoarthritis
• Excessive hair growth	• Rheumatoid arthritis
• Hunchbacked	• Rough, dry, brittle, crooked nails
• Lordosis (abnormal convex curve of lumbar spine)	• Shortened height
• Spinal misalignment	• Spinal misalignment
	• Spontaneous fractures

5.9a Causes of Marrow and Nervous System (Majja) Disorders

- Any doshic irritation which over stimulates or in any way affects the nervous system
- Artificial substances & drugs: alcohol, tobacco & other medications
- Cerebral concussion or compression
- Heavy metal toxicity
- High fever
- Lack of sleep
- Physical trauma, such as a bone fracture
- Radiation poisoning
- Viral or bacterial infection
- Spiritual possession or energy field difficulty
- Unhealthy & unbalanced diet- particularly excess Vata irritating foods: dry foods, beans, & leftovers
- Unhealthy food combinations
- Emotionally: stress, conflict & hectic lifestyle, unresolved emotions

5.9b Signs and Symptoms of Marow and Nervous System (Majja) Disorders

Increased Tissue	Decreased Tissue
• Excess sleep • Heaviness of eyes • Pineal & pituitary tumors • Sluggish & heavy throughout body • Tumors on the peripheral nerves	• Anemia • Attention Deficit Disorder (ADD) • Epilepsy • Insomnia Neurological problems • Lack of Understanding • MS, Parkinson's • Neurological problems • Osteoporosis • Osteoarthritis • Poor Communication • Rheumatoid arthritis • Sexual debility • Stroke paralysis

5.10a Causes of Reproductive Tissue (Shukra and Artava) Disorders

- Engaging in intercourse at midday or midnight
- Experiencing a few orgasms during one night
- Experiencing sex during menses
- Experiencing intense sex while under the influence of intoxicants or drugs
- Experiencing violent sex in the unhealthy position
- Genetic predisposition to reproductive imbalances & diseases
- Gonorrhea, syphilis, or herpes
- Over indulgence in sexual activity
- Physical or surgical trauma
- Practicing Tantric sexual practices without proper guidance
- Retention of ejaculation
- Unhealthy & unbalanced food combinations
- Use of chemical spermicides
- Emotionally: stressed & worried

5.10b Signs and Symptoms of Reproductive Tissue (Shukra and Artava) Disorders

Increased Tissue	Decreased Tissue
• Increased desire for sex • Preoccupation with sex • Male Reproductive Only: Excess semen flow with increased prostatic secretion but low sperm content • Premature ejaculation • Prostatic calculi • Female Reproductive Only: Multiple cystic ovary • Premature orgasm • Sterility	• Fear of sex • Low libido • Pain during coitus • Sterility • Male Reproductive Only: Low sperm count • Impotence • Female Reproductive Only: No ovulation • Primary sterility

Dhatus & Malas

5.11 Dhatus and Malas

Tissue Support (Dhatu)	Tissue Supported (Upadhatu)	Function	Waste (Malas)	Dosha with which Associated
Ingested Food			Urine and feces	All three doshas
Plasma & Lymph (Rasa)	Breast milk and menstrual secretions	Nourishment	Mucus (Kapha)	Kapha
Blood (Rakta)	Blood vessels, tendons	Invigoration	Bile (Pitta)	Pitta
Muscle Tissues (Mamsa)	Muscles, ligaments, skin	Coating of the skeletal system	Ear wax, nose mucus, navel lint, smegma, etc.	Kapha
Fat (Media)	Omentum	Lubrication	Sweat	Kapha
Bone (Asthi)	Teeth	Support	Nails, body and beard hair	Vata
Bone Marrow & Nervous System (Majja)	Head hair	Filling of the bone marrow	Lacrimal secretions	Kapha
Reproductive Tissues (Shukra & Artava)		Reproduction		Kapha (Male) Pitta (Female)

Malas: Waste Products of the Body

In addition to the doshas and the dhatus described above, malas (the waste products) are the other constituents of the body. The word Mala comes from the root "mal", to darken, stain or harm. Unlike the bodily humors they do not have a constructive function in the body, but like them, they do assist to maintain body function in their process of discharge.

Mala is more an impurity, yet each Mala has a nutritive function. The malas are the byproducts of the various dhatus present in the body. The chief malas are urine; feces; and perspiration. Other malas are: fat or secretion of the genitalia and secretions of the various orifices of the body such as the ear, nose, mouth, and so on. Malas play a supporting role while they are in the body. They are eliminated once their supporting role is finished.

The concept of malas, both as supportive and excretive products of the body, is important to understand. An example from modern medicine would explain it thus: when red blood cells get old, they are destroyed and may be considered as malas. The malas perform a supportive function when the iron content of the destroyed red blood cells is reabsorbed and utilized by the body directly. Another example is with the secretion of bile. Bile content is passed on as bile by the liver into the duodenum, where it aids the absorption of fats. Thereafter, it is excreted in the feces as a Mala or waste product. It is in this way that malas perform a dual role.

Eliminating waste is crucial to good health, but dosha imbalances stifle the flow of the malas, creating a toxic internal environment. If you are not eliminating malas, it means you are accumulating Ama somewhere in your system and you may have to undergo Ayurvedic cleansing to get rid of these toxins from your body.

Malas: Waste Materials

As a consequence of foods that we take into our bodies from the external world and the normal biological processes that take place internally, we generate different kinds of waste materials, or malas, which must be excreted. Ayurveda generally recognizes two kinds of malas:

- Ahara mala or wastes from food
- Dhatu mala or wastes from the tissues

The ahara malas include feces (purisha), urine (mutra), and sweat (sveda). These are the three main malas. The dhatu malas include the various secretions of the nose, eyes, ears; lactic acid, carbon dioxide, and other metabolites of cellular respiration; exfoliated hair, skin, and nails. Although these are all waste products, they serve a role in maintaining health as long as they are normal in their quantity, qualities, and function. However, if the malas become abnormal in some regard (i.e. increased or decreased) they become a factor in creating disease. The malas are composed predominantly of different elements. Feces are composed mainly of Earth element; urine, mainly Water and Fire; sweat, primarily Water. Of course all five elements are contained in every mala.

The following chart summarizes the effects of increased or decreased malas:

5.12 The Three Malas Chart

Mala	Increase	Decrease
Feces (Purisha) **Element: Earth**	• Heaviness • Flatulence • Abdominal discomfort (generalized)	• Bloating • Abdominal pain (mid) • Low back pain • Weakness • Asthma • Osteoarthritis • Hypoglycemia
Urine (Mutra) **Element:** **Water & Fire**	• Urinary frequency • Bladder dysfunction • Urinary tract infections	• Reduced urine • Chronic thirst • Renal stones • Abdominal pain (lower)
Sweat (Sveda) **Element: Water**	• Perspires easily • Fungal dermatitis • Low body temperature • Constipation • Body odor • Itching • Constipation	• Decreased perspiration • Dry skin • Burning sensations • High body temperature

Mala Locations

Each mala is located in the membrane structure that surrounds the channels of elimination.

5.13 Bodily Wastes

Rasadhatu and rasagni	Kapha (mucus/ phlegm)
Raktadhatit and raktagni	Pitta
Mamsdhatu and manisagni	Excretas of ear, eye, nose, mouth, hair follicles and genitals
Medadhatu and niedogni	Sweda (sweat)
Asthidhatti and asthagni	Hair, beard, nails follicles, nails
Majjadhatu and majjagni	Lubrication of eye, faces, and skin
Shukradhatu and shukragni	Ojas (Vital essence)

The process of transformation is brought about by the action of the Agni dhatu resulting in:

- A fine essence that fosters nourishment to the next dhatu.
- A supplementary support that is not subjected to any transformative change representing final formed product or products (updhatu).
- A by product that is the representative waste product of the dhatu.
- A component that retains its own material and nourishes its own similar constituent within the body.

In the process of transformation: each dhatu provides a healthy environment that nourishes the next successive dhatu in order of Rasa to Rakta, Rakta to Mamsa, Mamsa to Meda, Meda to Mafja and Majja to Shukra in the one or the combination of three ways.

- By the actual transformation of one dhatu into another.
- By serving as a conduit for nutrition to the next dhatu.
- By providing the charger or activator to the next dhatu.

The Energy Channels: Srotas

Tissues of the body interact with one another via srotas, which are sometimes described as being "ducts", but basically represent areas where blockage can occur. A srota is like a river. Just as there are streams that turn into rivers; rivers turn into lakes or oceans, so to in our body, a small srotas will turn into larger srotas, the largest of these srotas is the gastrointestinal tract.

There are 14 srotas (two of them in females only) affecting the physical structures: those involving the respiratory system, the digestive system (upper portion), the water system (intake and distribution), the lymphatic system, circulatory system, muscular system, adipose system, skeletal system, nervous system, reproductive system, sebaceous system, excretory system (intestines), urinary system, menstrual system, and lactation system.

The srotas are:

Three srotas to receive Prana, Water and food

Seven srotas to nourish the seven tissues

Three srotas to eliminate urine, feces, and sweat

The other srotas include lactation and menses

The last srotas works with the mind and emotions

The whole concept of srotas is both structural and functional. Each srota may be affected by a deficient flow of substances (in which case, the system to be nourished is weak), an excess flow of substances (in which case the system being nourished usually shows agitation or one will observe excessive drainage), a blockage of flow (often creating a mass), or a bypass (overflow) which usually manifests with substances appearing where they should not normally appear. In addition, the mind is considered to have a srota (mandvaha srota) that affects the flow of emotions, sensory impressions, and thoughts in a manner parallel to that of the physical srotas.

There are three main srotas that bring in nourishment. These channels receive: food, Prana and water. These channels are connected to outside energy.

In some ways, the srotas are like the Chinese meridians (jing), in that the types of disorders that can occur (deficiency, excess, blockage, and overflow) are similar in nature and the concept of forming connections is similar. While the Indian system has a separate depiction of flow pathways (nadis), the early conception of the Chinese meridians, which was as blood vessels, seems closely allied with the broader Indian conception of srotas, seen as narrow passageways through which substances flow.

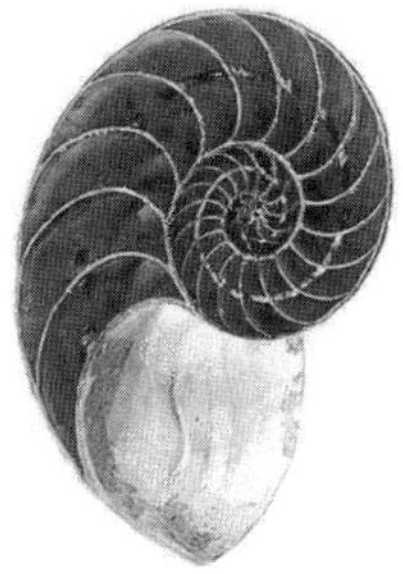

PART FOUR

The Fire

6 Digestion: The Cornerstone of Health

- The Fire
- The Cornerstone of Health
- Agni: Digestive Fire
- The 13 Main Forms of Agni
- Agni and Pitta
- The Four Varieties of Agni
- Agni Sources
- Enzymes and Agni
- Agni, Prana and Oxygen
- Seven Principle Causes of Indigestion
- Agni: Enzyme-Rich Foods
- Agni: Digestion and the Tissue Enzymes
- Rekindling Your Digestive Fire
- Stoking Your Fire — An Agni Program

The Fire

The ancient healing art of Ayurveda describes digestion as a sacred Fire, personified in the Indian tradition as the god Agni. The digestive Fire in the belly consumes our food and transforms it into the elements of the body, mind, emotions and spirit.

The tongue is our direct link to our Fire. The Fire of transformation, which occurs in the core of the belly, is our greatest link to strength and vitality. Without Fire, we cannot absorb nourishment into our being. No Fire-No Life.

When we feel hunger, this is a sign that the digestive Fire is radiating brightly. When our hunger lags and the Fire diminishes, then our digestion suffers, food is not assimilated and toxins accumulate in the body. According to Ayurveda, the condition of the digestive Fire determines the health of our entire being.

Making sure that Agni, this sacred fire, stays strong and healthy is the first step. By supplying the right amount of fuel and not overloading our stomach by overeating or drinking too much at meals our fire stays strong.

Keeping in mind that hunger is the sign of a healthy digestive fire, rather than constantly snacking, we can wait until the level of hunger is high, before we eat. Only then do we make our offering to the flames.

In India, as in many traditional cultures, meals are a time of sacred offering. Prior to eating, the food is offered to the divine power with humility, reverence and gratitude. The food itself is considered sacred and is prepared, handled and served as a precious gift. Many traditional cultures attach rituals to the act of eating to acknowledge its divine nature. This spiritual practice nourishes the body as well as the spirit.

In many parts of Western culture, however, this reverence for food and eating has faded, or vanished completely. Grace may still be said at the dinner table, but for the most part, food is eaten with very little thought of where it came from and an absence of sensitivity to the condition of the digestive fire. Who among us takes a moment of reverent silence before eating when we are dining on fast food? And, with jumbo portions being the typical amounts, how often do we over-eat, despite the discomfort that may follow?

The consequences of eating in this unconscious fashion, year after year, is destructive, and explains, in part, why people in our modern-day culture suffer so much from obesity, heart disease, high blood pressure, to name a few. These are all diet-related disorders and diseases and the answer, the way to prevent them, is also related to the diet - what we eat and how we eat it.

When our digestive Fire is strong, we thrive. When it is weak, we suffer.

Digestion: The Cornerstone of Health

"The Body is Nothing but Fire."
— Dr. Robert Svoboda

According to Ayurveda, digestion is the cornerstone of health. Healthy digestion nourishes the body. What you eat is a major factor to the quality of health. There are two aspects to food and nutrition in Ayurveda. One is the physical food you eat, digest and assimilate. In this process, the organs of the digestive system are involved. The second aspect is what you consume through your mind-body. What you see, hear, taste, smell, feel and think, are all important for your well-being and health. For example, it is common knowledge now that stress plays a key role in the health of an individual. Ayurveda had recognized the importance of environment to one's health. Remember, everything in your environment is composed of the five elements that are constantly interacting with your own doshas. We are all affected by everything else that goes on in this universe, as you are part and parcel of this cosmos. Ayurveda is concerned with the "big picture," so that we may function from a truly "wholistic outlook."

"Due to the purification of the body, the capacity of digestion and metabolism is enhanced, normal health is restored, all sense organs start working with vigor, old age is prevented and diseases are cured."
— Ca.Su. 16. 17/19

Agni: The Digestive Fire

Agni

The word Agni means fire, spark and digestive fire; "Ignite" and "Agni" have the same linguistic root.

Qualities:

Hot, Light, Dry, Sharp, Penetrating, Pungent, Luminous, Transforming

Functions:

The functions of Agni are absorption, assimilation, metabolism, digestion, perception, taste, touch, hearing, vitality, clarity, alertness, regular appetite and combustion. It includes the digestive function, sense perception, cellular metabolism and mental assimilation. Note the link between mental well-being and digestive health (and vice versa). It gives immunity, a sparkle in the eyes and luster to the skin.

Emotions:

When Agni is balanced it causes emotions that are beneficial to health: courage, cheerfulness, lucid, intelligence. When Agni is out of balance it causes emotions that are destructive to health: fear, anger, confusion, idiocy.

Constitutional digestive fire is responsible for digestion. It is the availability of fire that determines the production of gastric juices: hydrochloric acid, bile, enzymes, in short, the caustic chemicals that are required for the breakdown of food and its conversion into micronutrients that can be assimilated by the body and bulk matter that needs to be eliminated. When this fire is weak, it means that there is not enough digestive power to metabolize food.

Agni is the metabolism within our body. It is that which governs living beings physically and mentally. It can be described as an element related to our general body metabolism. Agni is the successor of Pitta (one of the Tridoshas) and Pitta is the successor of Divine Fire. Agni plays a vital role in the creation and maintenance of body tissues.

Agni is related to both the body and the mind. It initiates digestive activities in the digestive tract and generates thoughts, emotions and decisions in our psyche. Agni contains heat that helps in the digestion of external elements that enter our body. The food that enters our digestive tract is converted into life sap with the help of Agni. This then goes on to ensure our survival, growth and recovery from illness.

The knowledge of the external environment that enters our body through our five senses is transformed into memories with the aid of Agni, which further initiates thoughts, generates emotions and helps in making decisions.

The 13 Main Forms of Agni

Digestion, assimilation and absorption occur throughout the body, from the immediate absorption that happens in the mouth, when chewing, to the subtle digestion that feeds each cell of the body. Agni can be compared to different types of enzymes responsible for digestion and metabolic activity. We will explore some of these different types of Agni.

According to Ayurveda, there are 40 types of Agni in the body that carry out different metabolic activities. The following are the thirteen forms of Agni in the body that are most generally recognized:

The One Digestive Fire or "Agni in the belly"- This is the main Agni that we are referring to in tongue diagnosis for this is the main power of digestion in the body. The tongue is the most direct and easiest way to see the Agni in the belly. The process of digestion brings energy to all secretions and enzymes.

The Five Elemental Fires - these are located in the liver. They transform food into the five elements required for building the bodily tissues. When these five elemental fires are not operating accordingly, then the respective element in the body will not be developed appropriately.

The Seven Tissue Fires - impart and are responsible for the proper formation of the tissue. There are seven Agnis for the seven different body tissues. If the Agni is low, too much tissue and tissue of an inferior nature will be produced. However, if the Agni is too high, not enough tissue will be formed.

Agni is present throughout the body, but, for us to better understand, Ayurveda has classified it into subtypes. As mentioned above, there are 13 main Agnis; the most essential Agni is the central Fire in the digestive system. There are an additional 27. Keep in mind that all types of Agni lead to the "Fire of Consciousness."

Agni also corresponds to maturation. The function of Agni is not only digestion, but also to bring maturation to the tissues. The actual tone of each tissue is maintained by its Agni.. The word "tonic" comes from tone, and most tonics kindle Agni.

When we harness and maintain a healthy and balanced Agni, we can live a long and healthy life.

In Ayurveda, the focus is on both the quality and status of Agni. If our Agni is robust and healthy, it brings fragrance to life. Such an individual does not need perfume, for there is a perfume in the body, a sweet aroma of the living healthy body - this is Agni. However if Agni is imbalanced or disturbed the opposite occurs, and there is an unpleasant scent from the body.

Agni and Pitta

In the body, there is no Agni without Pitta and there is no Pitta without Agni. Pitta is the container and Agni is the content. Comparatively, Pitta is the matter and Agni is the energy. On a subtle level, Agni is matter and Tejas is pure essence of Agni. To explain this in other words, Pitta is the gross matter, Agni is the energy or subtle matter and within Agni is the subtler energy of Tejas.

The activity of Agni varies throughout the day. Agni's daily rhythm rises and falls through the course of the day. The time of day when Agni is the strongest is when the sun is at its peak at midday. This is the time when your appetite and hunger should be at its peak as well. When your stomach is empty, Agni renews your appetite once again. Maintaining the strength and natural ebb and flow of your digestive fires is needed for good digestion, good immune function, and resistance to disease. Agni is needed to form Ojas.

Agni kindles all the biological processes of life; it is the fire that powers the transformation of one substance into another. As well as promoting digestion, Agni is an essential aspect of our appearance, body temperature, auto-immunity, awareness, understanding, intelligence, our health, our energy and our lives. Many diseases are connected directly or indirectly to an abnormality of Agni. Agni is responsible for neutralizing toxins, bacteria, and viruses, which can disrupt our immune system.

<u>When Agni is healthy</u>, there is excellent digestion, normal elimination, proper tissue formation, good circulation, high energy, strong immunity, good complexion, pleasant body odor and breath, intelligence, enthusiasm and perception.

<u>When Agni is unhealthy</u>, digestion is inefficient and incom-

plete and all the functions mentioned above are disturbed. Most importantly, when Agni is disturbed, incompletely digested food forms an internal toxin known as Ama. This substance can further putrefy and ferment within the intestinal tract and can spread throughout the body to cause disease. Thus, the care of Agni is central to maintaining health and treating diseases.

The Ayurvedic texts mention factors that disrupt Agni. These include eating at inappropriate times, overeating, eating devitalized foods, eating before the previous meal has been digested, excessive sleep, anger, grief, immoral behavior, consumption of excess fluids or frequent changes in dietary habits.

All three doshas can affect Agni when aggravated. Lifestyle habits, dietary choices, unhealthy food combining and repressed emotions are all factors in creating dosha imbalance. When this occurs, Ama begins to accumulate. One of the first signs of Ama accumulation is a coated tongue and aches, pains and stiffness throughout the body.

Agni is classified into four categories according to how they manifest in the human being: regular, irregular, hypermetabolism and hypometabolism.

6.1 The Four Varieties of Agni

Balanced Metabolism – Balanced Agni	Balanced; Tridoshic
Irregular Metabolism – Irregular Agni	Irregular; usually associated with Vata
Hypermetabolism – Sharp Agni	Sharp; usually associated with Pitta
Hypometabolism – Slow Agni	Dull/slow; usually associated with Kapha

Balanced Metabolism

Metabolism is balanced in individuals who are eating the proper amounts of food for their metabolism, having adequate exercise and rest. Digestion, absorption and elimination are normal. An individual having balanced Agni can eat a wide variety of foods when they are in season without any negative sensations or symptoms. This is a healthy sign - a state of excellent health. One sees normal appetite, satisfaction surrounding meals, normal bowel movements, endurance **Emotional Signs**, mental clarity and emotional stability. They have a calm, quiet, loving mind and great clarity of awareness and good immunity.

Tongue Signs: The tongue will have all the signs of a healthy and vibrant tongue.

Irregular Metabolism

Irregular metabolism can promote irregular appetite, with intense periods of hunger alternating with lack of interest in food. There is often intestinal bloating, gas, constipation, abdominal discomfort or abdominal distention and colicky pain. Even a small quality of food turns into gas. It may lead to diarrhea, a feeling of heaviness after eating and gurgling of the intestines. Those individuals with an irregular metabolism may have strong cravings for hot, spicy food. Immunity is often diminished, especially with regard to the nervous system, bones and upper respiratory tract. Other symptoms that may appear are dry skin, cracking joints, sciatica, low backache or insomnia. The main reason many people lose their Agni is due to irregularity. If we throw off our schedule from the rhythms of nature, our body becomes confused and appetite and digestion begin to overlap. Emotionally, this can result in **Emotional Signs** anxiety, insecurity, fear and other neurological or mental problems. Not surprisingly, this type of Agni is common in Vata constitutions.

Tongue Signs: Eventually Ama is created and a brownish-black coating appears on the tongue especially in the Vata zone or back part of tongue. The tongue, as well as the mouth, may become dry with receding gums. If the Vata is extremely unbalanced, there may be cracks down the middle of the tongue.

Hypermetabolism

Due to the hot, sharp and penetrating attributes of Pitta, Agni can become intense when Pitta dosha is increased. Over-active or sharp implies strong digestion, circulation and immunity. Impurities, if they accumulate, tend to do so in rasa, plasma and the formed blood cells. The individual can have strong desires to eat large quantities of food frequently. Acid indigestion is common along with symptoms of heartburn. The liquid, sour and hot qualities of Pitta may produce hyperacidity, gastritis, hypoglycemia, colitis, diarrhea and dysentery. Other conditions that may occur are liver congestion, nausea, vomiting and numerous inflammatory disorders. This is a common sign in Pitta constitutions.

Emotional Signs that may develop are anger, envy and hate. The individual may also become critical and judgmental towards people and events.

Tongue Signs: The tongue becomes inflamed in appearance, having an overly bright red color especially in the middle section of the Pitta zone.

Hypometabolism

An excess of Water and Earth accumulation begins to show up as Kapha symptoms. This is due to the heavy, slow and cool qualities of these elements. The most common symptom with a hypometabolism is that the individual cannot digest even a normal diet properly. Even if the individual is not eating, there is heaviness in the stomach. There are also symptoms of congestion, cough and feeling cold. Under-active or mild usually manifests as slower digestion, low appetite, cravings for heavy or sweet foods and a tendency to carry excess body weight. Over-salivation, loss of appetite, allergies, nausea, and mucoid vomiting can result. Circulation may be slow and excess secretions often form. Some individuals may have edema, obesity, hypertension and diabetes. There will be lethargy, excessive sleep, cold clammy skin and generalized weakness of the body. The individual may have cravings for hot, sharp, dry and spicy food. This is usually seen in Kapha constitutions.

Emotional Symptoms: the individual may have behaviors that are signs of greed, attachment and possessiveness.

Tongue Signs: The tongue becomes very coated with a white film and lots of moisture and salvia on the tongue and throughout the mouth.

Agni Sources

1. Balanced intake of all six tastes (according to your constitution, time of day, year and your life).

2. All food should be freshly prepared, tasty, nutritious and appetizing.
3. Simplify, Simplify, Simplify.
4. Leave 4-6 hours between meals with no snacking.
5. Eating in between meals weakens the Agni.
6. Eating foods with cold, wet and heavy qualities weakens the Agni.
7. Agni is increased by pungent, sour and salty flavors.
8. A low dosage of bitter taste taken before a meal increases the secretion of hydrochloric acid in the stomach.
9. Agni stimulating and increasing herbs are ginger, black pepper, cayenne pepper, cinnamon. Use a small dose (1-2g) before meals to kindle the digestive fire.
10. Treat Agni with occasional fasts; use a mono-diet.
11. Drink warm lemon water and a seasonal cleanse to stimulate Agni.
12. Increase warming herbs, culinary seeds and spices.
13. Ginger is one of the best Agni spices.
14. Fermented and cultured foods (sauerkraut, miso, kim-chee, vinegars, seed and nut milks).
15. Food should be body temperature, not too hot or too cold.
16. Fresh sour fruits and berries.
17. Freshly made juices are high in life force (Prana), enzymes (Tejas) and water (Ojas).
18. Blender soups made from fresh produce that comes out of your garden.
19. Eat your largest meal of the day when the sun is at its highest.
20. Breath in a relaxed way during the day especially at meal time.
21. Relax and enjoy the meal.
22. Eating in stillness, relaxation and awareness encourages digestive fire.

23. Most of Cabbage Family is packed full of the warming mineral sulfer.

24. Eat whole, fresh, sun-ripened, enzyme-rich, organic, plant foods.

Avoid

24. Canned foods and leftovers.
25. Fried foods.
26. Cold foods and drinks.
27. Reduce or eliminate dairy products.
28. Old and aged foods and drinks.
29. Refined sugars.
30. Processed flour and grain products.
31. Animal products especially red meats, pork and beef.
32. Hot or cold foods are harder to digest.
33. Roasted, salted nuts and seeds.
34. Alcohol and artificial stimulants and colorings.
35. All preservatives, chemicals and artificial food enhancers.
36. Synthetic vitamins, minerals and chemically altered herbs.
37. Chemical fertilizers or sprays.
38. Eating on the run.
39. Eating at erratic times.
40. Eating when we are upset.
41. Exercising right after eating.

> *"The sign that the previous meal is digested is when the breath is fresh."*
>
> — Dr. Stone's *Health Building*

> *"Food must be digested just as fuel must be burnt, or clinkers remain. If the good reader ever fired a furnace or a boiler in a power plant, he learned a few very valuable lessons."*
>
> — Dr. Stone's *Health Building*

1st – Not too much shoveled in at once,

2nd – Spread the coal thinly over the hot embers,

3rd – Regulate the draft,

4th – Select the fuel which will burn best - leaving the least amount of clinkers - with the least fumes and smoke.

Diagnosis of the Power of Agni

- No discomfort after a desired quality of a healthy meal.
- No belching or flatulence.
- No feeling that the stomach is stuffed shortly after eating.
- No digestive symptoms during the passage of food through the small intestines.
- No undigested material or Ama in the fecal matter.
- No mental desire for sense gratification.

If any of these digestive symptoms are present, the power of Agni is low.

Enzymes and Agni

> *"The length of life is inversely proportional to the rate of exhaustion of the enzymes of an organism."*
>
> — Dr. Edward Howell, *Enzyme Nutrition, 1985*

Enzymes are the spark of life. Much research is occurring these days giving us vital information about the important part that enzymes play in our overall health. There is much written in Ayurveda literature to help understand the full meaning of our digestive power and Agni. Agni is present in all metabolic processes of digestion. Metabolism is the sum of all the biophysical and chemical processes through which living organisms function to maintain life. This includes both anabolic and catabolic activity.

Enzymes are the catalysts that support all functions of the body. Enzyme rich foods are those that have not been heated to high temperatures, processed, "pesticided" or "herbicided," microwaved, irradiated or genetically engineered. They represent an unbroken wholeness that is the original creation of Mother Earth and the nutritional gift of the Divine.

Enzymes - Natures's Chemists

Enzymes truly are Nature's chemists for they bring fruits and vegetables to maturity. Under refrigeration, their activity is slowed down. Enzymes are sometimes referred to as "ferments" because, as they die, they cause food to become hot, to ferment, decay and spoil. That is the main reason why food processors will cook, heat, pasteurize or add chemicals to food products. In doing so, the enzymes are killed, preventing foods from spoilage.

Enzymes: The Spark of Life

Life's miracle would be impossible without enzymes. Enzymes are at the heart of all biochemical functions, from digesting the food we eat to enlivening every metabolic reaction in the body. There are an estimated 50,000 enzymes active in the human organism. Each organ has its own set of enzymes. Of the 50,000 plus enzymes, about 25 of them are digestive enzymes. This is Agni at work.

Technically, an enzyme is a protein structure that carries an energetic charge while performing a specific metabolic function. However, it is the energy behind this protein structure that makes enzymes different than other protein-based substances. It is this energetic "life principle" that animates all living forms and "runs the whole show" we call life. When we process our foods in anyway, we are altering and destroying some of the electrical energy - the life-giving properties.

Altering Food Chemistry

Enzyme research has revealed the importance of fresh life-giving foods in the diet. The enzymes in fresh food help start the process of digestion and reduce the body's need to produce digestive enzymes. All enzymes are deactivated at a wet-heat temperature of 118 degrees Fahrenheit and a dry-heat temperature of about 145 degrees. It is one of those designs of nature that foods and liquids at 118 degrees can be touched without pain, but liquids over 118 degrees will burn. Thus, we have a built-in mechanism for determining whether or not the food we are eating still contains its enzyme content.

Modern day food preparation practices (from microwaves to high heat cooking) disrupt the food molecular structure and destroy all the enzymes. These enzymes are the indispensable catalysts that allow the body to utilize vitamins and minerals. Enzymes are extremely heat-sensitive and thus do not survive in heated foods.

Plant Enzymes Survive Gut and Support Digestive Fire

Enzyme research is one of the newest areas of research in nutritional medicine. With any new research there is controversy. Less than one fifth of all medical schools in the United States teach even the elementary aspects of nutrition. Of those that do, the true role of food enzymes are rarely addressed. According to the prevailing accepted dictum, enzymes found in foods are damaged by the hydrochloric acid of the stomach and are of almost no use in the digestive system. However, Dr. Howell has shown that as quickly as a particular food is masticated in the mouth, the enzymes initiate the break down of the food. This has been confirmed by Finnish Nobel Prize winner Artturi Virtanen.

When the food reaches the first part of the stomach, (upper cardiac stomach) the food enzymes are still energetically working. It takes at least 30 minutes for the hydrochloric acid level to rise to the critical level where the acidity of the hydrochloric acid could inactivate the food enzymes. Until this level is reached, enzymes are at work. What is more, not all foods kindle substantial amounts of hydrochloric acid. Foods like fruit, sprouts, grasses and many fresh vegetables do not cause hydrochloric acid production to rise rapidly or to any great measure. In this atmosphere, enzymes have a longer time to do their work. All foods in their natural state contain exactly the right amount of enzymes required to split every last molecule into the basic building blocks of metabolism: Amino acids (from protein), glucose (from complex carbohydrates) and essential fatty acids (from unsaturated vegetable fats).

Agni, Prana and Oxygen

Fresh foods are full of oxygen, especially green leafy vegetables, which contain an abundance of chlorophyll. Chlorophyll is high in Prana according to Ayurveda, because it has more of the Air and Ether elements. The chemical structure of chlorophyll is almost identical to the hemoglobin in our red blood cells. The only difference is that the hemoglobin molecule has iron in its nucleus and the chlorophyll molecule has magnesium. Chlorophyll detoxifies the bloodstream and every other part of the body better than anything else you could eat. When you eat fresh green chlorophyll foods, you oxygenate the blood.

A healthy breathing practice is another essential principle in maintaining an acid/alkaline pH balance. The power of our breath is a major factor in changing and acid internal environment to a healthy alkaline terrain. A person's body, though young, may die unexpectedly due to acidity. A body low in oxygen becomes low in Agni- leading to disease. We maintain the proper acid/alkaline carbon/oxygen equilibrium in our blood through relaxed breathing.

Our breath brings life to every cell of our body. This is one of the reasons that oxygen is one of the most essential nutrients to life. Each moment you take a breath in- you are taking in Prana and you are saying, yes to life.

Seven Principle Causes of Indigestion

- Excessive coldness in food, water and environment.
- Unhealthy food combining.
- Over consumption of liquids.
- Irregular eating habits.
- Disturbed sleep.
- Restraint of natural urges.
- Excessive indulgence in sex.
- Mental factors.

Agni Enzyme-Rich Foods

Agni enzyme-rich foods will give your cells the enzymes they need to digest and eliminate foods properly, helping to keep you youthful. A diet high in fresh, enzyme-rich fruits, vegetables, nuts, seeds, sea vegetables and sprouted whole grains, when eaten according to your constitution, can deter or heal many illnesses and help the body to make more of its own digestive, life-extending enzymes and digestive Agni. When we eat enzyme rich foods, the body does not have to draw on its own reserve source for proper digestion; the food itself is the source.

Fresh Fruits and Berries

Ayurvedic theory states that when one's digestive power is limited, one must get the needed nutrition from foods that are the easiest to digest. The easiest foods to eat are foods that have a watery content, are sun-ripened, enzyme-rich, high in organic trace minerals and natural occuring acids. Less hydrochloric acid is needed. Sour foods, berries and naturally fermented foods are also excellent.

Warming Carminative Herbs, Culinary Seeds and Spices

Warming herbs, culinary seeds and spices help to make food more digestible. First, when food is prepared in spices, as with a curry, the spices are absorbed by the food in such a way as to almost predigest the food. Second, spices stimulate the secretion of saliva and digestive juices. If people really do not have the capacity to produce these conversion chemicals, the spices will not excite what cannot respond to the stimulus, but the food itself is nevertheless easier to digest. It is important to use spices that have not been irradiated and chemically treated.

Whole Grains, Nuts, Seeds and Legumes

Organic grains, nuts, legumes and seeds are rich in enzymes, as well as other nutrients, but they also contain enzyme inhibitors. Unless deactivated, these enzyme inhibitors can put a strain on the digestive system. Sprouting, soaking in warm water, sour leavening, culturing and fermenting are all processes used in traditional societies to deactivate enzyme inhibitors, thus making nutrients in grains, nuts and seeds more readily available. As we have discussed earlier high heat will deactivate the enzyme inhibitors, however in the process will damage the enzyme spark, which support Agni function.

Satya Sai Baba, one of India's spiritual teachers shares his wisdom, perspective and essential point on why people may be slow to make their diets higher in nature's life-giving foods. He says:

"Out of all the species... Man alone tries to cook and change his food. A seed when planted will sprout to life... but when cooked, the life is destroyed... it is man alone who is subject to the most health trouble...The reason is, man does not like to partake of food as God created it. He is the victim of his tongue, which he wants to be satisfied in terms of taste, and so his own likes and dislikes come in the way of what he should eat. Man seeks to change the foods available in nature to suit his tastes, thereby putting an end to the very essence of life contained in them. Because he is exterminating the life-giving forces in the food available to him, he is increasingly subjecting himself to disease. So, it follows, again, that if man were to eat foods in their natural states, he certainly would not be subject to disease. "

"Our main object is to keep the mind in a tranquil condition. So we use the aid of everything in our daily lives to retain that tranquility. Therefore, food is taken into serious consideration. Rajasic food also includes meat and flesh. Animal food or flesh is already dead matter. Anything that is dead will begin to decompose immediately- it decays. So, you are eating dead matter, whereas a vegetable is still a living organism. Take a potato, eat half and cut the other half into ten pieces. If you plant the pieces, you get ten potato plants. Vegetables, while they may get dehydrated, never decompose. Also, as doctors agree, animal fat leaves more toxins in the system than vegetables and a lot of purin which gives rise to cholesterol."

— Sri. Swami Satchidanandaji Maharaj, Light Eating for Survival 1977 by Marcia Acciardo

Life-Giving-Life

Eating healthy means giving your body power foods. What are power foods? Power foods are those in their natural state – fresh, organic, live-foods. These are the same foods that are easily assimilated bringing regeneration and rejuvenation. Life comes from life. Enzyme-rich foods have the spark of Agni and balanced Agni yields health and longevity.

Agni: Digestive and Tissue Enzymes

The entire range of digestive and metabolic activity of the body takes place with the help of the biological fire of Agni. Agni can be termed as the various enzymes present in the elementary canal, liver and the tissue cells. The energy, or the heat element, exists in the body in the form of Pitta (i.e. various enzymes). Health, vigor, strength and life itself depends on the digestive and tissue enzymes. Abnormal activity of these enzymes leads to disease while cessation of activity leads to death. A person with good digestive power has a good appetite without having any symptoms of indigestion.

AGNI ENZYME DEFICIENCY

Although our bodies make most of the enzymes we need to survive, poor diet, illness, injury and genetics can wreak havoc with the body's enzyme systems, causing enzyme digestive secretion depletion, an Agni deficiency in Ayurvedic terms. For instance, some people do not have the necessary enzymes to digest certain foods. Lactose deficiency is a good example. Lactose is an enzyme that breaks down sugars in milk and other dairy products. Individuals whose bodies don't produce lactose suffer from diarrhea, gas, bloating and other intestinal discomfort whenever they eat or drink dairy products.

When food is not digested, it is broken down by fermentation rather than digestion. This produces gases. Worse, the gases are absorbed by other tissues of the body that become both toxic and spastic. In Ayurveda, as in all approaches to eating, it is not just what we eat that counts, but it's also what we assimilate.

ENZYMES AND ENLARGED PANCREAS

According to Dr. Howell, one of the world's most respected authorities on enzyme research, a diet devoid of enzymes can cause enlargement of the pancreas. In addition, it stresses the endocrine glands, such as adrenals, pituitary, ovaries and testes. The human pancreas is three times larger, as compared to total body weight, than that of any other animal in the wild. The fascinating fact is that when mice are feed processed foods, the ratio of their pancreas weight to total body weight becomes approximately that of a human's, three times larger. However, when their food is switched back to their natural live-food diet, their pancreas shrink to normal size. The conclusion is that the pancreas becomes hypertrophied, or enlarged, due to it being forced to keep up a high digestive enzyme output. Hypertrophy will in time lead to early exhaustion or burnout - no fire. The body has to work much harder when food is deficient in life-giving nutrients.

All of these factors are important for building and maintaining our life force energy and health. The statement *"the whole is greater than the sum of its parts"* fits in perfectly here. Why destroy the enzymatic activity, the fire within your food. Mother Nature and the power of the sun have presented us with wholesome food, in an "unbroken" way.

Rekindling Your Digestive Fire

Vata Indigestion

- Digestion tends to be <u>variable and often delicate</u>.
- Needs to rekindle the Agni once a month.
- Juicing program one day a week.
- Diet: light or no food if not hungry, then use sprouted grains made into a gruel, season with warming spices.
- Tastes to use: sour, salty and pungent.
- Herbs to use: ginger root, dill or fennel.
- Fast for 24-48 hours.
- Liquids - warm water or weak tea with ginger.
- Sunbathing is recommended.
- Exercise mildly and fluidly.

Pitta Indigestion

- Digestion tends to be <u>strong and intense</u>.
- Needs to rekindle the Agni twice a month.
- Juicing program three days a month.
- Diet: a light diet or fasting until appetite returns.
- Tastes to use: bitter, astringent and sweet.
- Herbs to use: ginger and fennel.
- Liquids: weak cooling tea of sandalwood.

- Sunbathing in moderation, semi shade.
- Walking near running water or a shady garden.

Kapha Indigestion

- Digestion tends to be <u>slow and often heavy</u>.
- Needs to rekindle the Agni up to once a month.
- Diet: a fasting program for as long as there is no desire for food.
- Juicing program one week a season.
- Tastes to use: bitter, pungent and astringent.
- Herbs to use: ginger, black pepper and garlic.
- Liquids: as little as possible by the teaspoon of weak ginger tea.
- Sunbathing: sit in the sun, well wrapped so the heat absorbed is retained within.

Constitutional Agni Programs

Vata: Follow the Agni Program for one week at a time.

Pitta: Follow the Agni Program for two weeks.

Kapha: Follow the Agni Program intermittently throughout the regimen.

6.2 Agni Signs – Ama Signs

Agni Signs	Ama Signs
• DIGESTION is strong without constipation or diarrhea.	• DIGESTION is weak, chronic constipation and /or diarrhea
• BREATH is pleasant sweet with and tongue is clear.	• BREATH is strong and unpleasant, tongue is coated in the morning.
• APPETITE is great and ability to eat just about anything.	• APPETITE is poor and food tastes bad.
• EYES & SKIN complexion has a glow and eyes are bright.	• EYES & SKIN are dark with no luster.
• URINE is clear and straw colored and not much of scent.	• URINE is cloudy, discolored and dark.
• FECES is normal without a strong smell.	• FECES has a strong offensive smell.
• JOINTS are pain free,	• JOINTS ache.
• FATIGUE - tons of energy, "energy to burn."	• FATIGUE is present, it takes effort to get thing done.
• DEPRESSION - none, happy and joyful as can be.	• DEPRESSION - it is hard to get motivated.

Stoking Your Fire - An Agni Program

The first step is to simplify and use foods that are easy to digest. By eating foods that are easy to metabolize, we allow our digestive spark to focus on burning accumulated toxins. By creating our internal "fires" to become strong, we can burn up everything we take in, creating abundant energy and vibrant strong tissues. However, if our digestion becomes delicate we will be unable to create the energy we need and want for our dreams to come true.

A Healthy Appetite

A strong appetite is a healthy appetite. This is the stimulus to produce and release salivary enzymes, hydrochloric acid and many digestive catalysts produced by the liver and pancreas. If you are not hungry, do not eat. Listen to the body's wisdom. This is one of the essential steps of building Agni.

Conscious Eating

Healthy eating is conscious eating. When we bring in consciousness we bring in the sacredness of eating. This is one of the best ways to enhance digestion. Bringing in joy and celebration enhances and optimizes the meal's nourishing value. Eating meals in a pleasant, uplifting environment is a way of honoring your body. Eating is a celebration. Remember that when creating a meal you are creating sacred space and sacred food. This is nourishment for the soul. Eating with consciousness reflects a deep respect and love of life. Every time you eat in this way you are saying Yes! to life.

7 Ama and Disease

- Ama Signs
- The Main Causes of Ama
- Ama and Dhatus
- Evaluating Your Ama Level
- Analysis of Ama Accumulation
- Seven Surefire Ama Bursting Approaches
- Ayurvedic Dhatu Balancing Recommendations
- The Power of the Sun

Ama

Ama, also spelled Aama (the first vowel is long, as in arm- the second, scarcely vocalized, as in across), is internal gunk, most often residue of partly digested food. At times it's spoken of as aamdosh, a type of stepchild fourth dosha after Vata, Pitta and Kapha, since if it's present to a sufficient degree, it may play a part in the creation and growth of disease that is equal to the other doshas.

Ama means immature, unripe, uncooked and undigested. In the medical context, however, the term Ama refers to events and factors that result as a consequence of Agni not functioning properly.

Ama is an essential factor in the development of pathology. The synonym of disease is said to be a condition produced by Ama. The term Ama possesses a unique significance in the context of pathology in Ayurveda and constitutes the most important causative factor of a great number of diseases, as described in the classical texts. According to Ayurveda, Ama is the beginning of the disease for all disease. It is the weakness of the digestive function due to a buildup of undigested food mass. This leads to a weakened immune system. No disease can take hold if our digestive fire is working optimally.

According to Ayurveda, due to the diminution of Agni the first dhatu, namely rasa, is not formed properly and the Anna rasa (food essence) undergoes fermentation and or putrefaction, being retained in the stomach, this state of rasa is Ama. So, the improperly digested rasa is Ama

Also, impaired Vata, Pitta and Kapha dosha when mixed with one another, lead, to the formation of Ama dosha. When Agni is inhibited, ingested food is not properly digested and the products that arise out of such an impaired digestion are being retained in the amashaya, they undergo changes and yield toxic substances, Ama. This may very well be compared with toxemia of different types.

Effects of Ama

According to Ayurveda, Ama produces obstruction of channels, loss of strength, heaviness, impediment to the flow of air, lethargy, indigestion, excessive salivation, obstruction of urges like stools, urine, flatus, etc., anorexia and malaise.

The formation of Ama is the first stage of dosha vitiation and can settle in different parts of the body.

The Main Causes of Ama

Following is a list of several of the major factors, both dietetic indiscretions and emotional stresses that contribute to the formation of Ama.

- Eating a large, heavy meal in the evening. This is the single, largest and most common mistake that the majority of individuals make. This habit is especially problematical once the person gets close to their Vata stage of their life (after 50) as the metabolism and digestion become slower. If you are overweight and over 50, it will be difficult to reverse a weight problem without cutting back large evening meals.
- Eating leftovers that have been in the refrigerator. Food that has been processed and then refrigerated is very high in Ama-creating qualities. Our diet should be fresh food freshly prepared for good health.
- Eating processed, refined foods made by man and not by nature. The more a food has been processed and fractions of

it isolated by chemical processes, the more it is high in Ama-creating quality. In Ayurvedic terms, processing destroys the inner intelligence and Prana (life force) of the food. Processed foods to avoid as much as possible include canned, packaged, microwaved, frozen foods and high-heated foods.

- Ingesting very hot or very cold foods and drinks. Extremely hot food is just as damaging to the digestive process as is cold food. They both depress the digestive fire and increase the likelihood that Ama will be created from that food.

Other factors that create accumulation of Ama:

- irregular eating habits
- poor food combinations
- heavy or indigestible foods
- over-eating, even of healthy foods, will create Ama
- ingestion of unhealthy or unpleasant tasting food
- foods that produces distension of the abdomen
- foods that are irritating and capable of causing inflammation of the stomach and intestines
- consumption of unclean and contaminated or infected food
- eating dried, fried or processed foodstuffs
- intense emotional stresses such as grief, anger, worry, fear, etc.

Ama Toxins

Ama originates from improperly digested toxic particles that clog the channels in your body. Some of these channels are physical and include the intestines, lymphatic system, arteries and veins, capillaries and genitourinary tract. Others are nonphysical channels called nadis (river or stream) through which your energy flows. Ama toxicity accumulates wherever there is a weakness in the body, and this will result in disease. Ayurveda offers ways you can cleanse the body of Ama such as Pancha karma. However, it's best to prevent it from forming in the first place. Symptoms such as a coating on the tongue or feeling tired all the time are signs of Ama.

SAMA AND NIRAMA DOSHA

Sama - in which dosha, dhatu and Mala become permeated with Ama. Nirama - in which dosha, dhatu and Mala are without Ama abnormalities.

Sama Vata

Signs and symptoms:

- obstruction of channels
- lack of appetite
- drowsiness
- edema
- pricking sensation
- pain in joints and all the body parts
- constipation

Treatment Plan - purification therapy by medicated enemas.

Nirama Vata

Signs and symptoms:

- clearing and cleaning of channels
- dryness
- mild pain.

Treatment Plan - purification cleansing breath practices.

Sama Pitta

Signs and symptoms:

- static
- foul odor
- acid eructations
- burning sensation in the throat and in the region of the heart
- green coloration and heaviness

Treatment Plan - purification therapy and purgation.

Nirama Pitta

Signs and symptoms:

- unstatic

- without bad odor
- pungent taste
- improvement in the digestive power

Treatment plan - removal of vitiated qualities of Pitta.

Sama Kapha

Signs and symptoms:

- obstructed channels
- appetite is nearly lost
- prevents normal belching

Treatment Plan - purification therapy, therapeutic emesis, fasting

Nirama Kapha

Signs and symptoms:

- regaining of homogenous consistency
- relieving from foul smell
- relieving from stickiness

Treatment Plan - removal of vitiated qualities of Kapha.

Sama Dhatu

When Ama comes in intimate contact with the dhatu, they become abnormal, both structurally and functionally. This is Sama dhatu.

Signs and symptoms of sama dhatu are specific to the respective dhatu and are observed independently. Nirama dhatu are normal, structurally and functionally.

SAMA AND NIRAMA MALA (feces)

Signs and symptoms:

- profuse in quantity
- very foul smelling
- sticks to the pot
- unformed
- sinks in water

Nirama Purisha

Signs and symptoms:

- normal in quantity
- well formed
- normal faucal smell
- not sticky
- floats in water

SAMA MUTRA (Urine)

Signs and symptoms:

- cloudy
- specific gravity and density is more than normal
- foul smell

NIRAMA MUTRA

Signs and symptoms:

- clear
- transparent
- normal color of urine
- specific gravity and density is normal
- urine has ferrous smell

The first and foremost treatment for Ama is fasting until normal Agni is maintained. Normal Agni reduces the obstructions in the channels and digests the Ama resulting in all signs and symptoms produced by Ama being reduced. When this has occurred, the indicated therapies are emesis and purgation. Herbs that help to combat Ama are ginger (Zingiber officinale) and most culinary seeds and spices.

Ama and the Dhatus

Our health depends on the body fire, Agni. If the body fire is in a properly maintained condition, if it is at an optimum level, then Vata, Pitta, Kapha are in a balanced state. Body tissues, dhatus, are also in order and waste products are eliminated properly.

An unhealthy diet or habits that are detrimental to health, an unsound lifestyle, seasonal changes beyond human limits, mental and/or physical stress and strain beyond personal capacity, all act as cause issues for creating an imbalance in the three body constituents. This further leads to derangement in body tissues, dhatus, which produces toxins, Ama, by affecting the body's fire, Agni.

Ama circulates throughout the body and accumulates in body tissues. It also chokes body channels. This could lead to irritable bowel syndrome, which can often lead to more serious illness. When Ama establishes itself in the body, it starts affecting the body and mind structurally and functionally and ultimately results in disease. Nature tries to eliminate Ama from the body by natural ways and means; however, when the body surrenders to disease, it has gone beyond the capacity of nature.

Ama refers to toxins, impurities and blockages that accumulate in the physiology. The localization of Ama in the tissues disrupts and confuses the delicate biochemistry of the body, resulting in a wide variety of symptoms. If Ama blocks the channels of circulation, like blood and lymph vessels, the body's ability to maintain homeostasis/balance in that area is lost and the fertile ground for disease occurs. When a person is unable to clear an existing disorder through proper medical or natural treatment approaches, then Ama is blocking the effect of your treatments. The first step is to remove Ama. This if done by:

1. Stopping the lifestyle mistakes that create Ama; and
2. Using natural Ayurvedic approaches to cleanse the body of Ama where it may have accumulated.

As Ama accumulates in the body, a wide variety of symptoms and disorders begin to appear. Localization of Ama results in stiffness aches and pains, heaviness, tiredness and dullness. Another whole set of symptoms and disorders get created as the body tries to fight the aggravating effects of Ama. For example, the result of this struggle between the body and Ama can result in the build up of excess tissue in the form of fibroids, cysts and a variety of tumors.

Another set of symptoms comes when the immune system

perceives Ama as foreign material and in its attempt to rid the body creates inflammation. This can further result in a mistaken or "auto-immune" response against the body's own tissues. Unfortunately, this can result in pain and/or swelling in that area. For example, conditions like arthritis, asthma and inflammatory bowel disease are created and aggravated by the accumulation of Ama.

Ama can come from environmental pollutants, mental and emotional disorders and a variety of other sources. However, Ama mainly comes from improperly digested foods. As a result of indigestion large, misshaped, molecules become absorbed into the bloodstream as they have not been broken down properly in the digestive tract. Because the various channels and openings of the body are structured for smaller molecules, the large Ama particles start to block the fine pores and channels within cells and throughout the body. Many symptoms result from this process.

For example, the area of accumulation results in cell blockage and this area will suffer from malnutrition as nutrients are shut out. As a result, even if a person eats a substantial, nutritious meal they will soon feel hungry again because certain tissues truly are starving. The person then eats more food to satisfy this false hunger, which in turn creates more Ama, and gets dragged into a downward spiral of increasing imbalance on all levels.

To reiterate, the body tries to maintain a state of health under normal circumstances. If circumstantial changes go beyond the body's capacity, accumulation of Ama begins. The body then works to reestablish a state of health, however, often fails to do so, in which case Ayurvedic procedures can assist in achieving the goal of heath.

Evaluating Your Ama Level

Consider these two lists and determine whether you have mainly symptoms of Ama-filled or Ama-free functioning.

7.1 Symptoms of Ama Accumulation

- You wake up tired even after a good nights sleep.
- You feel lethargic.
- Your tongue is coated especially upon awaking in the morning.
- You don't feel hunger even when you haven't eaten for hours.
- You have generalized aches and pains. They often are noticed the day after eating certain heavy foods, like meat, cheeses, desserts and fried foods.
- You lack mental clarity and energy.
- You have a sense of heaviness in the abdomen, legs or body as a whole.
- You feel weary and unenthusiastic.
- You experience frequent indigestion such as gas bloating and or heartburn.
- You feel blocked anywhere in the body, including constipation, sinus congestion and difficulty breathing.

7.2 Symptoms of an Ama - Free Physiology

- You feel fresh, rested and even blissful upon awakening in the morning.
- Your skin has a healthy glow.
- Your tongue is pink and clear.
- Your body feels light, regardless of your weight.
- Aches and pains are disappearing.
- Your abdomen feels light and balanced.
- You feel energetic during the day.
- You feel enthusiastic.
- Your mind is clear.
- Your weight is normal, for you.
- You look healthy and vibrant.

Analysis of Balance and Ama Accumulation in Your Tissues

7.3 Analysis of Balance and Ama Accumulation in Your Tissues

BLOOD PLASMA (RASA) -
the clear portion of the blood

_____ dry skin

_____ vaginal dryness

_____ excess mucus or respiratory congestion

_____ fatigue/tiredness

_____ ovarian cysts (female) or hydrocoele (male)

_____ underweight or early wrinkling of the skin

_____ TOTAL

RED BLOOD CELLS (RAKTA) - red blood cells and bile

_____ hot flashes or frequently feeling hot

_____ heavy menstrual bleeding or nose bleeds

_____ skin rashes or acne

_____ gallbladder problems

_____ endometriosis

_____ excessive thirst

_____ TOTAL

MUSCLES (MAMSA) - muscle tissue

_____ muscle aches or pains

_____ easily fatigued muscles

_____ itchy ear canals or eczema of ear canal or excess ear wax

_____ fibroids of the uterus (female) or enlarged prostate (male)

_____ fibrous tumors of the breasts

_____ dry, cracking lips

_____ TOTAL

FAT AND HORMONES (MEDA) - fat, hormone and carbohydrate metabolism

_____ weight gain

_____ diabetes or insulin resistance

_____ high cholesterol or triglycerides

_____ malodorous sweat or body odor

_____ fatty cysts under the skin, scalp or in the breasts

_____ coronary artery disease

_____ TOTAL

BONES (ASTHI) - bone, cartilage, hair and nail tissues

_____ low bone density (osteopenia or osteoporosis)

_____ hair breaking or split ends

_____ hair with dryness or lack of luster

_____ nails breaking

_____ joint pains or osteoarthritis

_____ deep pains in the bones

_____ TOTAL

BONE MARROW (MAJJA) - the central nervous system tissue and immune system

_____ frequent or recurring infections

_____ excess secretions of the eyes

_____ dryness of the upper portion of the eyelids (not inflammation or blepharitis)

_____ immune system disorder

_____ pain in the tendons, easily injured tendons or tendonitis

_____ tendency for fainting, light-headedness or spacey-ness

_____ TOTAL

REPRODUCTIVE ESSENCE (SUKRA) - The egg and its supportive tissues

_____ absence of libido or impotence (impaired erection or ejaculation)

_____ severe vaginal dryness

_____ lacking overall sexual attractiveness

_____ dull eyes, lack of clarity of the eyes

_____ infertility

_____ history of more than one miscarriage

_____ TOTAL

If you scored 4 or higher in any one tissue category, that tissue is being affected to a significant degree by Ama accumulation.

If you scored 2-3 in any tissue category Ama is beginning to form in that tissue.

Six Surefire Ama-Busting Approaches

- Eat fresh food, freshly prepared.
- Favor warming enzyme-rich foods.
- Eat the largest meal of the day at lunch when digestion is strongest.
- Avoid consumption of large quantities of acid-forming cheese and heavy meats.
- Sip warming herbal-spice teas and warm water throughout the day.
- Spend at least 20-30 minutes in the gentle glow of the morning or evening sun.
- Exercise and deep belly breathing daily.

Ayurvedic Dhatu Balancing Recommendations

If your scores indicate Ama is starting to accumulate in a specific dhatus, it is important to pay attention to the many areas of lifestyle, diet and eating behavior that have been described here.

7.4 Ayurvedic Dhatu Balancing Recommendations

Dhatu	Factors that Disturb the Dhatu. Reduce these factors if you have this dhatu imbalance.	Lifestyle and dietary factors to favor that balance the dhatu.
Rasa (blood plasma)	• Rasa is imbalanced by factors that disturb digestion • low water intake • fasting • irregular meal times • eating excessive quantities of dry foods • excess salt • eating before the previous meal is digested • overeating • Rasa is also disturbed by: Staying up late at night Insufficient sleep Mental stress, worry & fear	• drink plenty of water • eat sweet, juicy, fresh fruits (pears, grapes, plums, oranges, melons) • eat juicy vegetables (zucchinis, squashes, cucumber) • get more sleep • manage stress, ideally through meditation • perform herbalized oil massage daily
Rakta (red blood cells)	• acidic foods like tomatoes, vinegar, fermented foods • alkaline (leavened with baking soda) • toxins like alcohol, nicotine, drugs, chemicals • frequent anger and frustration • hot, spicy foods • artificial colors, preservatives, pesticides • aged cheeses • violent movies or news shows • late bedtimes	• more neutral taste diet, less spices • plenty of water intake • good quantities of fruits and vegetables • meditation • go to bed before 10:00 pm • reduce anger • don't skip meals, have regular meal times • drink 1/4 cup of aloe vera juice daily • include rose petal water in your diet

Dhatu	Factors that Disturb the Dhatu. Reduce these factors if you have this dhatu imbalance.	Lifestyle and dietary factors to favor that balance the dhatu.
Mamsa (muscles)	**Mamsa is disturbed by factors that create dense, sticky Ama** • old foods and leftovers • cheese, cold deli foods, ice cream • leftover or impure meats • overeating • deep fried foods • cold drinks • eating meat or cheese late in the day	• yoga, stretching • exercise • vegetarian diet • amla berry preparation • eat 1-2 dates a day and buckwheat at least once a week • strictly avoid red meat, pork and cheese
Meda (fat & carbohydrate metabolism & hormones)	**Meda is disturbed by factors that clog and slow metabolism** • overeating fats, refined sugar foods, deep fried food and high calorie food • large evening meals • excess meat and cheese • impure cooking oils like non-organic, refined vegetable oils • snacking late at night	• increase in fiber-rich foods • eat organic foods • use organic, unrefined olive oil • eat whole sprouted grains, especially barley and quinoa, marinated, green leafy vegetables, and sprouted legumes • increase exercise
Asthi (bones, cartilage, teeth, nails)	**Asthi is most easily disturbed by factors that aggravate Vata dosha** • late nights • mental stress • irregular meals • smoking • toxins especially mercury and lead	• adequate dietary calcium • vitamin D rich foods • calcium rich foods like sesame seeds, tahini, broccoli, soaked almonds, kale, fresh asparagus • 30 minute walk in the rising sun without sunscreen if tolerated (sunscreen blocks vitamin D production)

Dhatu	Factors that Disturb the Dhatu. Reduce these factors if you have this dhatu imbalance.	Lifestyle and dietary factors to favor that balance the dhatu.
Majja (bone marrow, immune system, brain and nerve cells)	• unnatural, unwholesome foods (junk food, processed food, fake cakes, genetically engineered food, food not ripened on the vine) • corticosteroids that decrease bone marrow production (consult your doctor before changing intake of any prescribed medicine) • mental stress • too much sunlight	• more rest • gentle but regular exercise • regular meditation • healthy, pure, wholesome foods • soaked almonds, walnuts, pecans, almonds and seeds • warm blended date/milk shakes • foods rich in calcium, magnesium, vitamin B6 and B12
Shukra (reproductive essence, sperm and ova)	• excessive sexual activity • frequent childbirth • carbonated beverages, baking soda, alcohol • mental and emotional stress • unwholesome foods lacking in nutrients • inadequate food intake • inadequate sleep	• practice moderation in sexual activity • go to bed before 10:00 pm • eat nurturing foods like date-nut-seed shakes, fruits and vegetables • fresh asparagus 2-3 times a week • mangoes in season • fresh sweet juicy pear or apple each day

Importance of the sequence of dhatu development

It is very important to remember that the dhatus get built up one to the other in the sequence rasa, rakta, mamsa, meda, asthi, majja, shukra. If a dhatu is disturbed early in the sequence, the others that follow will be weakened. For example, often an asthi imbalance (osteoporosis) is created by a meda (fat and hormone) imbalance. Balance the first dhatus in the sequence to strengthen the later ones.

The Power of the Sun

The sun is the source of all life on this planet. Without the power of the sun there is no life. While we may give little reverence to the sun in our culture, at a primordial level, we are completely connected to the sun. Without the sun our bodies and spirits would wither.

Sunfoods

All plant foods carry the life force of the sun. When a food has been denatured by human technology, it losses some of its life force. Foods that have the warmth and the qualities of the sun, can be called "sun foods." The closer they are to being ripened naturally by the sun the more enzymatic activity they have within them, meaning the more Agni potential they have. These foods carry within them the full sun's energy. They are alive!

Think of it. We are the only creatures on this planet that destroy and devitalize our nourishment through cooking and processing. All other living creatures thrive healthily on a natural diet. When we manipulate our foods we actually destroy the gifts of the sun. With the loss of connection with nature and the cosmos has come a loss of connection to natural order of things and we have forgotten where true nourishment comes from - the sun and the elements.

A Make-Sense Approach

Eating foods that are full of life is a make-sense approach to eating. Many feel that we need to process our food to improve their digestibility. If this is true, then why is it that humans are the sickest creatures on this planet? Animals that live on foods that have been ripened by the sun, without having to change them, have amazing vigor and vitality. They are able to live outdoors in the elements. This is why many animals, once domesticated and fed processed, cooked foods, are showing up with the same diseases as humans.

This is a make-sense approach to eating because we are constitutionally created to eat sun-ripened foods in their natural state. When we do, not only will we feel healthier but we become in tune to the natural way to life.

When the life force has been taken out of foods, the food is essentially dead. To expect this food to enliven our organism is impossible. Life yields life. Dead foods will yield a decaying organism. Our research has shown, without a doubt, that eating fresh, whole, sun-ripened, enzyme-rich, organic fruits, vegetable, seeds and nuts is the original way of eating. Our bodies and our digestive system are designed to accommodate these foods. Try it for yourself. See how you feel after eating denatured and processed foods for one week. Then for the next week see how you feel after eating whole sun-ripened foods in their natural state. The difference is remarkable.

The life force factor is not something scientific. Science can provide us with some valuable but limited knowledge of the creation process. If we could measure the life force in food with a scientific method, we would realize the abundance of life force that is present in nature's fresh plants, and how denatured and processed foods are devoid of this life force.

Denatured Foods Destroys the Patterns of Nature

From Ayurveda we know that nature forms everything with a unique blueprint pattern of energy and life. These patterns are usually circular or spiral shaped like those found in flowers, leaves, stems, branches and roots of plants and trees. These patterns are found in every cell, right through to the molecule and DNA patterning.

The act of denaturing our food changes and destroys what nature has formed on a cellular and molecular level. Nature has created food to nourish our bodies with every nutrient and intricate molecular pattern to sustain us in health. The food is given to us in a perfect wholesome state, ready for consumption. When food is consumed in an unnatural or denatured state, we are eating food that is no longer what nature created, but is now foreign and unnatural. A denatured food is food in which the molecular structure has been altered and in some instances the molecular structure is so deranged that you would not be able to find this shape or pattern in nature. This means that when we take in this food, we are deranging our cellular and molecular structure, which in turn means that the body can no longer hold its healthy shape and pattern. This is when disease begins to set in.

Mother Nature has provided food and nourishment for all her creatures, which includes us. Of the 23 million creatures that share our home planet, we are the only ones who alter our foods. All creatures have a natural diet just right for their unique body structure and physiology. How might we be an exception to this natural way of life? How have we lost our way? All that we need for nourishment comes to us from the natural green world of trees, plants and herbs, without needing to alter or change them in any way. The dance of the elements and the sun provides us with the best gifts that nature can give us. These are the foods that we are naturally attracted to and find the most pleasing, both in sight and taste. We each have an instinctive knowledge that knows this. When we choose whole, fresh foods, we are choosing Life!

Transformation Value of the Living Cuisine

The greatest value of the living cuisine of life-enhancing foods is its transformational power. For when you begin to consume more life-enhancing foods, you become a new and more radiant person. You don't just stay the same old person, only a little bit healthier. You actually become, to a great extent, a new being with new passions, a new philosophy and outlook on life, with new goals, dreams and desires. You become more of your true essence, your true and natural Self. You become a person who is more a part of the one great life of Nature and less of the confused human world.

You become less of the World and more "of the Earth."

Such transformations of course are almost impossible to imagine before you have actually experienced them yourself.

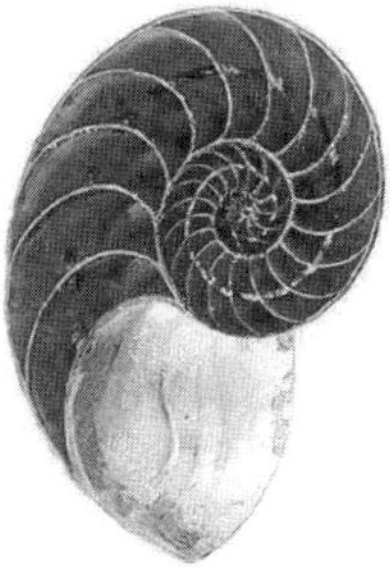

PART FIVE

The Diagnosis

We have explored the importance of knowing the type of seed you are born as - your Prakruti. We then explored the terrain, the present conditions that the seed is living in - your Vikruti. The third section explored the key to the health of the seed - the Fire/Agni. Now let us explore the diagnosis. Here we will bring all three aspects together - the seed, the terrain and the Fire. These together reveal a complete picture of the life of an individual. Now it's time to get into the heart of this work, to discover the present state of ones digestive system as well as what is currently taking place through the whole body, and how well a person is being nourished. Remember the tongue is the most direct way of seeing the state of your Agni. The tongue is also the easiest way to see changes taking place; in other words, it can reveal how well the health program is working.

Diagnosis in Ayurveda works at the energetic levels. We are

checking for the energetic flow of the elements. We are seeing if the elements are in the right proportions to support one's Prakruti. The body is constantly changing and balancing to adjust to the ever-changing fluctuations of the elements. With every breath, with everything that we smell, taste, hear, see and touch the body re-organizes itself to adapt to the changing stimulus. We are being shaped by what enters us through the senses. The sense of taste is the closest link we have to the tongue and the digestive system. We will cover this in-depth in this chapter.

The diagnostic process is very much like tending to the needs of a plant. You have already determined the type of plant it is, as well as the environment, composition of soil, etc., which it now lives in. The next step is to monitor how well it is doing. By checking on the plant and giving it the nourishment it needs, the plant can reach its full potential and beauty. As we check and monitor the internal environment, we can determine what needs to be added or taken away to successfully help the body to heal and flourish. Tongue Diagnosis is truly one of the best ways to monitor the progress of an individual's health journey.

8 Tongue and the Taste Buds

- Taste Fundamentals
- Taste Buds
- The Six Tastes
- Tastes and the Elements

"The taste of things remains poised a long time, like souls, ready to remind us..."
— Marcel Proust

"The tongue is a contortionist, an accomplished small-muscle and athlete. Anchored to the floor of the mouth, it searches, explores, snicks and sweeps about. It narrows and sticks out, it flattens and retracts, it curls, it manipulates food, wipes the lips, and licks the fingers. It clicks against the lips and teeth and palate, making the consonants of speech. It participates in kisses of passion."
— Jillyn Smith, 'Senses and Sensibilities'

8.1 Receptors for Tastes

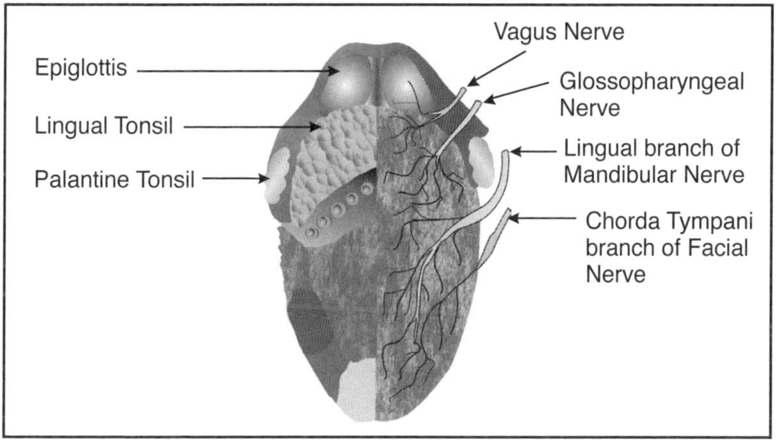

8.2 Tongue Organ Map

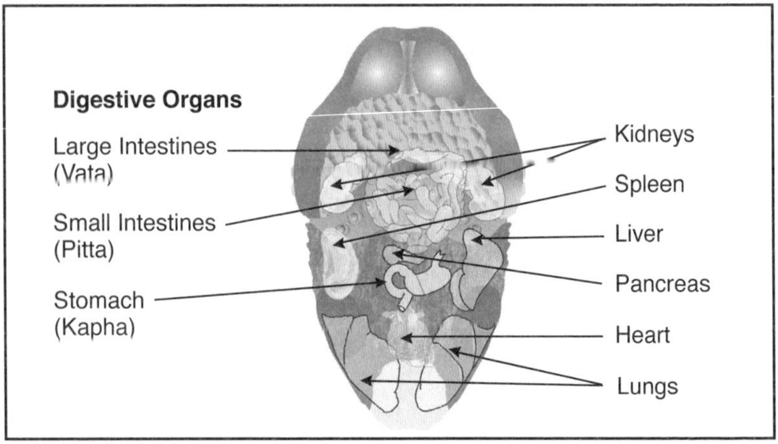

The Tongue

The tongue is an incredible sense organ that detects the taste of all nourishment we take into our bodies. The tongue aids in eating and in speech. Through the tongue, the sensory system judges the appropriate tastes and qualities to be consumed, thus protecting the body and aiding it to maintain balance.

Anatomy and Physiology of Gustation (Taste)

Mammals' taste buds are aggregations of 30-100 individual elongated "neuroepithelial" cells (50-60 microns in height, 30-70 microns in width), which are often embedded in specializations of surrounding epithelium, termed papillae. At the apex of the taste bud, microvillar processes protrude through a small opening, the taste pore, into the oral milieu. Just below the taste bud apex, tight junctional complexes join taste cells.

Regional Localization of Taste on the Tongue

There has been some controversy as to whether the taste maps of the human tongue, which appear in every textbook, are correct. Taste sensation can be localized on the tongue, but does the tongue have regions that are more sensitive to one taste modality than another? Fungiform papillae are concentrated on the anterior tip of the tongue and anterior lateral margins in humans and it has been demonstrated that NaCl (sodium Chloride) threshold was inversely related to the number of fungiform papillae (more papillae = more sensitivity, lower threshold). In a study of human fungiform papillae it was found that taste buds could respond to NaCl only or to both NaCl and sucrose. The responses to NaCl and sucrose occurred in different cells within the taste bud. Thus, one can infer that fungiform papillae are salt-sensitive but this does not mean they are insensitive to other tastes. Bitter receptors are not uniformly distributed over the tongue. In rats, the bitter receptors are expressed in a subset of taste cells in all papillae, but they are more concentrated in foliate and circumvallate papillae situated at the sides and the back of the tongue. Furthermore, alpha-gustducin, which is the G-protein coupled to the T2R bitter receptors (see below), is expressed more in circumvallate than fungiform papillae in the rat. One rather more empirical approach to resolving this question is to stimulate the different areas of the tongue directly. Thermal stimulation of the anterior sides of the tongue in humans (fungiform papillae and the chorda tympani nerve) evokes sweet and salt / sour taste. While thermal stimulation of the rear of the tongue (foliate / circumvallate papillae and glossopharyngeal nerve) causes a different relationship between temperature and taste to the anterior stimulation. One can conclude that the classical "taste map" is an over simplification. Sensitivity to all tastes is distributed across the whole tongue and indeed to other regions of the mouth where there are taste buds (epiglottis, soft palate), but some areas are indeed more responsive to certain tastes than others.

Taste Fundamentals

The basic tastes, Salty, Sour, Sweet and Bitter, stimulate the brain. These are registered via a series of chemical reactions in the taste cells of the taste buds. The five biochemical pathways underlying each taste quality are depicted here in separate taste cells solely for clarity. In reality, individual taste cells are not programmed, or "tuned" to respond to only one kind of taste stimulus.

SALTS, such as sodium chloride (NaCl), trigger taste cells when sodium ions (Na+) enter through ion channels on microvilli at the cell's apical, or top surface. (Sodium ions can also enter via channels on the cell's basolateral, or side surface).The accumulation of sodium ions causes an electrochemical change called depolarization that results in calcium ions (Ca++) entering the cell. The calcium, in turn, prompts the cell to release chemical signals called neurotransmitters from packets known as vesicles. Nerve cells, or neurons, receive the message and convey a signal to the brain. Taste cells repolarize, or "reset," themselves in part by opening potassium ion channels so that potassium ions (K+) can exit.

ACIDS are the sour taste because they generate hydrogen ions (H+) in solution. Those ions act on a taste cell in three ways: by directly entering the cell; by blocking potassium ion (K+) channels on the microvilli; and by binding to and opening channels on the microvilli that allow other positive ions to enter the cell. The resulting accumulation of positive charges depolarizes the cell and lead to neurotransmitter release.

SWEET STIMULI, such as sugar or artificial sweeteners, do not enter taste cells but trigger changes within the cells. They bind to receptors on a taste cell's surface that are coupled to molecules named G-proteins. This prompts the subunits of the G-proteins to split and which activates a nearby enzyme. The enzyme then converts a precursor within the cell into so-called second messengers that close potassium channels indirectly.

BITTER STIMULI, such as quinine, also act through G-protein-coupled receptors and second messengers. In this case; however, the second messengers cause the release of calcium ions from the endoplasmic reticulum. The resulting buildup of calcium in the cell leads to depolarization and neurotransmitter release.

AMINO ACIDS (UMAMI STIMULI), such as glutamate, which stimulates the umami taste, are known to bind to G-protein-coupled receptors and to activate second messengers. But the intermediate steps between the second messengers and the release of packets of neurotransmitters are unknown.

All Other Tastes

All other tastes come from a combination of these four basic tastes. Different parts of the tongue can detect all types of tastes.

The simple tongue "taste map" described in Ayurveda and Chinese medicine shows the different zones and corresponding body part.

8.3a Taste Buds

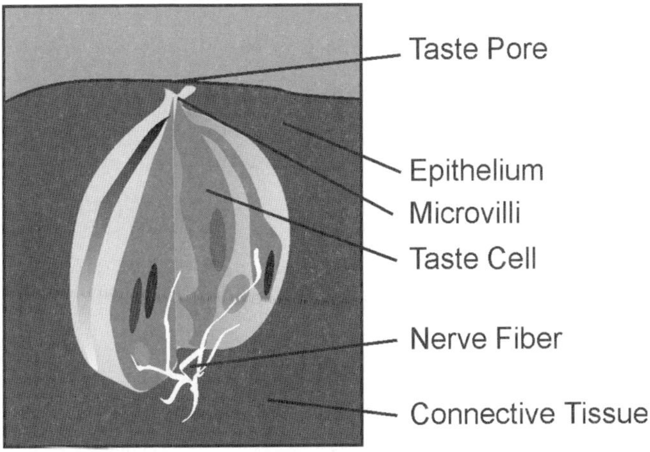

8.3b Taste Buds

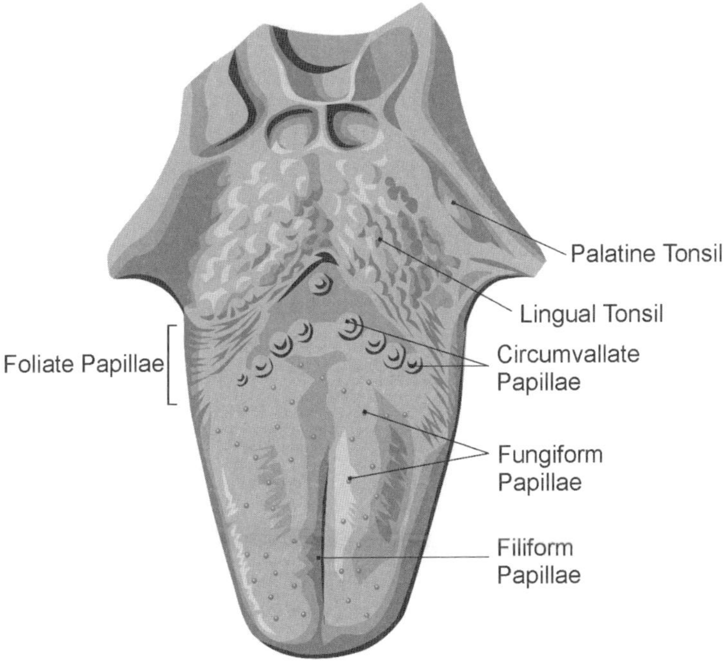

Taste Buds

In 1867, the taste buds were discovered. Taste buds are the receptor organs for the sensation of taste. A healthy human being has approximately 10,000 taste buds that are located along the tongue, palate, pharynx and larynx. The structure of each taste bud resembles that of a citrus fruit with 20-50 receptor cells forming each of the segments of the fruit. Each receptor cell projects cilia onto the surface of the tongue via an opening in the taste bud. Adjacent taste cells form tight junctions along their borders, thus preventing the flow of saliva into the taste bud itself. Because of this arrangement, the dissolved chemicals remain on the surface of the taste bud where the cilia are able to encode their qualities. Taste receptors are modified skin cells. They are, however, similar to neurons and have excitable cell membranes. These excitable membranes release neurotransmitters that in turn excite the adjacent neurons of cranial nerves. The cranial nerves then convey this information toward the brain. The mouth is a very busy place. We are unable to taste our food until it is dissolved by saliva, of which we produce around 10,000 gallons during a lifetime. It assists the appetite; the body's crying-out for energetic nourishment. The average life span of a sensory cell can extend from a few days to a month but most of them only live seven to fourteen days.

Taste buds consist of a cluster of receptor, or "taste" cells and supporting cells. Projecting from the top of a receptor cell are tiny taste hairs that are exposed to salvia that enters through taste pores. A substance taken into the mouth and dissolved in salvia interacts with receptor sites on the taste hairs, thus generating a nerve impulse that is transmitted to the brain.

Eating engages all the senses in some way. We see an apple, touch it and hear it crunch as we chew. The taste buds respond to apple chemicals, among them malic acid and the sugar fructose. Stimulation of the taste buds is joined by the stimulation of other receptors in the mouth- receptors for pressure, heat and cold. Vaporized chemicals from food enter the nasal passages, both through the nose and via the back of the mouth, and stimulate the olfactory processes. Pain receptors are sometimes stimulated. The flavors of taste are actually a combination of all these sensations. Taste, in the narrow sense, is categorized into the four basic sensations of the tongue map: Sweet, Sour, Salty and Bitter.

8.4 Papilla

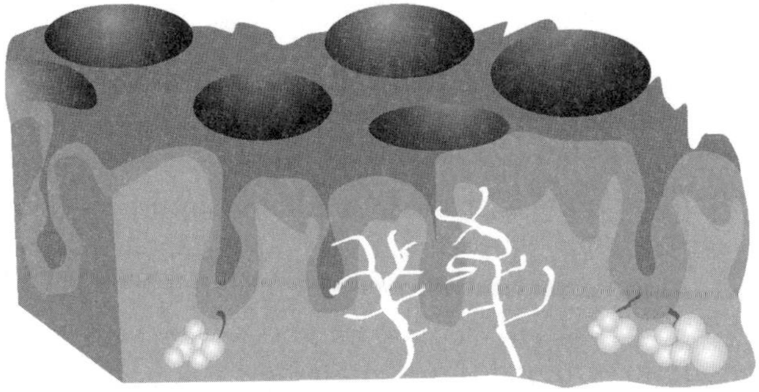

8.5a Circumvallate Papilla

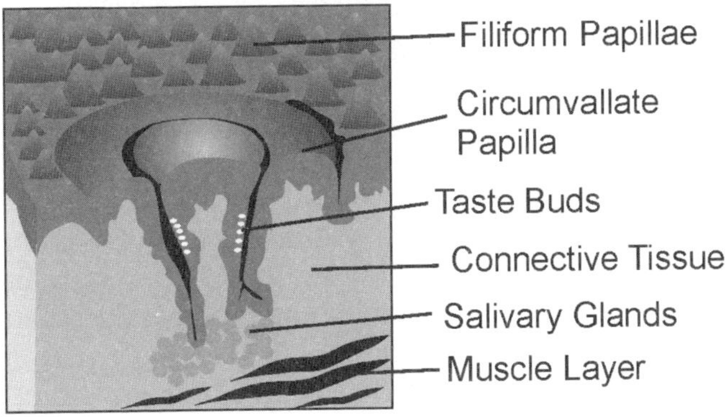

"Sensation is not only our link with the outside environment but also provides the body with important data about the internal world within."

— W. Cookery

8.5b Sensory Nerve Fibers

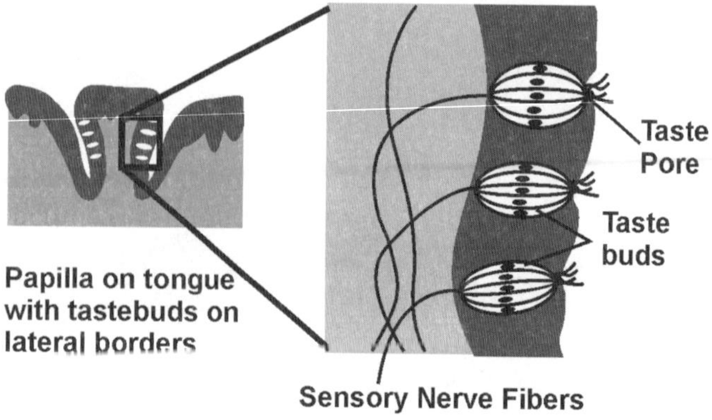

Receptors for Taste

The tongue is covered with a mucus membrane folded on the upper surface to form little peg-like projections known as papillae (from the Latin for "nipple"), which in turn contain the taste buds, the receptors for the chemical sense of gustation. The taste bud- containing papillae are three types: fungiform, vallate and foliate.

The fungiform papillae are mushroom shaped and are spread over the upper surface of the tongue. They appear as small red dots because of their rich blood supply.

The vallate papillae are flat shaped mounds surrounded by a furrow. They are fewer in quantity than the other types of papillae. Human beings have only eight to twelve of them, limited to an inverted V-shaped region obliquely across the back of the tongue close to its foundation.

The foliate papillae are few in quantity and are arranged as leaves or folds along the back edges of the tongue. There are less of them in adults than children.

Each papilla contains several taste buds. They are located on the tops of the fungiform papillae and on the sides of the vallate and foliate papillae. The roughness of the tongue that expands the surface area of the tongue and gives protection to the tongue is the fourth type of protection and is called the filiform papillae. These papillae are most numerous on the central part of the tongue, the area with the least amount of taste buds and sensations.

Taste buds or receptor cells are located mainly within protuberances called papillae on the surface of the tongue. Some buds are also on the palate, throat, and epiglottis. Taste buds on the different parts of the tongue respond more strongly to the four basic tastes: sweet, salty, sour and bitter. The other more subtle taste sensations are made possible by the combination of these tastes in association with taste stimuli, such as odor.

A substance must be dissolved in water to stimulate the taste buds. No moisture, no taste. Nothing is tasted until the tongue starts leaking water into the mouth. The "detection threshold" is the minimum concentration in water at which a substance can be tasted and the intensity is a measure of the strength of the taste sensation. Individual tastes and thresholds vary over time but, in general, substances with a bitter taste are detected at very low concentrations. The thresholds for common simple sugars are higher than those for synthetic sweeteners. Synthetic sweeteners are many times sweeter than natural sugars and are detected in minuscule amounts; the threshold concentrations for salty or sour are about the same as those for sweet.

The activity of taste receptors during the chemical encoding process has been defined with varying detail. The most fundamental of the responses belongs to the saltiness receptor cell. Sodium chloride basically breaks down into its component ions with the "salty" sodium ion directly entering the receptor membrane to induce depolarization, the same basic mechanism underlying the initiation and propagation of an action potential. The higher the concentration of sodium, the greater the receptor response. The saltiness receptor is also responsive to salts containing metallic cations (Na+, K+, Li+) bonded to small anions (Cl-, Br-, SO42-, of NO3-). Molecules that have a common structure stimulate the sweetness receptor cell; a hydrogen ion that is located 0.3 nanometers from a site that seeks to bond with another hydrogen ion. Molecules configured in this manner stimulate an increase in the levels of cyclic AMP within the receptor cell. The cyclic AMP stimulates the opening of calcium channels and neurotransmitters are then released to stimulate a cranial nerve. Sour receptor cells are stimulated by the hydrogen ions found when acids are in solution. Hydrogen cations bond to the receptor membrane and, along with an undefined mechanism involving the anions that are also in solution, close the potassium channels. The closing of potassium channels prevents potassium efflux and the build-up of a positive charge within the receptor cell induces depolarization and an action potential. Molecules that contain both a positively charged side group and a hydrophobic side group stimulate bitterness receptor cells. These side groups activate an enzyme, phosphodiesterase, which breaks down cyclic AMP within the receptor cell. The decrease in cyclic AMP results in the closing of potassium channels and depolarization of the receptor cell occurs. Finally, some sweetness and bitterness receptor cells function as metabotropic synapses. At these receptors, the stimulating chemical bonds to a membrane site that results in the activation of a G protein called gustducin. As is characteristic of metabotropic synapses, the G protein induces the release of a second messenger in the receptor cell and an action potential occurs. Some of the stronger tastes, such as the pungent flavor of spicy food, come about through stimulation of pain-sensitive nerve endings in the tongue.

The Six Tastes

According to Ayurveda there are six tastes. These are an important part of understanding the world we live in. Essentially, how we absorb our world is determined by how we "taste" it. Taste is obviously an essential part of understanding tongue diagnosis. First, let us explore the taste regions and the taste pathways.

Taste Regions

Sweet taste is linked with the tip of the tongue and salty to the backside of the tongue, sour with the sides and bitter are particularly linked with papillae that are located across the back of the tongue.

Taste Pathways

Taste signals from the various areas of the tongue are picked up by nerve fibers from one of four cranial nerves. The impulses then travel to the brain.

The healthiest food, spices or herbal medicines in the world, will turn into poisons in the body if they are not appropriately digested and assimilated. The digestive process begins in the mouth the instant the tongue tastes the food. All digestive organs must be ready by the time the food reaches the stomach. The tongue is the transmitter. It transmits the food's tastes directly to the brain. The brain determines, from this indication, what type of protein or carbohydrate has been ingested and what type of juices are required to be secreted for optimal utilization.

Taste is in actuality present in the mouth, not in the food. A food that is described as sweet is, for example, a food that is experienced as sweet by most healthy individuals under ordinary conditions. To an unhealthy individual, the same food may taste sour, astringent, bitter, or even have a harsh pungent taste.

A Taste Experiment

Take a pleasantly sweet apple and cut it in half; eat one half, then take a teaspoon of honey or maple syrup. Now eat the other half of the apple. It will not matter how pleasantly sweet the first half seemed, the second half of the apple will taste less sweet and more sour. The apple did not transform its taste, what did change is your sense of taste. When you ate the second half of the apple, your tongue and taste buds ignored the taste it had plenty of and selectively experienced sour, the apple's secondary or subtler taste. The sweetener momentary satisfied your tongue and taste buds capability for sweet.

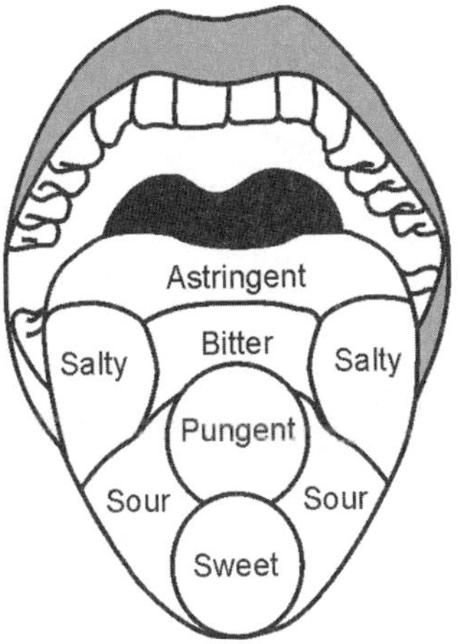

8.6 The Tongue Taste Zones

8.7 The Elemental Zones

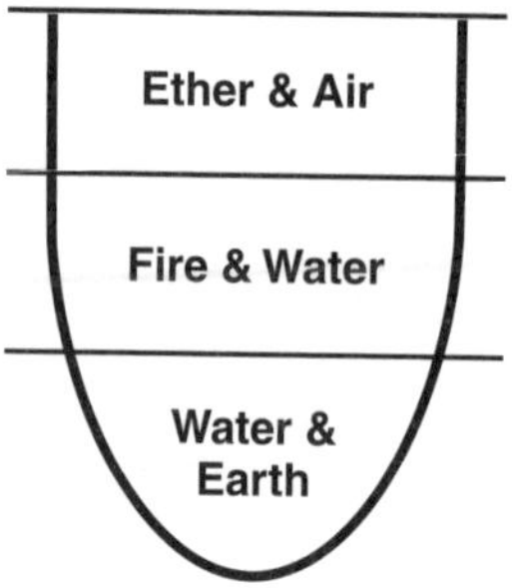

The Taste Buds and the Elements

The body has an innate perception or wisdom regarding food selection that functions through the sense of taste. The body favors those nutrients and foods that reflect its specific elemental make-up. The sense of taste gives us an indication of the elemental composition of the food and thereby protects us from ingesting substances that may distress the natural balance of the elements in the body. When we are offered unusual food or herbs, we will first take only a small amount to ensure that the food is good for us. We will instinctively choose a bowl of fresh fruits before a bowl of cayenne pepper, a strong pungent tasting herb.

The body contains only a small amount of the fire element Agni but it does contain a large amount of the water element. The body more readily accepts the sweet flavors since they are closely associated with the water element. To ingest a large amount of fire Agni, in the form of a hot spice like cayenne pepper, would greatly disturb the natural balance of the elements in the body. The human body is composed of the five elements but some elements exist in greater proportion than others. The six tastes arise out of varying predominance of the five elements that compose that food or herb substance.

9 Ayurvedic Tongue Diagnosis

- History of Tongue Diagnosis
- The Tongue Maps
- The Relationship of the Tongue to the Body
- Topography of the Tongue
- Tongue Diagnosis: A Four-Step Procedure
- The Healthy Vibrant Tongue
- Constitutional Tongue Diagnosis
- Tongue Diagnosis and the Body Organs
- Other Tongue Signs
- Constitutional Tongue Examination
- The Primary Factors to Observe:
  a) Body Color and Tongue Spirit
  b) The Body or Size, Shape and Movement of the Tongue
  c) The Tongue Coating
  d) The Amount of Moisture on the Tongue
- Tongue Diagnosis Signs
- Tongue Diagnosis: An Overview
- Comparative Clinical Significance in Ayurveda, TCM and Western Medicine
- A Tongue Diary
- Salvia pH Testing

History of Tongue Diagnosis

There has been much written about tongue diagnosis through the ages. Traditional Chinese Medicine (TCM) has the most information from which we can draw. Records from around the world indicate that the Traditional Chinese healers did the most extensive studies of the tongue and its diagnostic value. Tongue diagnosis dates to the Shang Dynasty which began around 1600 B.C. and ended c.1000. What we know of these two ancient healing models, the Traditional Chinese Medicine and Ayurvedic Medicine, indicates a great deal of similarities.

The tongue offers us two perspectives. First, it assists us in determining the individual's Prakruti. Looking at the color and shape of the tongue body does this. This indicates their Prakruti - something about the general tendencies of the individual. Secondly, the coating is more directly related to a person's Vikruti and current digestive process. It's considered to be a kind of "smoke," so to speak, that results from the metabolism activity of the food once it is in the stomach, duodenum and spleen.

For thousands of years, visual inspection of the tongue has been a unique and important diagnostic method of Ayurveda and Traditional Chinese Medicine (TMC). Observing the abnormal changes in the tongue proper and the tongue coating can aid in diagnosing diseases. Since the early 1980s, medical professionals in China have systematically studied the relationship between various cancers and tongue signatures. Their results have been published in national medical journals. For instance, China TCM Society, China Cancer Society and TCM Diagnosis Association conducted a national project that included cases of 12,448 cancerous patients, 1,628 non-cancerous patients and 5,578 normal patients [TCMA, 1987]. The results statistically showed that there are significant changes of color, coating, shape and dorsum shape of the tongues of cancerous patients versus those tongues of non-cancerous patients or normal subjects.

Visual inspection of the tongue offers many advantages. It's a non-invasive diagnostic, simple and inexpensive method. However, the current practice in Ayurveda and TCM is mainly experience based or subjective. The quality of the visual inspection varies between individuals, and although there are a few experts successfully diagnosing cancers based on inspection of the tongue, their skills are not easily transferable to other professionals. Their expertise is limited to qualitative descriptions, not to quantitative or mathematical formulations. To circumvent this problem, there are numerous practitioners that have been developing an imaging system for the tongue diagnosis.

9.1 History of the Healing Tastes

600 B.C.	Alcmaeon, the Greek physician believed that the tongue admitted tastants to the "sensorium," the seat of sensation, through tiny pores.
460-370 B.C.	Democritus described taste as resulting from the shapes of things making up what was being tasted. He explains sweetness as round particles; sourness as angular particles; and bitterness as round particles covered with little hooks that snagged the tongue.
384-322 B.C.	Aristole listed seven tastes: sweet, sour, salty, bitter, pungent, astringent and harsh.
180-200 A.D.	Galen, the Roman physician, agreed with Aristole's interpretation.
980-1037 A.D.	Avicenna, the Muslim physician, listed the four basic tastes: sweet, sour, salty and bitter, plus he added insipid.
1497-1588	Jean Fernel, the French physician, added fatty to the list.
1737-1798	Luigi Galvani formulated the scientific study of taste.
1745-1827	Alessandra Volta experimented with the production of taste sensations by touching a piece of zinc and a piece of copper (the founding of conducting electricity).
1801-1887	Gustav Fechner, psychophysics, a combination of physics and psychology, is born.
1883-1920	Wilhelm Wundt, in Germany stimulated the taste senses electrically and reported psychological effects.
1930-1940	Helmut Hahn, experimented and studied 15,000 thresholds for 108 taste substances on 43 individuals and measured the effects of adaptation on taste thresholds.

"It was interesting to notice how the tastes literally "felt" as they were being washed over the tongue. Salt and sweet were warm and pleasant; sweet was the most relaxing and salt was exhilarating. Bitterness curls the edges of the tongue. Sour felt icy and caused the surface of the tongue to contract."

— A time magazine food critic, reminiscent of Democritus's words

The Tongue Maps

9.2 Tongue Map (this diagram is a mirror image)

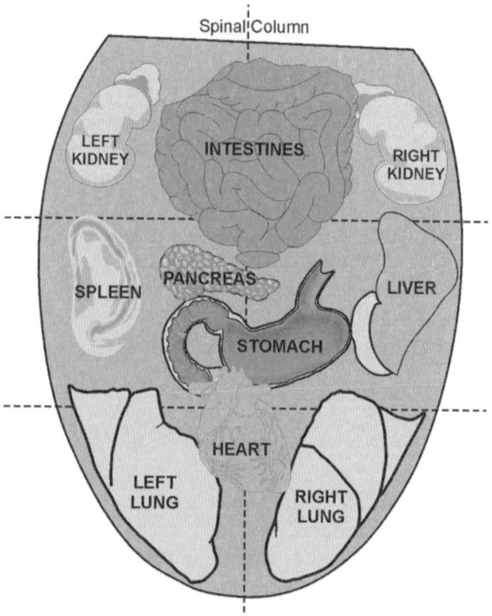

Tongue diagnosis, in combination with the constitutional questionnaires contained in this book, will help you determine your Prakruti and Vikruti constitutions. You are encouraged to study other Ayurvedic diagnostic techniques to confirm your results.

The Pluses of Tongue Diagnosis

- The tongue body color is one of the most reliable diagnostic tools, revealing, in most cases, one's true digestive capacity as well as the Prakruti and Vikruti states of the individual.
- The tongue's appearance is the most valuable measurements

for monitoring the positive or negative development of the individual's state.

- The tongue's topography reveals to us the body systems and organs that are imbalanced, although, if possible, it is helpful in know which areas of the body are in need of attention prior to diagnosis.
- Tongue diagnosis is comparatively objective in evaluation with other diagnostic procedures.
- Tongue diagnosis is one of the easiest diagnostic skills to learn, both for the layperson as well as for professionals.

A discoloration and/or sensitivity of a particular area of the tongue indicates a disorder in the organ corresponding to that area. A whitish tongue indicates a Kapha derangement and mucus accumulation; a red or yellow-green tongue indicates a Pitta derangement; and a black to brown coloration indicates a Vata derangement. A dehydrated tongue is symptomatic of a decrease in the rasa dhatu (plasma), while a pale tongue indicates a decrease in the red blood cells.

The Tongue Map

9.3 Tongue Interior and Exterior Map

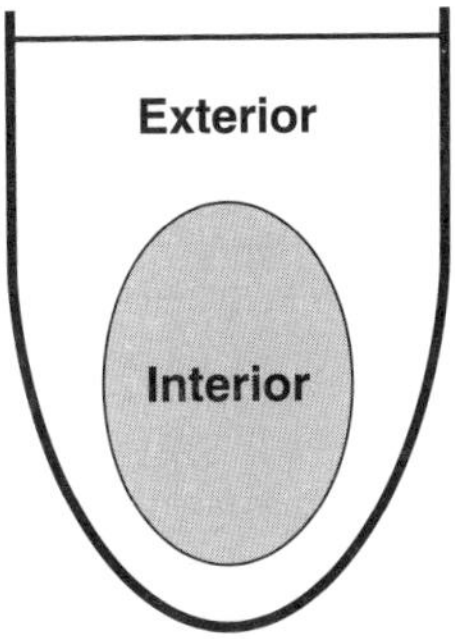

9.4 The Tongue Dosha Zones

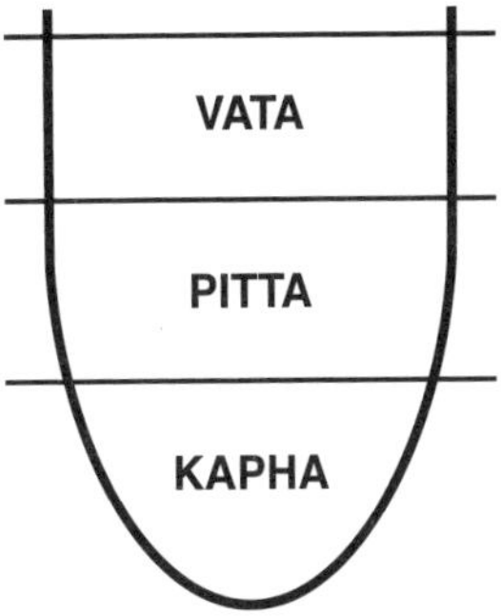

The interior of the tongue is where Agni is located; it covers the three main digestive organs of stomach, small intestines and large intestines.

The exterior is where the other bodily organs are located;

the heart, lungs, thyroid, liver, spleen, pancreas, gall bladder, adrenals and kidneys.

The tongue is your window to your digestive Fire - to your metabolism. It is the only internal organ you can see directly. Its color, shape and mobility indicate your vital energy and blood production. This affects the capacity to digest food, breathe, remove toxins and immune function. Your digestive fire points the way to your potential in health.

9.5 The Tongue and Its Reflective Organs

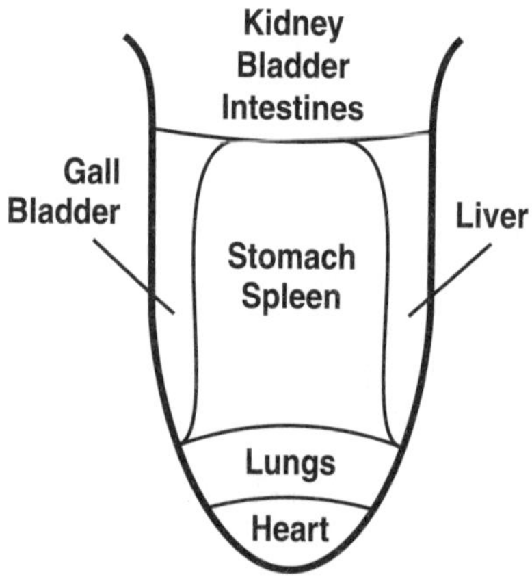

The Tongue and Its Reflective Organs

As with all diagnostic tools, there is a map. As we have mentioned, there are three zones relating to the three doshas, Vata, Pitta and Kapha. Besides these three doshas, we also have a mapping of the internal organs. For this we will divide the tongue into five sections: the tip, front sides, the center, the sides and the back.

When we are using the tongue as a diagnostic tool, it is a good practice to confirm tongue signs through other diagnostic tools such as pulse, iris and facial features. This is especially important if the condition is serious.

Acute and Chronic Disorders

A large, pale tongue, which is whitish in color, could indicate that the adrenals are exhausted. If the whole tongue is of this nature, it is associated with low Prana and chronic circulation problems and heart disturbance. If there is chronic fatigue, there may be a connection with a sluggish metabolism.

9.6a Tongue Organ Positions

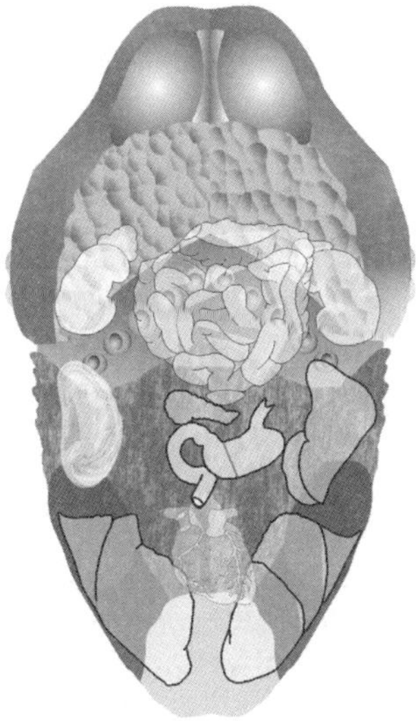

9.6b Tongue Organ Positions

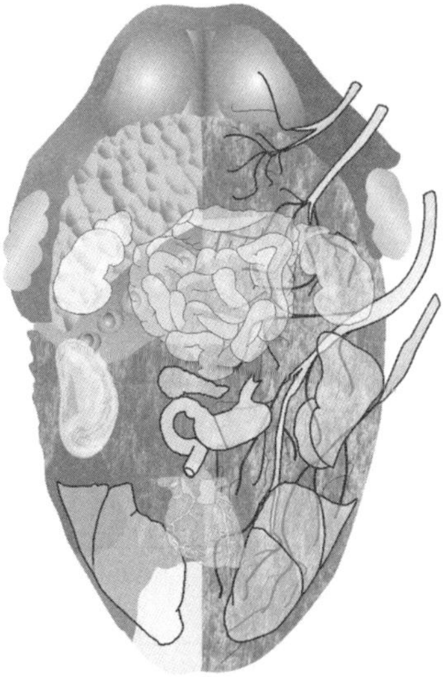

9.6c Tongue Organ Positions

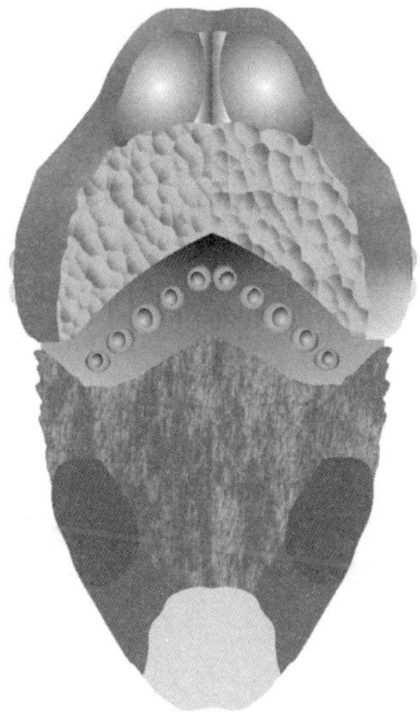

THE TIP- Heart and Thyroid

The front tip of the tongue corresponds to the heart area. Heart weakness, either inherited or a congestive heart disorder, shows up as a crack at the tip of the tongue. If the internal organs are inflamed, this is an indication of infection or dehydration that shows up as a dry and cracked red tongue. A tongue with a grayish mucous coating or a protruding red colored tip is revealing a very inflamed heart or thyroid.

THE FRONT SIDES - Lungs

The area between the center and the tip of the tongue corresponds to the lungs. The tongue will appear coated and discolored for individuals who are heavy smokers or suffer from emphysema or a persistent dry cough. If this area of the tongue is dry and cracked, it indicates dehydration and possible lung tissue injury.

THE CENTER AREA - Stomach, Pancreas and Spleen

The center of the tongue is the key area to check for digestive or metabolism problems. The stomach area of the tongue corresponds to the line from the back of the tongue through the center. When the digestive system is over acidic, such as with ulcers, the line may appear as dry, cracked and dark or bright red. Stomach ulcers appear as a burned area in this line along the center of the tongue. Other signs of a sluggish digestive system are cellulite, excess fat or weight problems.

THE SIDES - Liver and Gallbladder

At the edges of both sides of the tongue are the sections that correspond to the liver and gallbladder. Problems with the liver show up as a grayish color, dotted, and/or cracked. If the liver is underactive or there are deficiencies of the liver, this would show up as scalloped edges. If, on the other hand, the liver has accumulated toxins, the body of the tongue will appear dark.

When there is stagnation of Prana energy, the color of the tongue will appear purplish. This can affect the whole tongue or just the sides. One of the many functions of the liver is to produce enzymes that support calcium absorption. When there is enough calcium in the body the heart can run smoothly. However, if the circulation is sluggish, healthy blood will not reach the tongue, resulting in a bluish-purple tongue.

THE ROOT - Large Intestines, Kidneys and Adrenals

The back section of the tongue represents the large intestine, kidneys and the adrenals. The kidneys and adrenals are located at the sides and the colon at the mid back section. This is the most difficult part of the tongue to see. This section of the tongue is also the most thickly coated and discolored. The colon, in many people, carries and holds years of accumulated toxins and undigested material. In Ayurveda, this is the birthing place of Ama - the birthing place of many diseases. Congestion of the colon leads to constipation and diarrhea, a perfect breeding ground for bacteria and viruses. There are numerous causes - shallow breathing, lack of movement, unhealthy or acidic food choices, eating too fast, stress, repressed emotions and lack of sleep and down time.

Label Tongue Taste Areas Diagram

The tongue is a strong muscle in the mouth that is covered with papillae (small bumps on the tongue) and taste buds (that sense bitter, salty, sweet, and sour tastes). The taste buds are clustered along the sides of the tongue.

9.7a Tongue Areas Taste Diagram

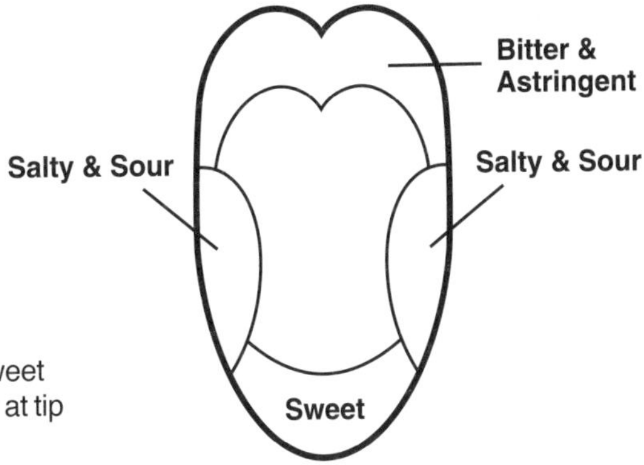

Sweet - Taste buds for sweet tastes are located mostly at tip of the tongue.

Salty - Taste buds for salty tastes are located mostly near the back sides of the tongue.

Sour - Taste buds for sour tastes are located mostly towards the front and middle sides of the tongue.

Bitter - Taste buds for bitter are located mostly towards the back of the tongue.

9.7b Tastes and Organs

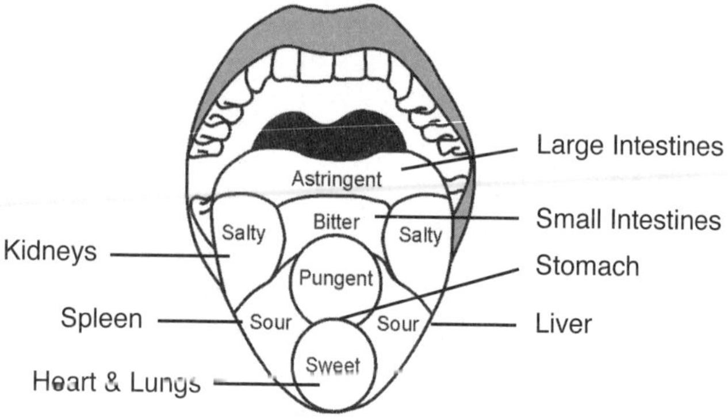

9.8a Sublingual Vein Extension on Underside of Tongue

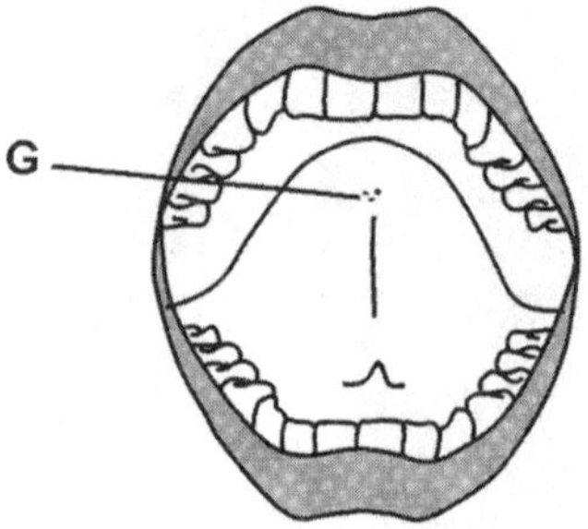

The Relationship of the Tongue to the Body

The tongue is a unique organ to study. It lies between the interior and the exterior and has a direct connection to the inner dynamics of the digestive system.

The tongue has a particularly close relationship to the digestive system and organs that correspond to the three doshas: stomach, Kapha; small intestines, Pitta; and large intestines, Vata. The liquids and solids are received by the stomach where they are transformed and continue through the small intestines and finally the large intestines. The stomach is regarded as the source of fluids, Kapha, and has the ability to produce fluids and is directly reflected in the tongue's moisture content. The vibrancy of the digestive fire and quality of the blood depends on the strength of the digestive fire to extract the essence from ingested foods. This contributes to the healthy, fresh, pale-red color of the tongue body.

All internal organs directly or indirectly supply the tongue through the nadis. As a result of these connections, the tongue can be used as a valuable source of information about the status of life force (Prana), blood quality (Tejas), and fluids (Ojas) in the body. The tongue is important for ascertaining the bodily humors and their Sama and Nirama states.

9.8b Typography of the Tongue

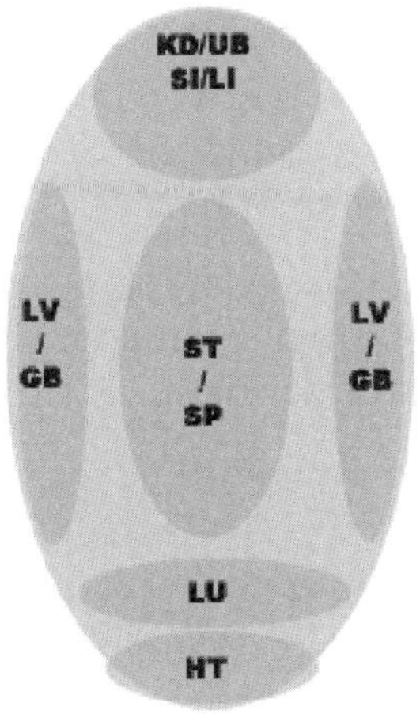

Topography of the Tongue

The tongue is divided into three areas or zones.

1. The first (anterior) third of the tongue reflects the dosha that correspond to Kapha (Earth and Water), which is called the upper burner in TCM. This includes the heart and lungs.
2. The second (middle) third of the tongue reflects the dosha that correspond to Pitta (Fire and Water), which is called the middle burner in TCM. This includes the spleen, stomach, liver and gall bladder.
3. The third (posterior) third of the tongue reflects the dosha that correspond to Vata (Air and Ether), which is called the lower burner in TCM. This includes the kidneys, bladder and large intestines.

Prakruti is seen in the tongue through the shape, tongue body color and general vitality of the tongue spirit.

Vikruti is seen in the tongue through tongue coating, movement and odor.

Tongue Diagnosis A Four-Step Procedure

When doing a tongue diagnosis, a clear understanding of the entire person and pathology is needed to evaluate either general or specific tongue signs. Here is a simple four-step process to determine the individual's Prakruti and Vikruti.

1. Get a general impression of the tongue by observing the tongue's vitality.
2. Collect and identify the individual's signs concerning the tongue's color, shape and coating. A topographic map of the tongue is essential for this step.
3. Examine the underside of the tongue. The best way to do this is for the individual to curl the tongue upward and gently rest its tip on the front part of the palate. Observe the size and color of the two veins on either side of the frenulum.
4. Reevaluate the general impression of the individual's tongue signs. This is the step that brings together the diagnosis to reach a conclusion of the treatment protocol.

A Step-by-Step Checklists for an Accurate Tongue Examination

Conditions for an Accurate Diagnosis

1. Observe and take notes immediately after reading the tongue.
2. Tongue should not be extended for longer than 20-30 seconds and with as little effort as possible.
3. The best lighting is natural daylight, second best is a halogen light.
4. Always try to maintain the same position and location when studying the tongue.

5. Inquire when the person ate their last meal or snack (some foods discolor the tongue).
6. Fatty foods will give an oily consistency.
7. Hot spices such as curry will have a yellowish discoloration.
8. Cigarettes or cigars have a drying effect upon the coating and give a yellowish discoloration.
9. Alcohol will give a reddening of the tongue body.
10. Intake of large amounts of fluids may lead to an increase in tongue moisture; conversely, a small intake of fluids reduces moisture.
11. Black tea or coffee may cause the coating to become a brownish color.
12. Check whether the person is taking any medications as some medications discolor the tongue body.
13. Check the thickness of the tongue coating.
14. The tongue should be held in a relaxed manner.
15. Inspect the tongue starting at the tip and finishing at the root.

The Normal Healthy Tongue

The tongue is a reflection of the energetic harmony within the individual's constitution. It reflects the harmonious balance and interplay of the five elements

The tongue of a healthy person would have a luster and shine with a fresh-looking pale red colour and a thin white coating (formed of the papillae on the surface of the tongue), which should be like "grass growing out of soil", that is, firmly rooted and not liable to be scraped off. The coating may be slightly thicker towards the back of the tongue but should otherwise not be uneven or patchy. Ideally, the tongue should be supple, free of cracks and not quiver or tremble. It should be slightly moist. Children's tongues are more likely to exhibit this state of health/perfection than adults. Variations from this give important information about the nature of a person's condition.

The Four Principles to Check in a Healthy Tongue

- The healthy tongue body color is pale-red.
- The healthy tongue body shape is neither too thick nor too thin.
- The healthy tongue coating is white and thin.
- The veins underneath the tongue are not distended.

1. SPIRIT - the healthy, normal tongue has spirit. Its color is vibrant and vital, especially on the root. When the tongue is full of vitality, it moves with ease and can protrude from the mouth without difficulty.

2. BODILY COLOR - the color is fresh, pale-red and vibrant looking. A healthy normal tongue texture is light reddish in color, not too pale and not too dark. This is because there is a healthy flow of blood reaching the tongue through the blood vessels under the mucus membrane and within the muscle structure. The blood penetrates the white, translucent tongue mucus membranes and appears reddish in color.

3. BODY SHAPE - is supple, neither too flabby nor too stiff, no cracks, does not tremble, is neither swollen nor thin, has no ulcers. As a general rule, the normal tongue shape changes only when pathology persists over a long period of time.

4. COATING - is thin and white, and slightly thicker on the root than elsewhere on the tongue. It is normal for the coating to be slightly thicker on the root zone of the tongue.

5. MOISTURE - is slightly moist, neither too dry nor too wet, yet with a luster indicating that the saliva is adequate.

6. SUBLINGUAL VEINS - the veins underneath the tongue are not distended, they are either barely visible or not at all. Their color ideally should be light and not a dark-blue or purple.

The most important characteristic of the tongue is the color of the body, as opposed to the color of any coating that may be present. Redness, compared with the healthy fresh pale red, indicates the presence of excess heat and a red tip may indicate persistent emotional problems. Red sides indicate excitation of the liver and a red centre shows heat. If the tongue body is pale this shows deficiency of blood or digestive fire, representing the moving, warming, defensive functions of the body. A bluish or purplish tongue signifies blood stasis.

The tongue coating relates primarily to the functioning of the stomach. Note that a healthy tongue should have some coating. Absence of coating, or a coating which is patchy or "rootless," shows deficiency. A thick coating results from excess. If the coating is thick and white it is cold in nature. If the coating is yellow, it is hot in nature. A greasy, slippery or sticky coating reveals a sluggish Kapha condition which can manifest as heaviness, abdominal bloating, poor concentration, difficulty getting going in the mornings, tendency to overweight, and symptoms such as depression or joint pain.

9.9 Healthy Tongue Diagnosis Chart

Aspect	**Specific Factor**	**Clinical Significant**	**Differentiation Prakruti & Vikruti**
Tongue Spirit		Healthy or Unhealthy Prognosis Prakruti	**Prakruti**
Tongue Body	Color Shape	Prana, Blood & Nutritional Quality	**Prakruti** Hot/cold Deficiency/excess
Tongue Coating	Color Thickness Distribution Root	Hot or cold disorders Strength or weakness of body's Prana or pathogenic factor Interior Environment: location of pathogenic factors Exterior Environment: progression of pathogenic factors Strength of body's Prana potential esp. the stomach and kidneys	**Vikruti** Hot/cold Deficiency/excess Deficiency/excess
Tongue Moisture		Health condition of bodily fluids	**Vikruti** Hot/cold

Constitutional Tongue Diagnosis

One of the greatest gifts of Ayurveda is its wholeness, expansiveness and embracement of all life. Ayurvedic tongue diagnosis helps us to look inside an individual.

In Ayurvedic medicine there are numerous methods of determining an individual's constitution. Most practitioners use more then one diagnostic tool to get the whole picture. Integrating a few basic skills such as tongue, pulse, iris, facial diagnosis and a through constitutional questionnaire can greatly enhance understanding the total picture. However, the best constitutional diagnosis in the world is not much use if we cannot tell the individual how to effectively treat their present condition. A thorough evaluation of the humors, tissues, channels, organs and waste materials of the body is essential in tongue diagnosis.

The main aim of Tongue Diagnosis is:

1. Constitutional Prakruti evaluation to determine inherited traits and tendencies.
2. Constitutional Vikruti evaluation of specific present imbalances and disorders.

The Vikruti is usually addressed first because this informs us of the symptoms and disorders that are causing discomfort and therefore need immediate attention. The Prakruti, on the other, tells us how to stay on a preventative path and the direction we need to take to maintain our optimal health.

Examination and Treatment

The aim of Ayurveda is to remove the root cause and give permanent relief. The treatment is mainly comprised of a healthy diet, powders, decoctions and medicated oils prepared from natural herbs and plants. The medicines are derived from natural sources and not synthetic and therefore they are accepted and assimilated in the body without creating any side effects.

If we know what to look for, our body and its waste products give us much information about the state of the body. Examination of our tongue, fingernails, skins, perspiration, eyes, lips, stools and urine gives an early indication of imbalance in our body. Different kinds of examinations are made to find out the root cause of a disease. The examination or constitutional diagnosis is the basis for protocol of treatment. Tongue diagnosis is an art with no set absolutes of doing it.

Steps in Tongue Diagnosis: Constitutional Prakruti

1. Examine the tongue body shape, color and tongue spirit
2. Examine and determine the condition of the metabolic digestive fire.
3. Examine by observation the general strength of the individual.
4. Examine by observing the emotional and mental nature, the state of Prana, Tejas and Ojas.
5. Determine the mental and spiritual nature according to the three Gunas.

Steps in Tongue Diagnosis: Constitutional Vikruti

1. Examine and determine when the imbalance started.
2. Examine and determine the fundamental dosha imbalance.
3. Examine and determine whether the present state is Sama or Nirama.
4. Examine and determine which of the six stages of disease is involved.
5. Determine if there are any psychological factors involved.
6. Determine if there are any environmental or lifestyle factors involved.
7. Determine the motivation and impulse of the individual versus that of the imbalance factor.

This is the basis of prognosis both for the Prakruti and Vikruti. From this conclusion, a treatment plan can be formulated. Remember that the initial diagnosis is a guideline for further treatment; it is not the end of the examination. As one of my teachers said, "The purpose of diagnosis is not necessarily to be able to reach a conclusion or to give advice, the purpose is to know what questions to ask next."

9.10 Constitutional Tongue Signs

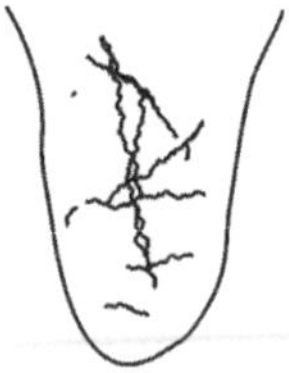

Vata Tongue

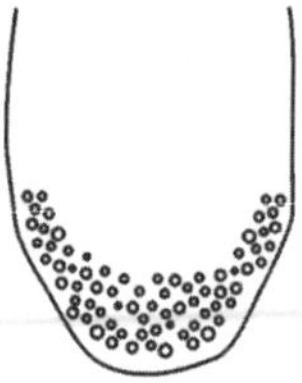

Pitta Tongue

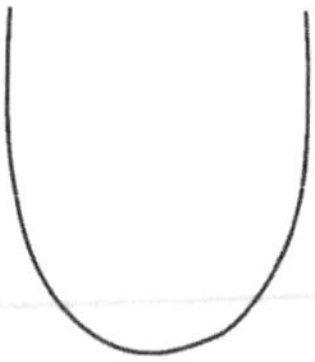

Kapha Tongue

Vata Disturbances on the Tongue

A thin trembling, pale tongue reveals a Vata constitution as well as the following:

- Dry, dark tongue
- Rough back area
- Small dark pimples
- Small cracks all over the tongue
- Coating over the back of the tongue
- Bumps on the kidney points or colon area
- Coating over the large and/or the small intestine

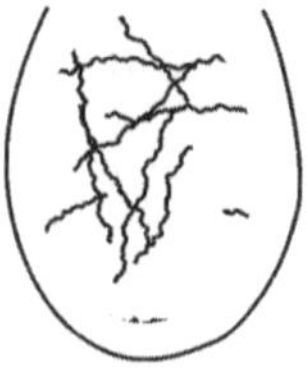

Cracks
Vata imbalances related to: nerves in the large intestines, sensitive nerves, nervous indigestion.

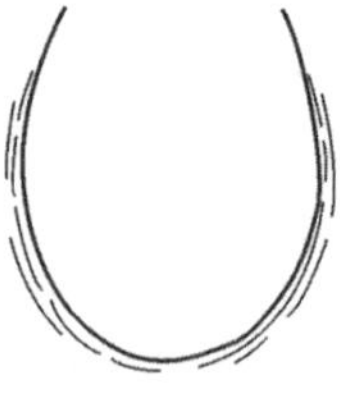

Tremors
Vata disorders related to: fears, insecurities and anxieties.

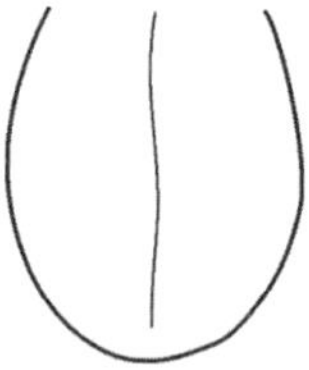

Midline Crack
Vata sign: Emotional disturbances and spinal column problems.

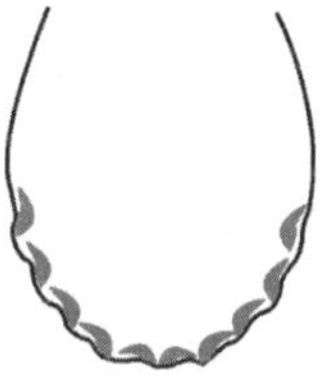

Teethmarks
Vata indication: Absorption and assimilation, problem absorbing and assimilating nutrients.

9.11 Vata Tongue Signs

Pitta Disturbances on the Tongue

A medium, reddish tongue reveals a Pitta constitution as well as the following:

- Red tongue
- White cold sores
- Yellowish-green coating on the tongue
- Coating on the middle section of the tongue
- Bright red patches over the digestive organs
- Bumps on the liver, spleen or pancreas points

9.12 Pitta Tongue Signs

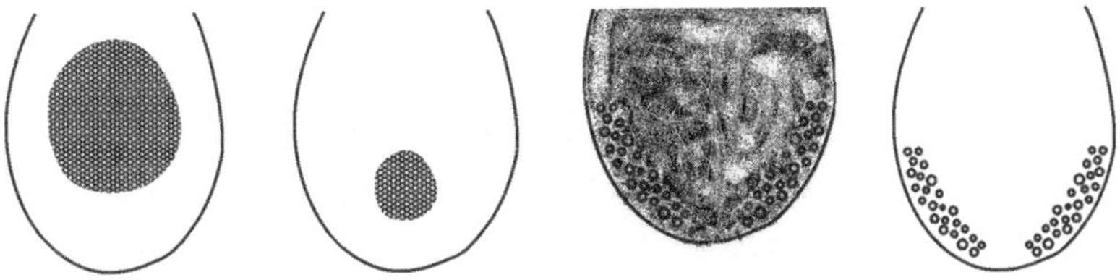

White with red perimeter
Pitta indicator: toxins and impurities in small intestines.

Reddish spot
Pitta sign: revealing a sensitive and delicate heart.

Red all over with red spots
Pitta imbalance: relating to disturbance in digestive fire.

Red spots
Pitta disorder: an imbalance of fire in the respiratory system usually infected or inflamed tissues.

Kapha Disturbances on the Tongue

A thick, roundish, pale tongue reveals a basic Kapha constitution well as the following:

- White tongue
- Oily coating on the tongue
- Depressions on the lung points
- Tip of the tongue whitish or coated
- White film or coating on the tongue
- Bump or depression on the heart point

9.13 Kapha Tongue Signs

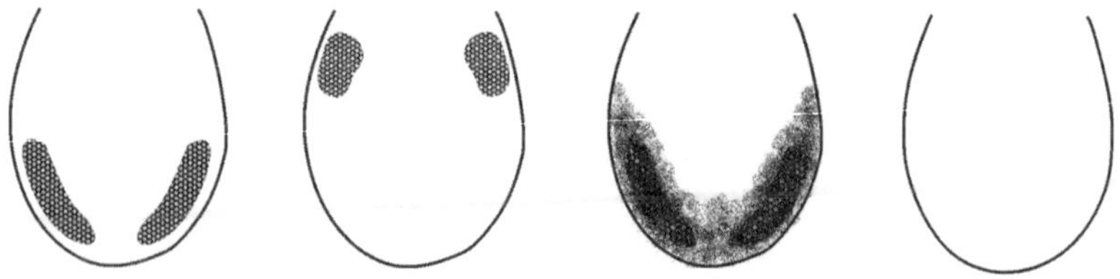

Frothy, either white or brownish
Kapha sign: lungs are congested, mucousy with bronchitis.

Discolored either white or off white
Kapha indicator: kidney problems or congested.

Brownish with dark spots
Kapha sign: pneumonitis if tongue is brown.

White coated tongue all over
Kapha disturbance: blood and tissues acidic.

Other Tongue Signs

General indicators of an accumulation of humors over a period of time are tongue cracks, thick coating and strong colors such as white, red and brown. Organ congestion, either over-performing or under-performing is revealed by cracks, depressions, or bumps.

- Bad breath is an indicator of low digestive ability, Agni. It is also indicator of toxic accumulation. Check root problem on the tongue for intestinal disturbances.
- Malabsorption of nutrients is revealed by teeth indentations on the side of the tongue.
- Cracks or fissures in the centerline reveal back problems.
- A deep line down the center of the tongue reveals repressed emotions or held nervous energy on the spinal column.
- Chronic disorders are revealed by extreme cracks, depressions or bumps.

9.14 Tongue Midline Cracks

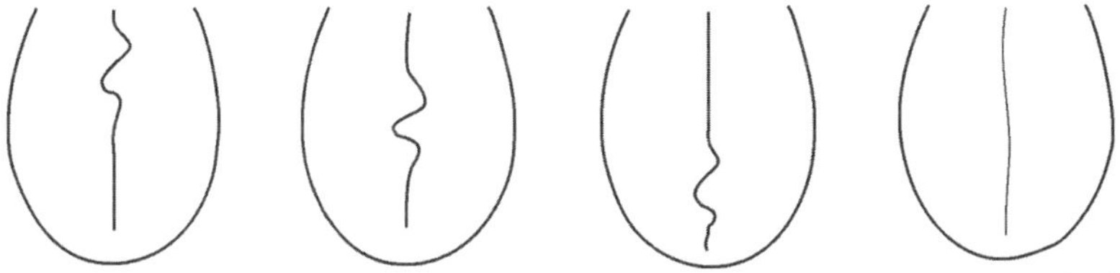

Crooked midline
Vata disturbance: in the Vata zone relates to lower back problems

Crooked midline
Pitta disturbance: in the Pitta zone relates to middle back problems

Crooked midline
Kapha disturbance: in the Kapha zone relates to upper back problems

Long vertical midline
Heart disturbance: the deeper the crack the more chronic the condition

9.15 Tongue Cracks

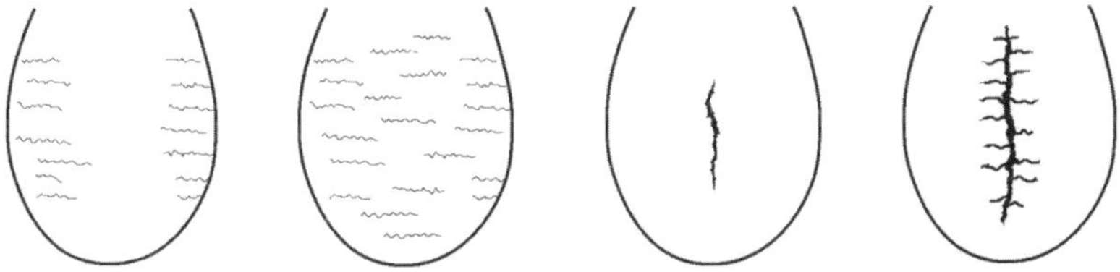

Transverse cracks on the sides of the crack
Liver and spleen disturbances: indicates a drying, contraction usually a deficiency sign.

Long or short horizontal cracks
Vata deficiency: Usually indicates a chronic deficiency of nutrients, digestive organs are depleted.

Short vertical crack in the center
Stomach under active and malnourished.

Deep central crack with small vertical cracks
Deep, long-standing emotional problem and overwork, stress and unhealthy eating habits.

9.16 Tongue Shapes

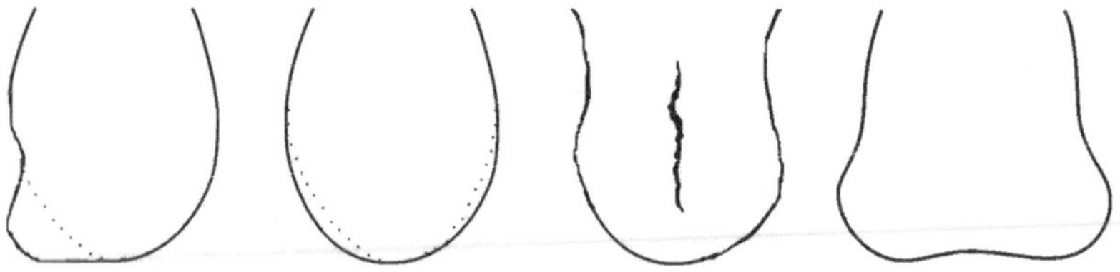

Swollen on half of the tongue Weakness on the side of the body, need of tonification and strengthening circulation.

Swollen sides Liver disturbance with irritability, headaches, vicion problems and dizziness.

Swollen along a central crack Heart indicator: symptoms of shortness of breath, constriction in the chest cavity.

Hammer shaped tongue Mental disturbance due to years of pathological stresses.

Tongue Diagnosis and Taste Preferences

VATA - predominate taste in the mouth is Sweet and Sour.

PITTA - predominate taste in the mouth is Bitter and Pungent.

KAPHA - predominate taste in the mouth is Salty and Sweet.

Constitutional Tongue Examination

1) Examine the individual's structure, the general condition of the limbs, along with complexion.
2) Determine the metabolic factors: appetite, circulation and condition of the waste materials.
3) Examine the strength and activity of the individual, including external aggravating factors.
4) Examine the pulse, tongue, iris and abdomen.
5) Determine the mental and emotional nature with respect to speech, sleep, memory, etc.
6) Examine the state of Prana, Tejas and Ojas.
7) Determine the mental and spiritual nature according to the three Gunas and their qualities.

Constitution examination should reveal the balance of the:

Three Humors - Vata, Pitta and Kapha

Three Gunas - Sattva, Rajas and Tamas

Three Subtle Essences - Prana, Ojas and Tejas

Disease Examination

1) Determine the time of onset of the disease, past history of both patient and family.
2) Examine whether the condition is Sama or Nirama, the state of vitality of the digestive system.
3) Determine the humoral imbalance and the main factors of the disease: fatigue, pain, fever, etc.
4) Examine what environmental and/or factors like diet, work or exercise may be causing illness.
5) Determine which of the six stages of disease is involved, along with the disease/stress cause.
6) Determine any mental or psychological factors involved.
7) Examine the strength and motivation of the patient versus that of the disease factor.

Tongue diagnosis is an art and a science - it will comprehend all the symptoms of a patient. The best diagnosis in the world in is not of much value if we cannot treat their condition effectively. Our diagnosis skills should be balanced with skills in the natural healing modalities. Each individual is a living organism, in constant flux. Observing our patient on a regular basis is key to achieving the results we want.

While making a diagnosis, an Ayurveda practitioner also takes into consideration the Prakruti; the body constitution of a person. This personal constitution helps an Ayurvedic practitioner to decide on a customized treatment protocol for the patient. Because no two persons' constitutions are the same, their body types are different and their response to a similar drug therapy would be different.

Besides the physical symptoms, the mental, spiritual and social aspects are also taken into consideration. The place of living, environment, work conditions, diet, life style, various seasons, family and social life; all play an important role in choosing the healing program. This information is important to establish an accurate diagnosis and treatment regimen.

Diagnosis and Patient Examination

In Constitutional Medicine, examination comes in many forms. Using all of our five senses will give us the most complete picture as to what is taking place for the individual. All the humors, tissues, channels, systems, vital and sense organs and waste materials of the body, as well as the state of the mind and the life force are examined in detail. Keep in mind that in Ayurveda the concern is with the vital life force, Prakruti. As we enliven the vital force, disease is treated.

A complete physical and psychological examination may aim at either:

- constitutional evaluation- the whole condition of the whole body is examined.
- treatment of specific disorders- we target the symptoms and syndromes of the disease.

The Three Stages of Investigation

Even though the Practitioners of Ayurveda may not use the sphygmomanometer to measure the blood pressure and the stethoscope to listen to the heart sounds, their methods of examination of the patient and their diagnosis of the disease are scientific. In fact, diagnosis in Ayurveda is more detailed and, therefore, more accurate. The texts lay down the various techniques for diagnosing disorders.

Three Stages of Investigation: Tongue examination is carried out in three stages: case history of the patient, objective examination, and inference.

Case History of the Patient: The patient is questioned in detail about his illness and any illnesses his family has suffered from. A general evaluation is then made in terms of patient's body constitution, somatic make-up, gastric capacity and capacity for exercise according to age.

Objective Examination: The next stage of examination entails a thorough examination of the patient's nails, eyes, eye lashes, eye brows, nose, teeth, lips, hands, feet, hair, pupils, urine, feces, shadow and skin luster. The entire body of the patient is then palpitated to find out its normal and abnormal condition. The physician determines which organs of the entire system are cold or hot, moist or dry, light or heavy, sensitive or insensitive, rough or smooth, rigid or loose, depressed or elevated. Body odors are paid special attention to. This pathological investigation helps in the assessment of the progress of the disease, its etiological factors, and the probability of curing the disease.

Inference: The third stage is that of inference in which the physician draws his conclusions based on the case history of the patient and the examination he has completed.

Identifying the Imbalance of the Body Constituents

On completion of his investigation, the physician can also conclude which particular dosha is responsible for the state of morbidity. Ayurvedic texts provide detailed descriptions of the symptoms that arise from the decrease or increase of the three doshas. As Charaka has laid down in his Samhita:

> *"The Tridoshas, when increased, manifest their characteristic symptoms in proportion to the intensity of their morbidity. When decreased, they cease to manifest their characteristic qualities and when normal, they perform the normal functions of the body."*

After determining the imbalance in the equilibrium of the three doshas, the Ayurvedic practitioner probes deeper still to identify the type of imbalance and describes it in the context of three phases: waning, aggravating and expanding.

Practitioners of Ayurveda are keen observers. They also study the state of the body fluids, blood, flesh, fit, bones, marrow, semen and the vital essence or Oja which, incidentally, is known as the vital force in the naturopathic system of medicine. They also try to find out whether the disease is curable or not. As Charaka has pointed out:

> *"The physician who knows the differential diagnosis between the curable and the incurable disease, conditions and begins treatment with full knowledge of the case, in time, obtains success for his effort without fail."*

Sushruta has also given his definition of disease:

> *"The person who has a normal equilibrium of the Tridoshas, the seven body constituents, and the body's waste products, as well as a normal appetite, and one who is more joyous in body, mind, and spirit is really healthy; and the person, otherwise, is called unhealthy."*

9.17 Tongue Diagnosis and the Body Organs Internal Heat and Cold on the Tongue

Organ -Chinese Elements	Area of Tongue	Internal Heat	Internal Cold
Tongue		red, dry, cracked, thick dark coating	pale, scalloped, excessive salvia
Heart - Fire	Tip	fast heartbeat, palpitation excitement	slow heartbeat, low energy, depression
Lungs - Metal	Near front sides	dry cough, thirst, laryngitis, anxiety	phlegm-like cough, shortness of breath, low energy, depression
Stomach - Earth	Center	ulcer, burning, excessive hunger, obsession	sluggish digestion, excessive mucus, hypoglycemia, overweight
Spleen- Earth	Center	craves sweets & sugary foods, obsessive & fanatical thoughts	lacks appetite, diarrhea, whining
Liver - Wood	Sides	insomnia, allergies, anger, red eyes, strong sexual drive, menstrual pain	nervousness, anemia, greenish skin, indecision, low enthusiasm
Kidney - Water	Root sides	dark urine, sparse urine, Strong sexual drive	clear urine, lots of urine, low sexual drive or strength
Intestine - Metal	Root	burning diarrhea, frequent urge pain, spasm	watery diarrhea with exhaustion, pain relieved with massage

Body Color and Tongue Spirit

The appearance of vitality indicates the health of an individual. This quality is referred to as the "spirit" of the tongue, denoting an apparent liveliness. Tongue "Spirit," as it is called in Chinese medicine, has no metaphysical significance. In this context, it is associated with vigor and well being. A tongue with a vital color is described as a "tongue of life" and a tongue with a dark and withered appearance as a "tongue of disorder." This simply means the relative seriousness of disease. In analyzing the vitality, observation of the root of the tongue is of particular importance. The root of the tongue is the Vata zone. If the root has a good vibrant color, the prognosis is good no matter what the illness or disorder may be. However, if the root has a dark, dry and withered appearance, the prognosis is poor.

A healthy tongue is understood to have spirit when it appears to be flourishing and energetic. An unhealthy tongue with no spirit on the other hand appears to be emaciated. Flourishing signifies possessing strength and brilliance. When the tongue is healthy and has spirit it is an indication of a condition that is easily treated with good results.

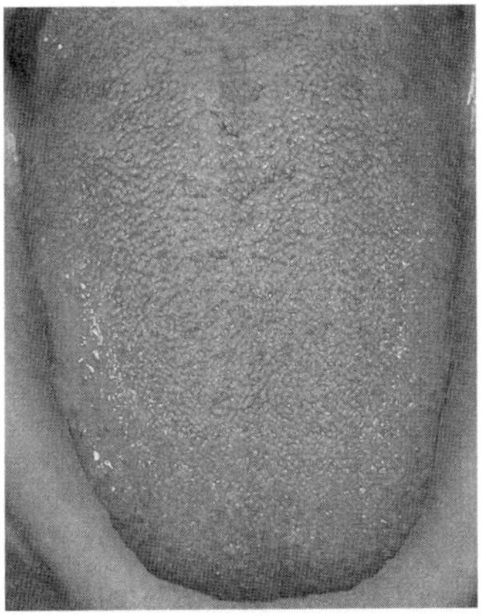

9.18 A Healthy Tongue

The healthy tongue shows a lively reddish color on the root or Vata zone. The root of the tongue reflects the health of the large intestines and the kidneys.

The tongue body color is an immediate indicator of the pathological condition. Whenever there is any doubt in diagnosing an individual's true state or Prakruti through the tongue, the tongue body color is one of the best and most accurate indictors. Prakruti we can see by the tongue body color and shape.

Tongue Body Color

The tongue body color is the color beneath the tongue coating.

Tongue body color, in almost all cases, reveals the true state of the body given that it is unchanged by secondary and short-term issues of Vikruti.

The tongue body colors can range from pale red to purple and even a bluish coloring. See tongue body color chart for specific details of color and indictor meanings. Keep in mind that an excessively red color indicates a more Pitta or Agni potential.

In acute conditions, the tongue body can provide valuable information regarding the quality and depth of infiltration of a pathogenic factor. For example, a continuing high fever lasting for days may change the coloration of the tongue body to a dark deep red color. On the other hand, as with a chronic condition, for instance cancer, the tongue body can reflect long-term pathological disharmony as well as constitutional tendencies and potentials.

Underside of the Tongue

The underside of the tongue is a valuable indicator, particularly the two main veins under the tongue on either side of the frenulum. The main area or zone it corresponds to is the Kapha zone. If one vein is distended, it signifies the blood stasis is mainly on one side of the body. Veins should be noted for their size. Examining this area of the tongue can be beneficial as an early detection of both blood and Prana imbalances.

- Dark veins indicate blood stasis, the darker the color the more severe the stasis.
- If the veins are distended but not dark, stagnation of Prana or Vata imbalance is indicated.
- Distended veins indicate a condition of excess - usually a Kapha sign.
- Thin veins indicate a condition of deficiency - usually a Vata sign.
- Reddish purple and shiny veins indicate Pitta
- White slippery veins indicate the presence of cold damp energy - usually a Kapha sign.
- If the veins on the underside are dark and the rest of the tongue body is dark, this indicates that the blood stasis is of

a short period of time, is not very severe and, for the most part, involves the Kapha.

Tongue Body Color Constitutional Indicator

VATA - if the tongue body color is purple or bluish, this indicates blood stagnation that is due to an internal cold environment. A dry tongue is another sign of an excess Vata, especially if located in the Vata zone, which is located at the root or the back of the tongue.

PITTA - if the body is red, it indicates the presence of Fire, an excess of heat and imbalanced circulatory system. A coating reveals excess heat, Fire, and no coating is due to the deficiency of internal heat, Fire. If there are red spots or points, this is an indicator of blood and heat stagnation.

KAPHA - if the body is pale and moist, it indicates a deficiency of heat and blood and a poor circulatory system. A pale tongue body may indicate kidney deficiency.

> *"A flourishing and moist tongue indicates a good supply of bodily fluids. A dry and withering tongue indicates the exhaustion of bodily fluids. Flourishing is called "to have spirit" and indicates brightness, clear color, freshness and a light red color. All these attributes indicate life; the absence of them indicates death. A bright moist and blood-colored tongue indicates life; a dark withered tongue with no blood color indicates death."*
>
> — A Guide to Tongue Differentiation (Bian She nan) (1920). Reference provided by Su Xin-Ming

The body color is the single most important aspect of observation. It is giving the true condition of the body, irrespective of temporary conditions resulting from recent physical exertion or emotional upset. The tongue body color is the definitive indicator for diagnosis.

Constitutional Tongue Color Indicators

Vata tongue color - is somewhat pale or dull in color.

Pitta tongue color - is red, can be blue or purple, as well as yellowish-green in color.

Kapha tongue color - is pale or white.

Normal tongue color is pink.

Red tongue indicates heat or fever.

Dark red tongue reveals the condition is certain to be one of intense heat in one or more organs.

Pale tongue, lips and complexion indicates anemia.

Pale white, the condition is indicating blood deficiency

Purple or blue tongue indicates stagnation of blood and liver disorders, particularly when there are purple spots on the tongue.

Redness on the tip of the tongue reveals heat in the heart, stress and anxiety.

A margin of the tongue- redness reveals an early stage or superficial heat or febrile condition.

Whole tongue redness reveals a more long term or long-standing heat condition.

Tongue Body Shape, Size and Movement

The tongue body shape is the next step in determining an individual's Prakruti. Tongue body shape includes the physical contours, consistency, texture and mobility of the tongue.

The tongue body shape tells us a lot about the health of the individual. To fully appreciate the information from the tongue shape we need to combine that information with the tongue body color. The reason being, changes in color in conjunction with shape will give you a more accurate diagnostic reading. However, in cases where the tongue body is healthy in appearance but the shape considerably irregular, the shape becomes a more essential factor to accurate diagnosis. Tongue shape will change only when pathology persists over a long period of time.

The healthy shape of the tongue is supple and soft without being flaccid. It is neither too slender nor too enlarged. Its surface is unbroken by cracks. Its form comes to a point towards the tip. When the tongue is extended it neither shivers nor shakes uncontrollably, nor is it involuntarily rigid or immobile.

Cracks, depressions and localized swellings on the tongue body are a reflection of the energetic disharmonies in specific areas of the body. An example of this is if the front third, the Kapha zone of the tongue, is engorged and puffy, this indicates retention of phlegm in the lungs and respiratory system. If the individual complains of a cough, attention should be given at once.

Vata - thin, long or small tongue and the tongue often trembles.

Pitta - medium size, but may also be sharply pointed.

Kapha - large, round, thick or fatty tongues with big lips.

Tongue Body Shape Indicators

The tongue's body shape indicates:

- the severity of the imbalance
- the length of time of the imbalance

The combination of tongue body and shape provides precise information about the condition and potential of Vata, Pitta and Kapha distribution.

Examination of shape reflects the state of the organs, blood and Prana (life-force) energy. It is most useful in differentiating conditions of excess and deficiency.

Examination of the tongue's body must include consideration of the shape, the features of the tongue surface and the texture of the tongue body as well as any involuntary movements of the tongue.

Examining for shape involves looking to see whether the tongue is thin or swollen, long or short and whether specific parts of the tongue are swollen. Large or flabby tongues with scallops, tooth prints or indentations around the margin of the tongue indicate chronic low Agni and weak digestive power.

Examining for features involves observing for aberrations as cracks and ulcers.

Examining for textures involves observing the extent to which the tongue body is supple or stiff.

Examining for movement involves watching for any movement of the tongue when it is extended. Movements may include trembling, quivering, side-to-side motion, curling in any direction or shifting to one side.

Check tongue shape chart for examples and indicator meanings.

There are times when the tongue does not reflect a pattern of disharmony. This seems to be the case involving the liver. To make an accurate constitutional diagnosis it is recommended that a person fill out a thorough Prakruti and Vikruti questionnaire and include pulse or iris diagnosis for a complete assessment. It is essential that one remember that tongue diagnosis is only one aspect, although a very informative and important one, of the entire diagnostic protocol in Ayurvedic medicine.

Tongue Coating

The tongue coating is one of our main diagnostic tools. It indicates a person's present Vikruti constitution and state of function of the digestive organs. From the Ayurvedic perspective, the tongue coating is related mainly to Agni and Kapha. The coating of the tongue is the result of a Kapha and physiological process and its presence on the tongue reveals the proper or improper functioning of the stomach. In ancient China there is an expression, "a healthy person should have a thin coating like grass growing from the soil," in the way the earth can be seen between the blades of newly-sprouted grass. A coating that is too thin is like a bare patch of lawn.

A healthy coating on the tongue is thin, slightly white and slightly moist. The thin coating is due to the small amount of turbidity that flows up from the stomach as a by-product of digestion. If the coating is absent, it indicates that the stomach's digestive capacity is severely damaged. However, if the coating is too thick or excessive it indicates improper functioning of Agni in the digestive system. An excessive coating is thick and covers all three zones of the tongue.

The home base of Kapha is the stomach, the origin of digestive fluids. When the stomach cannot digest foods properly and stagnation builds in this region, the tongue coating will become wet and slippery in appearance.

One of the key aspects to observe in the tongue coating is the distribution of the coating. Usually there is a slight progression of coating in different areas of the tongue surface. The natural progression of the coating should be - the thinnest on the tip and edges, a bit thicker towards the middle and even more so around the back area of the tongue. A thick coating will be found in the central surface area of the tongue since this is the zone that corresponds to Kapha and Pitta, where the stomach organs are found. The root of the tongue corresponds to the large intestines, the Vata zone, which is also involved in the digestive process. Since the large intestines are the last process of the digestive system, this is where the thickest coating will be found.

The tongue coating provides valuable information about the state of the bodily fluids. It indicates retention of undigested food matter, excessive amounts of phlegm and dampness and the degree of heat or coldness in the digestive organs. It also indicates the strength and depth of pathological causes and conditions.

Tongue coating indicates Ama, the by-products of indigestion, an indication that the bodily humors are accumulating.

Constitutional Color Signs

Vata - a brown or black tongue coating more pronounced at the back.

Pitta - a yellowish tongue coating.

Kapha - a white tongue coating often with a layer of mucus on top of it.

Absence of tongue coating shows a Nirama condition.

White thick tongue coating shows accumulation of Ama.

Yellowish, thick or greasy coating shows inflammation due to the fermentation of the Ama.

Black tongue coating may occur after a febrile disease owing to burning out of the body fluids.

Tongue Coating Indicator Check List

Things to look for when checking the tongue coating:

- coating with or without root
- presence or absence of coating
- coating thickness
- coating distribution
- coating moisture
- moldy or greasy coatings

Tongue Coating Vikruti Constitutional Indicators:

- Externally contracted disorders in the early phase - the tongue coating assumes major significance.
- Internally generated chronic disorders - the coating is of secondary importance relative to tongue body color and shape.
- Indicates the deficiency or excess quality of a present imbalance.
- Indicates a quick change, as a result of treatment or pathological process.
- Indicates the present state of health of the internal Pitta digestive organs, especially the stomach.
- Absence of coating indicates deficiency.
- Thick coating indicates excess.
- A greasy, slippery, or sticky coating indicates the presence of phlegm or a damp-wet condition.
- Indicates the heating or cooling characteristics of a condition: white means cooling, yellow means heating.

Tongue Moisture

A healthy tongue coating will be slightly moist, indicating a good supply and movement of the bodily fluids. Coating moisture provides an indication of the state of those fluids. If the coating is excessively moist, it indicates excessive fluids or stagnation of fluids. This is caused by a Kapha excess or an Agni deficiency. If, however, the coating is dry, it indicates that the fluids are insufficient causing a Vata imbalance.

The examination and evaluation of the tongue moisture provides an indication of the status of the body's fluids. In terms of differentiation, tongue moisture reflects the relative state of the twenty attributes such as hot/cold, dry/wet, etc.

Vata - a dry, coated tongue that is cracked indicates a nerve disorder.

Pitta - a moist tongue in Sama conditions but a red and dry tongue in Nirama conditions.

Kapha - a moist or wet tongue with possible mucus and excess salivation, frothy or foamy salvia or bubbles, indicates Kapha and weakness of the lungs.

A slightly moist tongue indicates a healthy and vibrant individual.

A moist tongue indicates the accumulation of fluids, phlegm or Ama in the system.

A dry tongue indicates dehydration or fever and insufficiency of body fluids.

An extremely wet tongue indicates the accumulation of body fluids.

Wet Coating

A wet coating is an indicator of some of the following:

- Kapha imbalance
- Pitta or Agni imbalance
- A wet, slippery, oily coating indicates low Agni

Dry Coating

A dry coating is an indicator of some of the following:

- An yellow coating on the tongue is an indicator of excess Fire
- A deficiency of Water element in the kidneys

9.19 Prakruti: Tongue Body Color Chart

Body Color	Significant Indicator
Pale	Slightly dry: Blood deficiency Wet: Pitta or Agni low
Pale, Bright and Shiny	Prana and blood deficiency, particularly of stomach and spleen organs
Red	With coating: excess heat in the blood Without coating: Kapha deficiency with Agni
Red and Wet	Heat with retention of dampness
Red and Dry	With coating: heat from excess burning body fluids Without coating: deficiency heat and exhaustion of body fluids
Red and Shiny	Kapha indicator- kidney and stomach imbalance
Red and Scarlet	Heart or nutrient deficiency
Red with Red Points or Spots	Heat in some areas and with some blood stagnation
Red with Prickles	Heat in the nutritive level or in the Vata or Pitta Area
Red with a Purple spot in Center	Blood stagnation and heat in stomach
Red and Peeled	Heat from stomach and kidney deficiency
Dark Red with a Dry Center	Stomach fire excess or stomach deficiency with heat
Reddish Purple	Heat and blood stagnation
Reddish Purple and Distended	Extreme heat with blood stagnation and toxin from alcohol injuring the heart
Bluish Purple	Blood stagnation from internal cold
Bluish Purple and Moist	Blood stagnation from internal cold stiffening the tendons and bones
Bluish	Severe internal cold with blood stagnation
Bluish Color with Coating	Severe internal cold with stagnation and exhaustion of blood; low stamina and vital energy

Body Color	Significant Indicator
Bluish Color in Central Surface	Pitta, Agni and spleen deficiency with retention of phlegm in chest
Bluish Color in a Pregnant Woman	Danger of a possible miscarriage
Distended Veins on the Underside of Tongue	Deficiency and stagnation of Prana If veins also dark: blood stagnation

9.20 Prakruti: Tongue Body Shape Chart

Body Shape	Significant Indicator
Thin	Kapha is low and deficient blood (tongue pale body color) Kapha is low (tongue red body color)
Swollen	Spleen and/ or kidney disturbance and und under active with wetness Agni is low, Kapha is high in stomach and spleen Heart and stomach have excess heat (tongue red body color) Alcohol toxicity (tongue red body) Toxin
Swollen Edges	Vata - Spleen imbalance
Swollen Sides	Pitta and liver imbalance
Swollen Tip	Pitta high and heart disturbance (tongue red body color)
Swollen between Tip and Center	Vata - Lung imbalance with retention of phlegm
Swollen along Central Crack	Pitta high with heart pressure (tongue red body color) Vata - heart imbalance (normal tongue body color)
Half Swollen	Nadi and srota channels are weak
Partly Swollen on Side	Vata is high with stagnation in the chest
Half Surface Swollen	Vata is high and lung disorders
Hammer Shaped	Stomach, spleen and kidney deficiency

Body Shape	Significant Indicator
Stiff	Exterior heat invading Pericardium (tongue red or dark red body color) Heat injuring body fluids (tongue red body color) Heart has excess fire
Flaccid	Vata disturbed and poor blood quality (tongue pale body color) Extreme Pitta injuring body fluids (tongue red body color) Kapha - kidney imbalance with high Pitta (tongue deep red body color)
Long	Pitta, Agni high with heart disturbance Phlegm - fire in heart
Short	Pitta - spleen disturbance, internal cold and sluggishness (tongue pale body color) Pitta high with insufficiency of body fluids due to excess heat (tongue red body with coating)

9.21 Vikruti: Tongue Coating Chart

Coating Color	Significant Indicator
White or White and Thin	Kapha- cold and/ or wet in the exterior region
White, Thin and Slippery	Kapha- cold and damp in the exterior
White, Thick and Slippery	Pitta zone is sluggish low Agni and high Ama; toxic buildup; cold, slow digestion especially in the stomach
White, Thin and Dry	Blood disturbances (tongue body color pale) Pitta sluggish and low Agni (tongue body color is pale) Lung fluids injured (tongue body color is normal) Exterior region is dry (tongue body color is normal)
White, Thick and Wet	Agni is low, Ama is high Exterior region is cold (body color normal) Pitta zone - interior region is cold and damp (tongue body color normal)
White, Thick and Dry	Interior region is hot with dirty fluids

Vikruti: Tongue Coating Chart (cont'd)

Coating Color	Significant Indicator
White, Thick and Greasy	Ama is high and Pitta is low with wetness and sluggish digestive system
White, Thick, Greasy and Slippery	Ama is high, Pitta and spleen is low and under active with coldness and wet phlegm
White, Thick, Greasy and Dry	Ama is high, exhaustion of body fluids due to excess dampness and heat
White, Rough and Cracked	Vata injured due to excess heat
White, Sticky and Greasy	Ama buildup, Pitta region is wet with phlegm; exterior region is wet and damp effecting Vata
White like Powder	Exterior region has excess heat (tongue body color is slightly red on tip or sides) Interior region has toxic buildup (tongue body color is red or dark red) Excess heat in all three regions
White like Snow	Ama is high, Pitta region and spleen are exhausted and under active with cold and wetness
White and Moldy	Ama is high, Kapha, stomach and kidney disturbances; interior is wet with toxins
Half-White and Slippery	Right side: pathogenic factor half-exterior, half interior Left side: heat imbalance in the liver
Yellow or Pale Yellow	Pitta region is wet and heat in the chest
Yellow and Slippery	Wet and heat throughout the body
Dirty Yellow	Kapha & Pitta organs stomach and small intestines are wet with heat
Yellow, Sticky and Greasy	Excess heat and phlegm disturbances throughout the body
Dry Yellow	Excess heat injured fluids, damaging internal organs
Yellow Root, White Tip	Exterior region pathogenic factor changing into heat and penetrating to the interior region
Bilateral Yellow Strips (remainder white)	Exterior region pathogenic factor penetrating to the interior region Excess heat in the stomach and intestines

Vikruti: Tongue Coating Chart (cont'd)

Coating Color	Significant Indicator
Bilateral Yellow Strips (remainder yellow)	Excess heat in the liver and gallbladder
Half-Yellow, Half-White (longitudinally)	Excess heat in the liver and gallbladder
Gray, Wet and Slippery	Ama is high, wet and sluggish spleen
Gray and Dry	Excess heat throughout the body
Black or Black, Slippery and Greasy	Ama is very high, cold in the stomach and intestines are cold and wet

9.22 Imbalance Between Tip; and Root and Left and Right Sides

	Tip-Root	Left-Right
Body Color	Tip and root of different color: stagnation of Prana or blood flow	Different coloration on left and right: stagnation of Prana
Body Shape	A) Whole tongue swollen; tip even more swollen: a long-term imbalance, B) Only tip swollen: overwork	Only one side swollen, with red points: malnourishment
Coating		Yellow coating on one side only: A) phlegm in the chest B) gallbladder heat imbalance affecting the stomach area
Moisture	Tip red & dry, root dirty & swollen; defective transformation of bodily fluids	One side wetter: movement of fluids in the chest; Lung disturbance

9.23 Digestive Fire and Efficiency

Appetite	Tongue	Condition
Strong	Clear	In general, healthy, ready to build or maintain-strong Agni
Strong	Coated	Digestive fire is fairly strong has some Agni, the digestive efficiency is probably foundering, possible causes is overeating or eating unhealthy food-combinations, not digesting well, the GI tract needs some support and attention
Weak	Clear	Need to build digestive fire
Weak	Coated	Need to eat more lightly, build digestive fire, and clean out GI tract, lots of Ama accumulation
Variable	Either coated or clear	Some Ama buildup, needs to develop a regular digestive fire

Tongue Diagnosis Signs

Channels of Flow or Srotas

In Ayurveda, channels throughout the body nourish the tissue with nutrients or remove waste products. When these channels flow unencumbered, all is in harmony. Problems arise when these channels are blocked, or there is an excessive flow, decreased flow, knotted or flow out into wrong channel. There are a total of 16 channels. The first three are: the Prana channel (Pranavah Srotas), food channel (Annavah) and water channel (Ambhuvah). These three are connected with nutritional intake and the environment. The next seven channels are: Rasa (Rasavah), blood (Raktavah), muscle (Mamsavah), fat (Medavaha), bone (Asthivah), marrow (Majjavaha) and reproductive (Shukravah).

The next three are the connection to the external world. They are: sweat (Svedavaha), feces (Purishavaha) and urine (Mutravah). Two additional channels are for females: menstruation (Artavavaha) and breast milk (Stanyavaha). The last, and one of the most important channels, is the Manovaha Shrotas. This channel connects to the nervous system and reproductive system.

Tongue Diagnosis

In Vata derangement, the tongue will be cold, rough and furrowed. In Pitta, it will be red or yellow. In Kapha, it will be pale and sticky. In depletion of Tridoshas, the tongue will be dark with the papillae raised and dry.

9.18 The Healthy Tongue

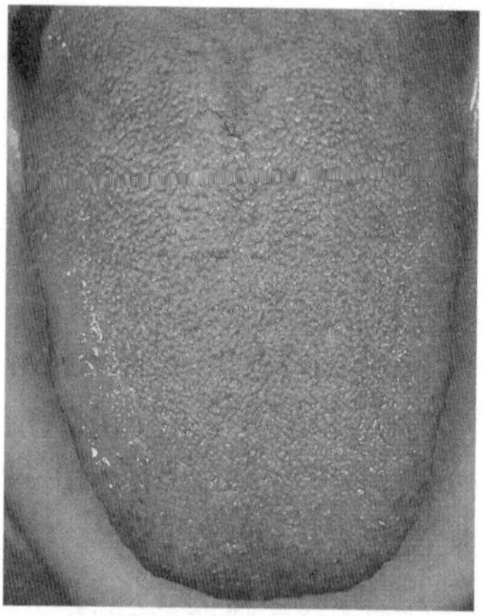

Prior to an examination, it is important not to eat or drink anything that will discolor the tongue and give a misleading impression to the practitioner.

9.24 The Unhealthy Tongue

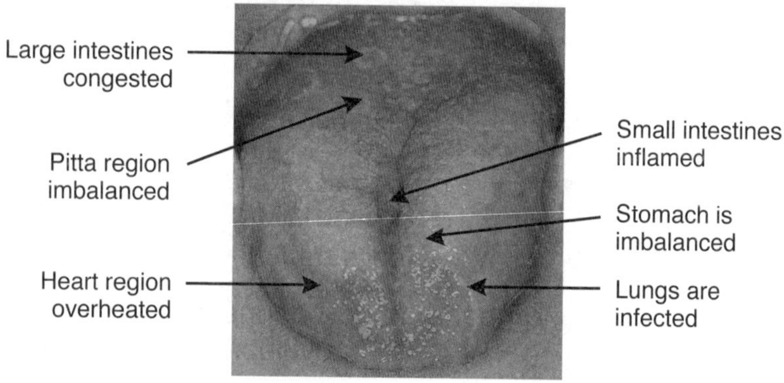

There are numerous colors, signs and markings that tell us that there may be imbalances and tendencies developing within the body.

Color of Tongue Body

Pale tongue: Indicating Pitta is low and/or blood deficiency.

Low Pitta could cause a hypothyroid condition or other metabolic deficiencies.

Blood deficiency may or may not be synonymous with anemia. In either case, there can be a lack of red blood cells, neurotransmitters, and/or hormones.

A vibrant pinkish-red tongue: Sign of a healthy tongue.

Slightly red tongue: See red tongue.

Red tongue: Internal heat or Pitta is high. Internal heat can be from one of two causes. It can be due to infection or illness that gives you a fever, or it can be due to a lack of Kapha in your body. Kapha is body fluids and they keep the body cool.

Purple tongue: Blood stagnation. Blood stagnation is poor blood circulation which can also cause prickly pain to be present. This can be due to local trauma after a long period of stress. Blood stagnation can also arrive after a period of blood deficiency in which case the tongue will be a very pale purple.

Observe the color of the tongue. Focus on the color of the tongue body, not the coating or shape, just the color of the tongue body.

9.25 Color of Tongue Body

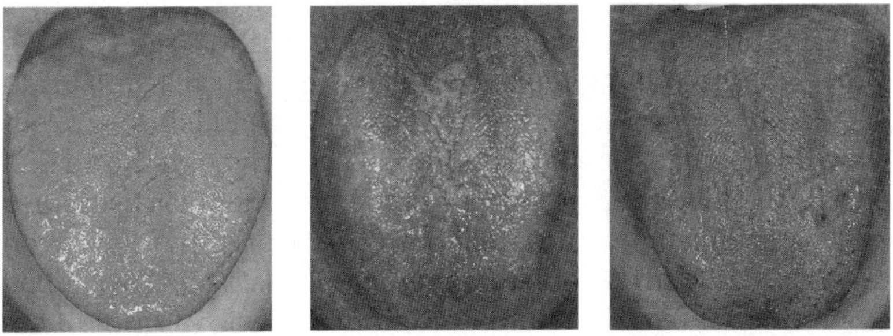

Pale white or pink | **Pinkish-red** | **Slightly reddish-purple**

Color of Tongue Coating

No coating indicates a Kapha imbalance. Kapha imbalance is due to a lack of fluids in the body. The tongue coating tells us about the fluids in your digestion specifically and, should there be no coating, we can assume that not only is there a deficiency of fluids in your stomach and intestines but elsewhere as well.

White coating: Normal or slightly cool and wet body environment.

Cool body environment: White tongue coating is thin, this is a normal sign. A thin white coating is defined as a white coating that is thick enough to see but thin enough to see through.

When the white coating is thick, this is cool body temperature indicator and occurs when either the energy of digestion is low or when the diet and foods being eaten are particularly difficult to digest.

Dirty white or light yellow coating: Cold internal temperature becoming hot.

Cold becoming hot occurs when a common cold is turning into a flu or a viral infection.

Yellow coating: Internal heat.

Internal heat occurs when you have a fever or metabolic functions are operating in some other state of hyperactivity.

Brown coating: Internal heat that is damaging the Kapha.

Internal heat damaging the Kapha occurs when a high fever, or other source of heat, cause a drying out of the internal tissues and organs.

9.26 Color of Tongue Coating

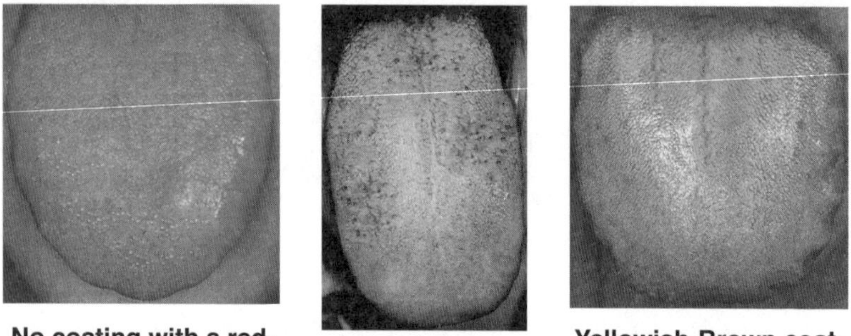

No coating with a reddish tongue body

Whitish-yellow coating

Yellowish-Brown coating

Thickness of Tongue Coating

No coating: Kapha deficiency or imbalance.

Kapha deficiency is a lack of fluids and / or cooling down in your body is taking place. When there is a lack of fluids in your stomach specifically, there is no warm fluid that arises to generate the tongue's coating.

Thin coating: A normal healthy sign or a slight Vata disturbance.

A normal healthy coating is what occurs when there are no other signs or symptoms of pathology.

Thick coating: accumulation of Kapha, wet, damp environment creating phlegm.

Dampness and phlegm indicates a fluid metabolism problem giving rise to any one of a number of moist, oozing or muggy pathologies.

Geographic coating: Stomach disturbance.

Stomach Kapha occurs if the fluids in the stomach and intestines become deficient causing symptoms such as heartburn, constipation and / or chronic hunger.

9.27 Thickness of Tongue Coating

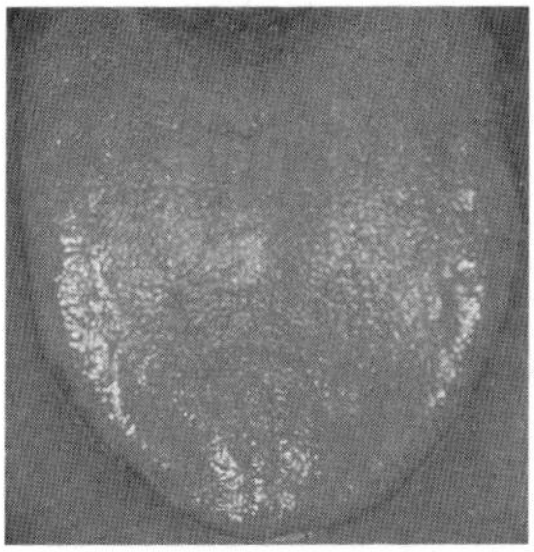

No coating

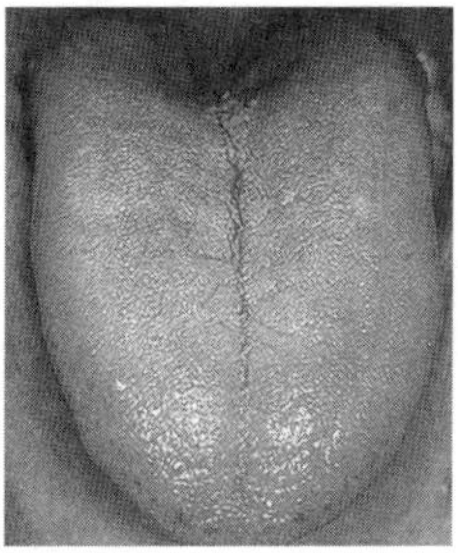

Thin coating

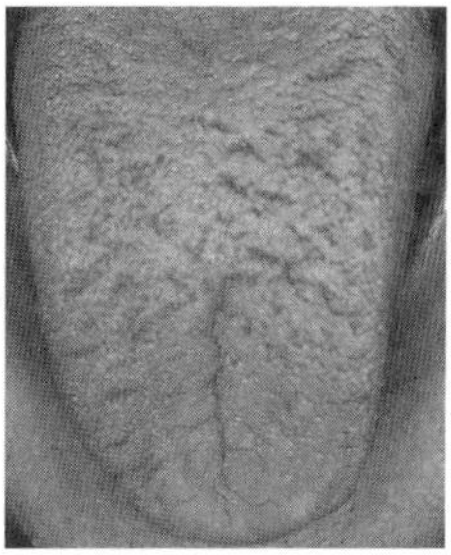

Thick coating

Location of Tongue Coating

Thin in front, thicker in back: Mucus and sluggish intestines.

Sludge is not an official Ayurvedic term, but it basically is sludge in the colon. Those who eat a lot of meat, fried foods or otherwise greasy, fatty, sweet, cold, dairy, develop this tongue indicator. Deep fried foods or cold ice cream build sludge quite quickly if the Agni is particularly low.

Damp heat in the Vata zone is another possible diagnosis associated with this tongue coating. Anything turbid, sticky, smelly or otherwise gross that comes out of the lower abdomen and digestive system is a sign of a sluggish digestive system. Indications from diarrhea to vaginal discharge are all possible symptoms.

Coating distributed over entire tongue: systemic wet phlegm.

Dampness is a wet damp pathology that arises from weak digestion or unhealthy diet. Phlegm can manifest as a foggy feeling, like heaviness in the limbs or a headache that feels heavy. Excess water or Kapha can clog up the channels giving rise to arthritis. Phlegm can accumulate and look like water in the body. Edema or water accumulations are good examples of systemic phlegm.

Phlegm occurs after dampness has had a chance to get thicker and stickier. Phlegm comes in two forms. Substantial phlegm is the substance that you cough up. Insubstantial phlegm can clog up your channels and give rise to neuropathies, forcing parts of your body to go numb. Menier's disease can be caused by excess phlegm.

Coating thicker in the Pitta region: occurs from phlegm and dampness in the central area of the digestive tract.

Dampness and phlegm indicate a fluid metabolism problem giving increase to any one of a number of pathologies indicated by moist, sticky and bodily discharges.

The Middle Pitta region reveals to us that the phlegm and dampness are limited in location to the digestive organs from which phlegm and dampness tend to arise. Key symptoms associated with this pathology include nausea, motion sickness, lack of appetite and weight gain.

9.28 Location of Tongue Coating

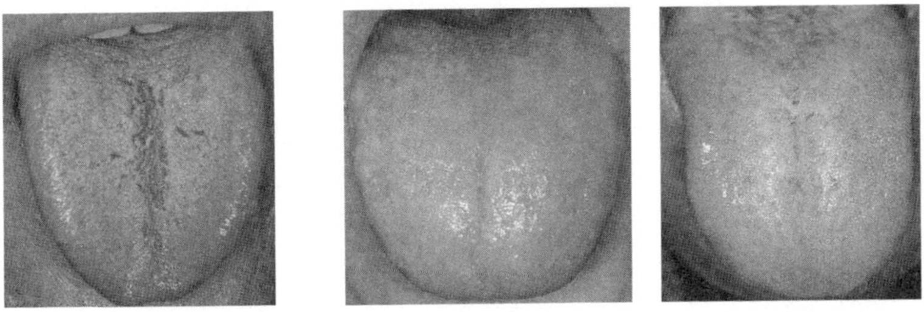

Evenly distributed everywhere | Thin in front, thick in back | Thicker in the middle, thin elsewhere

Cracks in Tongue Body

No cracks: Vata and Kapha are healthy.

Kapha is all of the substance of your body. There's substance and then there are all the functions. Kapha is substance. Pitta is metabolism function. We tend to deal typically with the fluid material. Once the fluids are working appropriately, they can give rise to denser things like organs and the skeletal system.

One crack down the middle: is an indication of Vata disturbance and a deficiency of Kapha in the stomach. Stomach Kapha disturbance occurs when there is a lack of fluids in the stomach or small intestines. If the crack extends to the tip of your tongue, your heart and lungs may be stressed. These tongue markings can develop from symptoms such as chronic hunger, constipation, heartburn, dry chronic cough and even insomnia. A crack down the middle of the tongue is an indication of a Vata nerve disorder. Numerous individuals have a crack down the middle of tongue indicating a wear and tear of the nervous system.

A few cracks: systemic Kapha deficiency and disturbed Vata.

Kapha deficiency and Vata disturbance indicates that there is a dryness going on in the body and the nervous system is depleted. Nourishing the Kapha and Vata of the body can successfully handle night sweats, hot flashes, bad temper, and restlessness and sleeping problems.

9.29 Cracks in Tongue Body

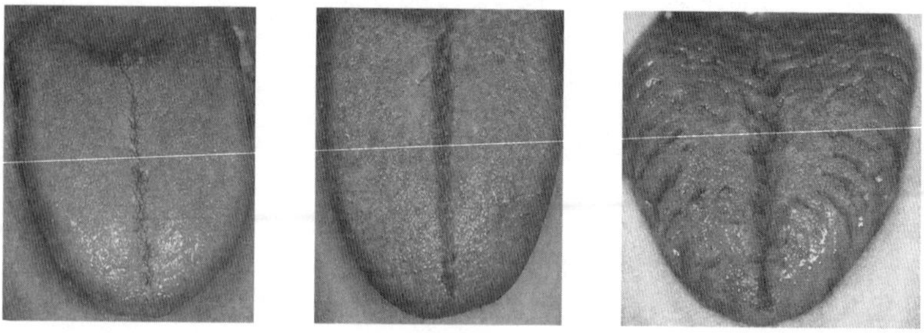

Slight crack | One crack in the middle | More than one crack

Teeth Marks around the sides of the Tongue

No teeth marks: Healthy sign.

Slight teeth marks: a Vata imbalance with an accumulation of stagnate energy.

Vata imbalance is how we describe nervous digestion or nervous indigestion. With a nerve disturbed digestion, there isn't much energy in the body to keep the digestive system calm. The tongue is a muscle, and when there isn't enough Vata in the body it loses its facility to retain its natural shape and takes on the grooves or notches of the teeth. Numerous complaints can occur from Vata imbalance such as headaches, migraines, clear emission fluid discharge, nausea, weight gain or loss and edema.

Heavy teeth marks: a Prana disorder or disturbance. Much the same problems as mentioned above, except more severe.

9.30 Teeth Marks Around the Sides of the Tongue

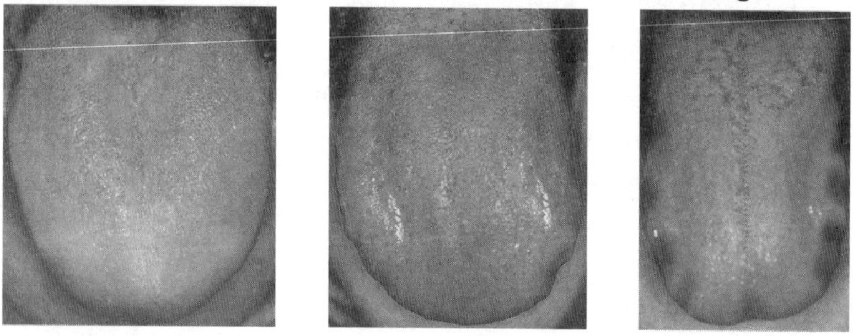

No teeth marks | Slight teeth marks | Heavy teeth marks

Spots on Tongue Body

No spots: A healthy sign.

Spots in the back of the tongue: disturbance in the Vata region.

Disturbance in the Vata region suggests that there is some sort of nerve disturbance or infection going on in the large intestines.

Spots on one or both sides: Liver imbalance.

Liver imbalance occurs when there's some sort of pain in the abdominal region, most likely connected with mood swings, irritability, red eyes or migraines. Liver disturbance may be the body working to move out some stagnant blood.

Spots evenly distributed: excessive or unbalanced heat in the body.

Excessive heat suggests an infection going on in the body, or some other cause of hyperfunction of the metabolism or other body system.

9.31 Spots on Tongue

* Spots can be white, pink, red or bluish-purple in color; they are usually raised and inflamed.

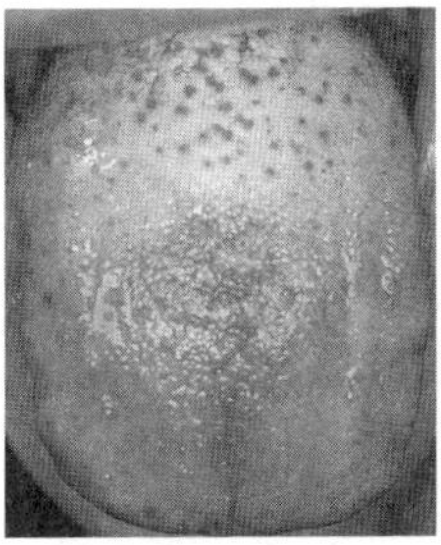

Spots in the back of the tongue

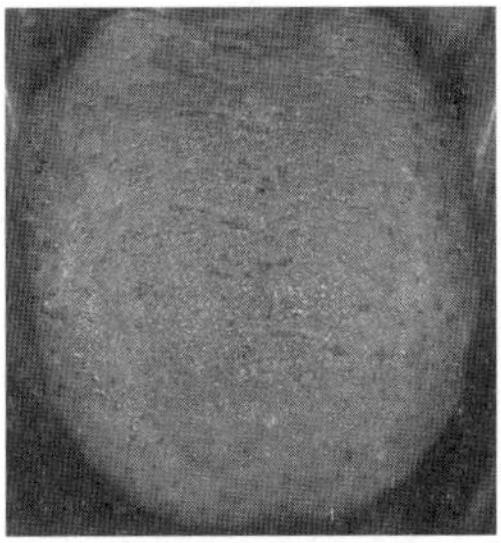

Spots on one or both sides

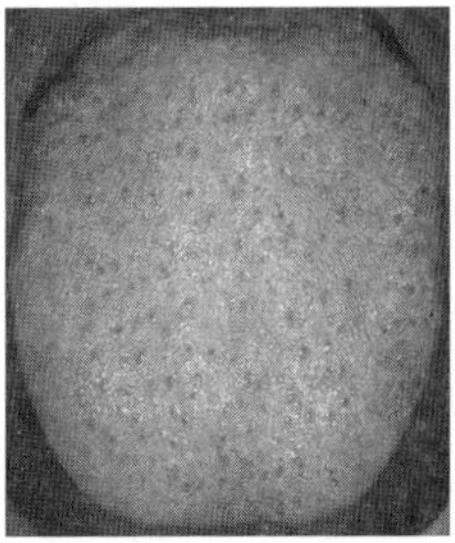

Spots evenly distributed through tongue

Sublingual Vein Extension on Underside of Tongue

Underside of Tongue Veins barely visible: Healthy, a good sign.

Veins extend less than 50%: Still a fairly good sign.

Veins extend more than 50% up tongue: Blood stagnation.

Blood stagnation occurs from unhealthy blood circulation with impurities and toxins. It can also cause prickly and stabbing pain. This is usually due to local trauma, as it can follow a long phase of nervous tension, anxiety or worry.

9.32 Sublingual Vein Extension on the Underside of Tongue

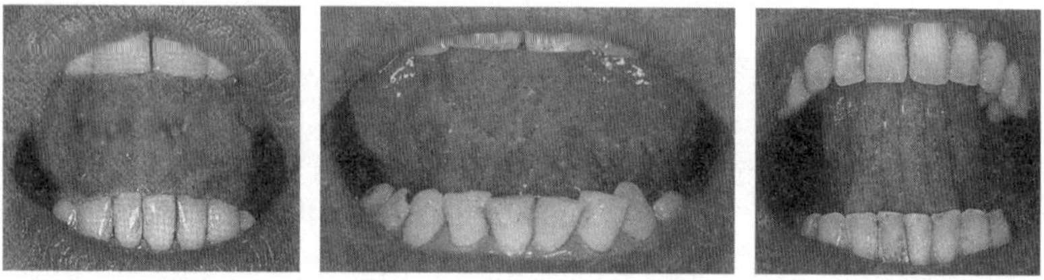

A healthy underside of tongue | **Veins extend half way up tongue or less** | **Veins extend more than half way up the tongue**

Tongue Diagnosis: An Overview

9.33 A 14-Point Checklist of Tongue Diagnosis

1. Tongue diagnosis is an external observation of internal processes.
2. To fully understand tongue diagnosis, knowledge of: The Five Elements, The Three Doshas, The Seven Dhatus, The Twenty Attributes, and The Six Tastes are necessary.
3. The tongue body and coating are affected mostly by short-term events and change constantly.
4. A normal tongue has a slight white coating and is a vibrant pinkish-red.
5. The shape is not as important as the coating.
6. The coating is a physiological by-product of the digestion of food and fluids depending on the digestive organs especially the spleen for transportation and the stomach for breaking down the food.

7. The tongue observation is a very precise indication of the source of the larger problem that the individual may be experiencing or have a tendency towards.
8. The most significant aspects of the tongue are the body color, shape and coating.
9. The external factors of food, juices, herbs and medication (if any) and self-care can also influence the tongue color and coating.
10. The center of the tongue indicates the most about the digestion history of the individual.
11. To understand the state of the heart, look way back at the tip of the tongue for redness.
12. If the tongue is very pale, it indicates a very high fever is imminent and the coating would be white.
13. The sides of the tongue are swollen, with crevices and red, indicating irritation on the extremities.
14. The tongue is a reddish purple especially around the tip, you question the individual further about his/her cardiac history.

Tongue: Related Tastes and Organs

According to Ayurveda, there are different regions that correspond to the six tastes and also to particular organs. There are also specialized taste buds on the tongue and, when we eat food, the Agni is awakened allowing us to experience its taste.

SWEET TASTE - corresponds to the tip of the tongue, which relates and activates the apical area of the lungs and the thyroid gland.

SOUR TASTE - corresponds to front sides of the tongue, which relates and activates the middle and lower lobes of the lungs.

SALTY TASTE - corresponds to the back sides of the tongue, which relates and activates the kidneys.

PUNGENT TASTE - corresponds to the middle frontal section of the tongue, which relates and activates the heart and stomach.

BITTER TASTE - corresponds to the middle back section of the tongue, which relates and activates the pancreas, spleen and liver.

ASTRINGENT TASTE - corresponds to the far back section of the tongue, which relates and activates the large intestines.

RELATION OF RASA TO TONGUE AND ORGANS - The taste buds have a direct connection to these various organs. This is the reason that there is an immediate reaction in the body right after eating a meal. For example, the moment you eat your meal, if you eat some bitter greens, your digestive organs, like the pancreas, spleen, and liver are stimulated through the taste buds. Another example is, the moment you eat something sour, a message is sent by the chemo-receptors in the lungs to create more bronchial secretions.

EXCESS OF TASTES DAMAGES
THE CORRESPONDING ORGANS

Excess of Sweet Taste - leads to obesity and sluggish, underactive thyroid.

Excess of Sour Taste - leads to pulmonary congestion.

Excess of Salty Taste - leads to water retention and weakened kidneys.

Excess of Pungent Taste - leads to burning sensations in the stomach and gastritis.

Excess of Bitter Tastes - leads to weakened pancreas, spleen and liver.

Excess of Astringent Tastes - leads to constipation in the large intestines.

9.34a Tastes and Their Related Organs

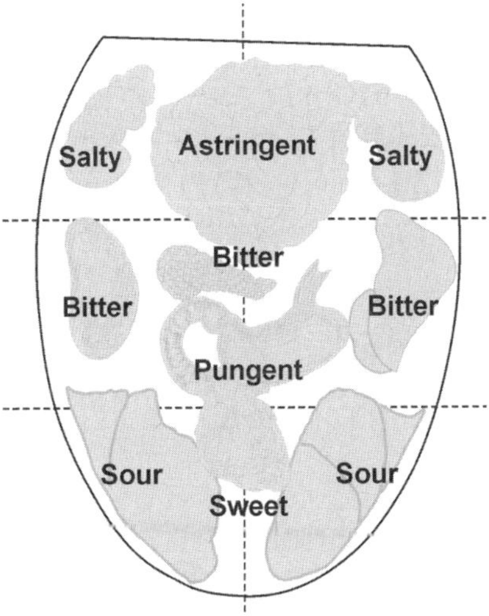

9.34b Tastes and Their Related Organs

Sweet	Thyroid and Upper Lungs
Sour	Lungs
Salty	Kidneys
Pungent	Stomach, Heart
Bitter	Pancreas, Spleen, Liver
Astringent	Large Intestines

The Seven Disease Tendencies

According to ancient Ayurveda, as explained by Edward F. Tarabilda, the Ayurvedic teacher and author of Ayurveda Revolutionized: Integrating Ancient & Modern Ayurveda, there is a theory that explains that disease can manifest through one of the seven tissues. This is fundamental in both preventing and treating disease. As stated in Ayurveda Revolutionized... "to isolate certain key attributes in relationship to the science of taste and diseases related to that taste. Thus, it is not enough to know if Vata is deranged; one must also know which attribute of Vata the primary one is causing the disease. For the purpose of Ayurveda is to be able to enhance our ability to prevent and treat disease with precision and effectiveness." The following Seven Disease Tendencies and Tongue Signs Chart shows which tissue corresponds to the disease tendencies along with the dosha and appropriate taste therapy. Hopefully this chart will aid in pinpointing where the imbalance may lie in the bodily tissues.

9.35 The Seven Disease Tendencies and Tongue Signs Chart

The Disease Tendency	Tissue	Dosha	Tongue Signs	Taste Therapy: Tastes to Avoid
Disease of Heat	Bone	Pitta	Red and at times swollen, particularly in the Pitta zone relating to the small intestines and heart. Also, the tongue may be dry and the individual, in severe cases, may experience thirst.	Pungent/ Fomentation
Disease of Coldness	Blood	Vata/ Kapha	Prominent papillae, tip is red and painful, white mucusy coating, teeth marks on the sides of the tongue, low Agni, cravings for sweets.	Salty/ Cooling
Disease of Lightness	Bone Marrow	Pitta	Due to excess Agni there may be very little or no coating. Tongue may appear red. An excessive appetite, poor digestion due to too much bile.	Bitter/ Lightening

The Disease Tendency	Tissue	Dosha	Tongue Signs	Taste Therapy
Disease of Heaviness	Adipose or Fat	Kapha	White coating on the tongue. Tongue may be swollen. Digestion will be slow. Sweet taste in the mouth, also cravings for sweets may lead to diabetes.	Sweet/ Nourishing
Disease of Dryness	Muscle	Vata	Dry, furrowed and red on margin. Difficulty sticking tongue out and it may be trembling. Tongue may appear slightly bluish or black color or furring.	Astringent/ Drying
Disease of Oiliness	Reproductive	Kapha	Strong metallic or slimy taste with an excess of salvia. There may be a contraction and a constant protrusion of the tongue.	Sour/ Oleation
Mixed Type of Disease	Lymph	Vata/Pitta/ Kapha	Dry, rough and hoarse with sore vocal cords. Speech difficulty due to trembling voice. Voice sounds weak and strained.	One or more of the above

The Six-Fold Therapeutics

The six major forms of therapy are mentioned in the ancient Charaka texts, these six therapies are as follows:

1) Bitter/Lightening Therapy- used to decrease body weight and purify the system. Pancha karma is seen as part of lightening therapy.
2) Sweet/Nourishing Therapy- used to increase body weight and nourish the system.

3) Drying Therapy- used to reduce body fat.
4) Sour/Oleation Therapy- used to promote unctuousness in the body.
5) Pungent/Fomentation Therapy- used to induce sweating.
6) Astringent Therapy- used to reduce the flow of fluids in the body.

9.36 Comparative Clinical Significance in Ayurveda, TCM and Western Medicine

Tongue Feature	Ayurveda	Chinese Medicine	Western Medicine
COLOR			
Pale	Low Prana	Deficiency of Chi & Blood	Anemia, Malnutrition
Red	High Pitta	Heat in Pericardium	Toxemia, Infectious disorders & Fevers
Purplish	High Pitta	High heat affecting Pericardium	Infections affecting: respiratory & circulatory systems
Bluish	Agni & Pitta out of balance, Kapha is high	Internal dampness & phlegm, cold liver & kidneys	Heart problems, respiratory & circulatory disorders
TONGUE BODY			
Contracted	Pitta & Agni disturbance	Heart-blood deficiency, internal heat affecting the tissues and muscles	Severe infections creating weakness and emaciation
Crooked	Vata high	Liver Wind	Stroke, or similar nerve damage, or over stimulation
Flaccid	Vata is high	Yin damage, Blood deficiency	Low thyroid, general fatigue, hypoglycemia
Smooth	Kapha is out of balance	Overeating, over consumption of Yin, Stomach Chi is exhausted	Malnutrition, anemia, atrophy of filiform and fungiform papillae

Tongue Feature	Ayurveda	Chinese Medicine	Western Medicine
TONGUE BODY			
Smooth	Kapha is out of balance	Overeating, over consumption of Yin, Stomach Chi is exhausted	Malnutrition, anemia, atrophy of filiform and fungiform papillae
Swollen	Kapha is high, Pitta is disturbed	Cold & heat dampness, phlegm over flowing	Edema, infections and congestions in the tissues
Protruding	Kapha is imbalance, Pitta is in oxcess	Phlegm, toxins & Heat in the heart	Fevers, toxemia
Trembling	Vata is high	Internal movement of Liver Wind	Often an indication of hyperthyroidism, poor health, & neurosis
Hyperactive	Pitta is high, Vata is disturbed	Excess or Weakness: heat in the Spleen & Heart	Can be a sign of anemia, exhaustion, or the after affect of a stroke or cerebral vascular accidents
TONGUE COATING			
White	Kapha is high	Febrile disorders	Early stages of febrile disorders; convalescence or chronic mild diseases
Yellowish-Orange	Pitta is high and out of balance	Excess heat affecting the whole digestive system	Constipation, Bacteria infectious disorders
Grayish dark color	Kapha is high with Agni imbalance	Febrile diseases, interior symptoms affecting internal organs	Acidity, dehydration, chronic digestive disorders
Black	Vata, Pitta & Kapha disturbed and out of balance	Interior- symptom complex; heat invading Blood level	Fungal infections, severe diseases at this stage

Tongue Feature	Ayurveda	Chinese Medicine	Western Medicine
CHARACTER			
Thin	Pitta is slightly high, Kapha is affected	Exterior symptom-complex in febrile disease	Mild pathogenic factors
Thick	Pitta is high, Kapha is high	Interior-symptom complex; excess heat, cold & phlegm	Pathogenic factors, affecting respiratory & digestive systems
Moist	Kapha is slightly high	Mild disorders that have not affected body fluids	Normal to excess salvia secretion
Dry	Pitta & Agni are high	High heat consuming body fluids	Dehydration, fevers, decreased salvia secretions
Greasy/ Slippery	Kapha is high	Dampness and disturbed Chi in Stomach, Spleen or Lungs	Sluggish digestion; unhealthy oral cleaning habits

A Tongue Diary

A Three-Day Tongue Journal

One of the best ways to learn about tongue diagnosis is through observation and study of your own tongue.

DAY ONE

1) Morning Observation - draw and describe
   Stick out your tongue, relax it and observe for these following qualities:

- Is it long or narrow?
- Wide or puffy?
- Does it have teeth, or rippled looking marks at the sides?
- Is the tongue pale or white?
- Is the tongue red or purple in color?

2) Late afternoon - draw and describe
Make a note of your level of energy or exhaustion in the afternoon.

- Does either the color or shape of your tongue change from morning to afternoon?
- Have the teeth marks changed in definition?

DAY TWO

1) Morning Observation - draw and describe
Observe the tongue coating before and after eating. Begin to be aware of what kinds of foods cause change in your tongue.

- Is the tongue the same shading and coloring as the previous day?
- Note the change on the tongue from morning, afternoon and before bed, how has it changed?
- What color is the coating: white, creamy, yellowish, grayish or black?
- How thick is the coating?
- Do you have lots of salvia or do you have a dry mouth?

2) Evening - draw and describe
During the evening, eat plenty of hot spicy, salty food. Note the changes of the tongue.

- How did it change?
- How different is the shading and coloring of the tongue?

DAY THREE

1) Morning Observation - draw and describe
Take notes on the color and coating of the tongue.

- Are there any other marks such as spots, grooves, bumps, cracks?
- Where are they located?

2) Before Bed Draw & Describe
Before bed, eat a bowl of fresh green vegetables, such as kale, collards, spinach or dandelion leaves without any seasoning or spices, or make some fresh green juice and drink it before bedtime.

- Does it change your tongue the next morning, if so, how is it different?
- What is the biggest difference that you see?

Acid-Alkaline pH Testing is another valuable tool to determine the state of one's digestive system and overall health. Please refer to pages 247-281 for complete information regarding testing your own pH levels.

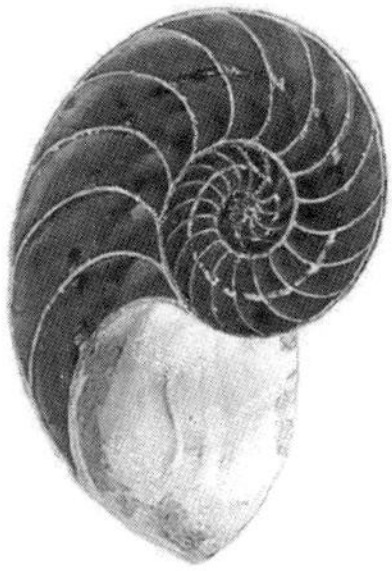

PART SIX

The Nourishment

10 Nourishing Wisdom

The Nourishment

We started our journey of exploring with the discovery of the type of seed you were born as. From there we discussed the terrain that the seed is growing in and how fertile it is to support and nourish the growing seed. Then we brought in the element of Fire, Agni, the spark that brings all life to flourish, without Fire there is no life. Then came the diagnosis, which brings in the seed, the terrain and the Fire all together so we can see the full picture.

The nourishment is the final stage of understanding tongue diagnosis. As mentioned earlier, tongue diagnosis conveys how well we are able to digest and assimilate the nourishment that comes to us through our senses. As long as our Prakruti seed is being nourished, our Vikruti terrain is fertile and our Agni fire is burning brightly and then our life will flourish.

This next section of the book is actually one of the most important. Now that you have found out who you are, the next question is "how do you stay healthy"? We bring in numerous skills and dietary wisdom from the ancient past of Ayurveda and we blend that in with modern nutritional medicine. Together we can begin to shape and put together a recipe of success in health.

In this chapter we will explore a variety of practices that we can incorporate into our lives, such as: eating and living habits, chewing, how to absorb the life force from food, food combining, fasting and purification processes, acid-alkaline balance and Rasayana Therapy.

Following this, we will continue exploring the six healing tastes in detail for physical, emotional, mental and spiritual well being. Then we conclude with what it means to incorporate a Sattvic approach to eating for a more vibrant and harmonious lifestyle.

The Six Stages of Digestions

"The person who always eats wholesome food enjoys a regular lifestyle, remains unattached to the objects of the senses, gives and forgives, loves truth, and serves others without disease."
— Vagbhata Sutrasthana

According to Ayurveda, there are six stages of digestion. It takes approximately six to eight hours for the digestive system to assimilate a meal. The six tastes each relate to one stage of the digestive process. Each taste nourishes the rasa tissue during its respective stage of digestion resulting in rasa tissue containing all six tastes. Within six to eight hours all six tastes enter plasma and lymph, the rasa tissue.

Phases of Digestion and the Doshas

Kapha Stage: predominant for the first 1-2 hours, nourishes all bodily Kapha

Pitta Stage: predominant for the next 2-3 hours, nourishes all bodily Pitta

Vata Stage: predominant for the final 2-3 hours, nourishes all bodily Vata

The Sweet Stage

The first hour of digestion is the sweet stage. This is when all of the tastes are present but the sweet taste is dominant. During this stage, Kapha secretions are released. The instant the food enters the stomach; the fundus of the stomach secretes gastric mucosal secretions. This is when the food is digested into smaller particulars allowing Agni to make contact with all food particles. During this digestive process, simple sugars are digested and released by the stomach for general circulation. This causes a rise in blood sugar. The elements of Earth and Water give a sense of satisfaction and fullness. The sweet taste of Kapha nourishes and gives a feeling of contentment.

The Sour Stage

The next stage of digestion is the sour stage. The food particles continue to get even smaller. During this stage the stomach feels lighter due to the increase of the Fire element. The food in the stomach becomes sour and lighter due to the secretion of hydrochloric acid, from the lesser curvature of the stomach, as well as other enzymes. The Kapha qualities that are present during this time help in protecting the stomach from these acids. Agni secretes sour taste into the rasa tissue. The hormone gastrin stimulates the release of pepsin, which is an enzyme that starts the digestive process of proteins. If there is an excess of sour taste in the body, it can aggravate any rashes, eczema and hives or itching. This is due to a build up in Pitta dosha.

The Salty Stage

The third stage of the digestive system is the salty stage. The elements present are Water and Fire. This stage occurs in the first section of the small intestine called the duodenum. When the pyloric value opens and food enters the duodenum, bile from the gallbladder and pancreatic enzymes mix with the food. The pancreatic secretions and bile are alkaline and the food coming from the previous stage in the stomach is sour, which is classified as acidic. The acid and alkali is salt and water. This action is causing the food to become salty. The salty taste has a buffering action, which assists the break down of protein and fats. The pancreatic juice releases numerous enzymes: amylase, lipase and trypsin. If there is low kidney function, swelling and edema can occur during this stage.

The Pungent Stage

The fourth stage, which is the pungent stage, occurs in the jejunum, which is the second part of the small intestines. The dominant elements during this stage are Air and Fire. The food during this stage becomes yellowish-brown due to the Fire component being present. The enzymes in this upper part of the jejunum have qualities that are hot, sharp and subtle. It also causes increased heat and circulation. The majority of assimilation occurs in the ileum and the large intestines, but the initial absorption of chyle occurs in the jejunum. If there is high Pitta, it can irritate skin rashes, bleeding disorders and hemorrhoids.

The Bitter Stage

The fifth stage is the bitter stage. This takes place in the longest and final portion of the small intestines. There is a continuing of the digestive process in the ileum where there is a presence of bile which is bitter in taste. The Air and Ether components of bitter taste create nearly all of the assimilation of food through the villi of the ileum wall. The presence of the Air element continues to stimulate and maintain peristalsis.

The Astringent Stage

The sixth stage of digestion occurs in the cecum. The cecum is a pouch that forms in the first portion of the large intestines. This is where the food becomes astringent and dry. The presence of the elements of Air and Ether support this drying up process. The liquid foodstuff becomes thicker, heavier and rougher and gives bulk to the stools. This final stage is necessary for the absorption of certain vitamins, minerals and water. This takes place in the ascending and transverse colon. The astringent stage stimulates mass peristalsis. This final stage is when true appetite returns and is due to the Air component of astringent taste stimulating Prana in the hunger center of the brain.

Final Stage

The timing and rhythm of the various tastes is not permanent. It will vary from person to person It will change according to time of day, time of year, time of life, and vary from one constitution to another.

The Six Stages of Digestion

10.1 The Six Stages of Digestion

Stage	Elements	Food Enters...	Digestive Juices & Action	Absorption of Food Stuff	Action	Timing	Tissues Nourished
Sweet Stage	Earth & Water	Mouth	Saliva	Simple Sugars	Promoting Energy & Content-ment	Within 6-8 hours	Plasma & Lymph
Sour Stage	Water & Fire	Stomach	Hydrochlo-ric Acid	Protein & Fats	Can exacerbate Pitta Conditions	Within 6-12 hours	Plasma, Lymph, & Blood
Salty Stage	Water & Fire	Duode-num	Alkali Pancreatic Secretions, Bile & Digestive Enzymes	Carbohy-drates, Proteins & Fats	Maintains water-electrolyte balance	5 days	Muscle & Adipose Tissue
Pungent Stage	Fire & Air	Jejunum	Intestinal Enzymes	Carbohy-drates, Pro-teins & Fats continue to be digested	Increases heat & circulation	After 5 days	Bone Tissue
Bitter Stage	Air & Ether	Ileum	Rapid Ab-sorption		Cools the body, calms Pitta symp-toms	After 7 days	Bone Marrow, Nervous & Connective Tissue
Ast-ringent Stage	Air & Earth	Cecum	Stimulating Peristalsis	Absorption of remaining minerals & liquids	Stimulating peristalsis & resulting in hunger	After 28 days	Repro-ductive Tissue

Process of the Digestive Phases

Food/Drinik - are Conveyed to Stomach by the "Life-Sustaining Air"

1) Approximately 1/2 hour after food intake, it is mixed by the "mixing phlegm"; the chime becomes sweet and moist, the Kapha in the entire body is increased.

2) Approximately 1/2 to 1 1/2 hours after food intake, the "digestive bile" is stirred by the "fire-accompanying air"; the chime becomes hot and sour; the Pitta and Fire Agni is increased.

3) Approximately 1 1/2 hours after food intake, the nutrient essence is separated from the excess matter by the "accompanying air"; the chime becomes bitter; the Vata in the whole body is increased.

10.2 The Determining and Energetic Factors of Food and Herbs

Taste Color Shape Texture Aroma Temperature/Season Size (Density/ Weight/ Buoyancy)
Air and Ether Foods Leafy greens and lettuce Cabbage family Bitter greens Nightshade family Most dry, compact legumes All dry, rough, old, stale foods Hollow vegetables with tiny seeds except for peppers, which are Fire/Air/Ether foods)
Fire Foods Sour and Pungent fruits and vegetables Warming spices Nuts, seeds and oily foods Pickles, vinegars and salty foods Sprouted whole grains Foods red in color All acidic foods and medicines
Earth & Water Foods Sweet, juicy fruits Salty and sweet watery vegetables Cool creamy foods Sticky, cooling foods

The Psychobiology of Chewing

- Chewing affects digestion and assimilation of nutrients.
- The way we chew affects our mood and our subjective experience of eating.
- Chewing is a learned process.

In a fascinating experiment, scientists deprived a group of test rats of the taste sensation. Another group was placed on a normal rat diet. Within a short period of time the taste-deprived rats all died and when they were autopsied the scientists could find only one cause of death, clinical malnutrition. The scientist came up with only one explanation - that there are important, yet unknown physiological connection between taste and health. What this means is that to be fully nourished by food we must experience it through tasting and chewing. Likewise, to be fully nourished by any experience in life, we must taste and chew it thoroughly.

The mouth is the first part of the digestive process. This is where the chemical digestion of carbohydrates is initiated. Enzymes then break down the carbohydrate molecules if the mouth is well salivated. The mechanical digestion of food is also commenced in the mouth with the process of chewing. The surface area increases as the food is broken down into smaller and smaller pieces. When the food reaches the stomach, the number of molecules exposed to the stomach's acid and enzymatic environment is maximized.

The following is the simple "Row, Row, Row Your Boat" melody with words to remind us to "Chew, chew, chew" our food.

Chew, chew, chew, your food,
Gently through the meal
The more you chew,
The less you eat,
The better you will feel!

Ayurvedic Dietary Suggestions

10.3 Constitutional Treatment Principles

	Vata	Pitta	Kapha
Tastes to Reduce Dosha	Sweet, Sour, Salty	Astringent, Bitter, Sweet	Bitter, Pungent, Astringent
Seat or Home Base	Large Colon	Small Intestines	Lungs/Stomach
Main Therapy	Oil Enemas	Purgatives, Laxatives	Emetics
Therapeutic Herbal Properties	Carminatives Adaptogens Warming Nutritives Nervines Demulcents Moistening-Tonics Antispasmodic Diaphoretics	Cooling: Alteratives Diaphoretics Astringents Hemostatics Febrifuges Antipyretics	Warming: Carminatives Diaphoretics Stimulants Expectorants Astringents
General Therapeutic Food Properties	Sprouted Whole Grains Sweet-Sour Fruits & Berries Sea Vegetables	Moist, Cool & Sweet foods, Fruits & Raw Honey, Leafy Greens & Bitters	Pungent-Spicy foods; Bitter, Astringent and Drying foods

Eating Behavior for Healthy Digestion

"Without proper diet, medicine is of no use. With proper diet, medicine is of no need."
— Ancient Ayurvedic proverb

Fundamentals of Healthy Eating

How we digest and assimilate our food is just as important as what we eat. If digestion is disturbed, even the best diet will not provide proper nutrition. The following points include a variety of recommendations to aid in the most complete digestion of food.

- Eat according to your hunger level.
- Eat at approximately the same time every day.

- Do not overeat. Eat to about 2/3 to 3/4 capacity.
- Food needs to be warm (ideally eaten fresh or warmed to body temperature).
- Food needs to be tasty and easy to digest.
- Foods need to work together and not contradict one another in their actions.
- Allow 3 - 6 hours between meals.
- Eat a balanced meal with all six tastes.
- Chew the food well. Digestion starts in the mouth.
- Eat fresh foods freshly prepared.
- Fresh fruit and vegetable juices are recommended as part of your daily diet.
- Eat organic food whenever possible. Ayurveda recommends a vegetarian diet as ideal but if you have been eating meat for many years the transition should be made gradually with great attention placed on having a balanced diet and variety.
- Eat sitting down and in a settled environment. Sip warm or room temperature liquids or teas between meals. This enlivens digestion and helps the food be better dissolved and absorbed. Sit comfortably for five to ten minutes after finishing the meal. This allows the digestive process to get well underway. If you immediately jump up from the meal, digestion will be disrupted and the food will be improperly processed.

Avoid

- Using a microwave as it can aggravate Vata in the food.
- Ice-cold liquids and foods with a meal as they suppress digestion.
- Snacks containing refined sugar. Instead have sweet juicy berries and fruits, soaked dried fruits, nuts and seeds, spices, and other wholesome foods.
- Leftovers.
- Reading, watching TV, using the computer or driving a car while eating.
- Leaving the table very hungry or very full.
- Eating before the previous meal is properly digested.

- Artificial foods, colors and preservatives.
- Genetically engineered or genetically modified food.
- Eating too quickly or too slowly.
- Eating when not hungry and do not delay eating when hungry.
- Carbonated beverages, they aggravate Vata as they are filled with air and destroy the foundation of Ojas.
- Cold foods. Cold food depresses digestion and clogs the physiology.
- Caffeine. Caffeine is very aggravating to Vata and Pitta and can significantly imbalance the physiology with overuse.
- Honey should not be heated in any way such as by cooking, baking or by adding it to hot beverages. Ayurvedic theory says that when heated honey is ingested it creates a toxic effect in the body. It can be added to herbal tea once the beverage has cooled down to body temperature.
- Mental and emotional temperament should be relaxed and pleasant.

10 Essential Points for Determining Healthy Foods

1) Constitution of the individual
2) Nature of the food
3) Method of food processing
4) Food combination
5) Quality of food
6) Climatic environment
7) Season and time of day
8) Age of the individual
9) State of mind of the individual
10) Principles of proper food intake

10 Principles of Healthy Food Intake

The following principles are stated almost word for word in the Caraka Samhita, in the chapter entitled Vimanasthana, section 1:24.

1) Food should be eaten when it is warm.

2) Food should be unctuous (moist and oily).

3) Food should be taken in proper quantity.

4) Food should be started only if the previous meal is completely digested.

5) Foods taken at the same meal should not have strongly opposite potencies.

6) Meals should be taken in a quiet, comfortable room that is used only for dining, equipped with proper serving and eating utensils.

7) Food should not be taken too quickly.

8) Food should not be taken too slowly.

9) Food should be taken with full concentration; there should not be excessive talking, laughing or emotion during meals.

10) One should take food in a prescribed manner with regard for one's specific needs.

Life Force in Food

The following is the hierarchy of food preparation starting at the top with no preparation, which leaves the food with its full nutrient content, and ending at the bottom with the most processing, rendering the food lifeless with little or no nutrient value retained. The way we determine the life force of food is by how the elements and the three vital essences, Prana, Tejas and Ojas integrate and remain intact. The question to ask is, "Have the elements and the vital essences been denatured?"

Prana - Has the life force of the element of Air, oxygen, been denatured?

Tejas - Has the fire force of the element of Fire, enzymes, been denatured?

Ojas - Has the lubricating nectar of the element of Water, fluid essence, been denatured?

Whole, Fresh, Sun-Ripened, Enzyme-Rich, Organic, Alkalinent Foods

- Consumed immediately because once the skin of fruits or vegetables is broken, Prana (life-force) oxygen combines with the enzymes and the decaying process begins this process is called oxidation.

Dehydrated or Dried

- Loses 2-5% of nutrient value
- Dried without chemicals or additives
- Commercial brands of dried fruit contain sulfur-dioxide; exception: raisins

Frozen

- Freshly picked and frozen immediately
- Loses 5-30% of nutrient value (use within 3-6 months, preferably within one year, before the next year crop is ready)

Steamed

- Loses 15 - 60% of nutrient value
- Steamed means the green bean is still a bit crispy (if it's limp, it's cooked). The longer the cooking time and the higher the temperature the more lose in life-enhancing qualities and nutrients.

Cooked (High Temperatures over 118 for 30 minutes)

- Baked, broiled, boiled, grilled, steamed too long, home canned
- The green bean is limp
- Loses 40 -100% of nutrient value, depending on how hot and how long it is cooked

Cooked Leftovers Microwaved

- Loses 90 - 100% of nutrient value

Commercially Canned Foods, Fried Foods and Foods with Additives

- These not only lose 100% of their nutrient value, but have toxins added to them

Six Types of Ayurvedic Nutritional Imbalances

1. Quantitative deficiency. This includes under-nutrition due to insufficient food.
2. Quantitative excess. This includes excessive amounts of any food and even water if taken in excess at the wrong time, or not appropriate for that person's constitution.
3. Qualitative deficiency. This includes wrong food combination, which results in malnutrition, toxic condition and lack of essential nutrients.
4. Qualitative excess. This includes emotional overeating of rich or high fat foods that can result in obesity and/or high cholesterol and promote hypertension, coronary vessel disease and stroke.
5. Ama-producing. Certain foods and food combinations lead to toxemia and to certain digestive disorders.
6. Prakruti. Foods not appropriate for one's constitution may reduce immunity and cause disease. These six factors are closely correlated with the strength of Agni (the gastric fire).

Ayurvedic Concepts of Food Combining

Food Combining

To create the most efficient digestive system and to be able to get the most nourishment, food combining is important. Part of creating a healthy protocol necessitates that we follow a few dietary guidelines.

The order in which we eat different classes of foods, how we combine them, and the amounts we consume will determine how well we digest and assimilate our vital nutrients. The better we digest and assimilate our foods, the less likely we are to form toxic substances, accumulate excess fat and crave unhealthy foods.

Within the various dietary approaches of both conventional and alternative medical nutrition, there is a great deal of controversy concerning food combining. This has led to a growing uncertainty among consumers as to which, if any, foods are best taken together or separately.

Ayurveda offers a rational and scientific approach for determining correct diet that is based upon an individual's constitution. Vata, Pitta and Kapha are the energies from which human beings are constituted. This energetic constitution is the basis of determining which foods are best for maintaining physiological balance for a given individual. This approach is quite different from the conventional view of a balanced diet that exhorts us, despite individual differences, to eat from the same basic food groups and nutrient pool. Ayurvedic wisdom takes into consideration one's individual constitution and such factors as age, sex, race, climate, digestive capacity, stress, immune status, strength, illness, emotions and adaptability.

According to Ayurveda, every food has its own taste (rasa), a heating or cooling energy (Virya) and post-digestive effect (Vipaka). When two or three different food substances of different taste, energy and post-digestive effect are combined together Agni (Fire), can become overloaded, inhibiting the enzyme system and resulting in production of toxins in the system. While it is true that an individual's Agni largely determines how well or poorly food is digested, food combinations are also of great importance. When foods (proteins, carbohydrates and fats) having different attributes, tastes, heating or cooling properties and post-digestive effects are eaten together, Agni will be slowed down. The foods can then remain in the stomach for seven to eight hours. These same foods, if eaten separately, might well stimulate Agni, be digested more quickly, and even help to burn Ama. Thus, according to Ayurveda, one should eat according to one's constitution and take fruits, carbohydrates, proteins and fats separately at different times of the day. Combining foods improperly can produce indigestion, fermentation, putrefaction and gas formation. This condition, if prolonged, can lead to toxemia and disease complex. For example, eating bananas with a protein food can diminish Agni and change the intestinal flora, producing toxins and possibly causing sinus congestion, cold, cough and allergies.

Ayurveda emphasizes that food should not be improperly combined because of early observations that certain combinations of foods caused many physical and mental problems.

These problems include: excess intestinal gas, constipation, diarrhea, abdominal pain, urinary retention, digestive fermentation, lethargy, sleep disorders, depression, anxiety, a confused mind, and ultimately—a decrease in the function of the entire physiology. These were the direct observations made by the ancient Indian physicians. Today we know that different classes of food require their own specific digestive enzymes. This may seem like an obvious fact to anyone who has taken high school biology, yet as a society we seem to have missed the vitally important implication of this fact. By consuming many different types of food at a single meal we place a demand on our digestive glands to manufacture and secrete many different digestive enzymes simultaneously.

The principles of Ayurvedic food combining are derived from written information left to us by Indian physicians living 100 A.D. The basic difference from how we eat today is that they only ate two or three kinds of foods at any one meal. We tend to have at least six or seven (if not more) types of food at most meals. Foods should not be too fancy. Gourmet foods with rich, refined sweet tastes will influence even the most strong-willed, health-conscious person to overindulge. Foods should be simple and naturally delicious. For thousands of years, mankind has prepared natural and unprocessed foods in simple ways. It is these foods that our physiology needs in order to flourish. For those of us who have become stressed or gained weight, returning to a more simple dietary style is the key to health and weight loss. It is also the best way to maintain health. Remember, eating only a few kinds of foods at each meal will not result in nutrient deficiencies if you eat a variety of foods based on what is in season in the country in which you live. A true Ayurvedic approach to eating will give anyone a sufficient variety of healthy, nutrient-rich foods for an entire lifetime.

Ayurvedic Food Combining Principles

- Avoid taking seed or nut milks or yogurts with sour or citrus fruits; the only exception would be soaked or sprouted seeds or nuts.
- Fruits and grains or other starchy foods should not be eaten together because the sugar will not be properly digested. Fructose (fruit sugar), as well as other sugars, is digested quickly,

whereas starch takes quite some time to digest.

- Avoid eating melons and grains together. Melons digest quickly whereas starchy grains take more time. This combination will upset the stomach.
- Melons should be eaten alone.
- Honey should never be heated. Honey digests slowly when heated and the molecules become non-homogenized glue that adheres to mucous membranes and clogs subtle channels, producing toxins. Natural raw honey is nectar.
- Nuts or seeds and fruit should not be eaten together. The action of hydrochloric acid in the stomach causes the nut or seed milk to curdle. For this reason, Ayurveda advises against taking nuts and seeds with sour fruits.
- Cold beverages should not be consumed during or directly after a meal as it reduces Agni and digestion. Small sips of warm or tepid water taken during the meal serves to aid digestion.
- While eating, one should properly masticate the food in order to soften it and ensure that it is thoroughly mixed with saliva.

Sattvic Foods

Foods that are classified as Sattvic foods are abundant in Prana - the universal life force. The ancient criteria for foods to be classified as Sattvic were quite simple:

- Foods grown on healthy fertile soil
- Foods that are attractive in appearance
- Foods that are protected from animals

A few points to add to this list from a modern concern are:

- Foods should be grown without pesticides, herbicides, chemical fertilizers, hormones, irradiation or anything unnatural or denaturing.
- Foods should be whole, fresh and as unrefined as possible. Modern methods of processing, refinement and chemical additives, besides adding toxic substances to our foods, depletes foods of their Prana, life force, creating a food that is heavy, impotent and lifeless.

- All food that is denatured and flesh food can be classified as dead food. It's Prana, vital energy, leaves it at the instant of death and the inert material left behind is devoid of life- supporting energy. All dead food becomes tamasic: heavy, dull, stagnant, obstructing and destructive. Fresh foods retain their Prana longer and efficiently preserve and transfer their living energies to the human.

The seeds from all foods are a testament to this living energy. Given water and a little warmth they will germinate and grow. Choose organic foods with their seeds and they will retain their vital energy along with their taste, smell and appearance for days afterwards.

Sattvic Foods, Prana and Water

Most Sattvic foods contain a great deal of water. Food, in its fresh form, contains from 75% to 95% water. When we are born our body is 98% water, this is the Kapha stage of life. By our mid life we are 75% water, this is the Pitta stage of life; once we are elderly, during our Vata stage of life, we are 65% water. In the aging process we are drying up. As Dr. Robert Svobada has stated, by slowing down the dehydration process we slow the aging progression. By consuming Sattvic watery foods we are nourishing all of our tissues.

Energy comes from Prana, which is found in oxygen in all whole, fresh food. Prana is lost and unabsorbed through digestion if our digestion is impaired or our food is denatured, dead, canned, stale and old or over cooked at high temperatures. Oxygen is lost in all foods that are denatured. A lack of oxygen makes people weak. Food lacking in oxygen will not give strength or energy. Anti-oxidant foods deactivate free radicals allowing us to live longer, overcome illness and maintain more acute mental and muscular faculties. Anti-oxidant foods are fresh Sattvic foods.

A free radical substance is the opposite of an anti-oxidant food that prevents oxidation. A free radical is an electron-deficient molecule produced from oxygen and heated fat or oil in the body. In seeking to acquire another electron, a free radical is capable of combining with and destroying enzymes, amino acids and other cellular elements. For health and longevity, we want to minimize oxidation in the body due to free radical damage. A high oxidation means that electrons are being stolen from the body by cooked oils. Fresh live plant foods and fats deactivate free radicals by giving them electrons.

Within the body there is a balance between Prana - Air and Water, which is a balance between dryness and wetness within the body. Without the right amount of lubrication and hydration of the tissues, the Prana cannot be absorbed. Water is an essential means of transportation for the absorption of Prana. Along with the Prana in food, water is also absorbed into the body. The Prana mixes with the water of the mucus membrane and is absorbed to conduct the Prana. Prana energizes the whole body. This is one of the main reasons that people with a Kapha constitution have a better holding capacity for Prana-vital energy. Their bodies have the capacity to hold more water.

Water-Rich Food

Everything that you eat has to turn into liquid for the body to assimilate it. When you consume a piece of toast, your body has to use an amazing amount of energy to break it down, and in most cases does not accomplish the full assimilation. However, when you consume a piece of ripe juicy fruit such as a sweet peach or a leafy green vegetable, which is mainly water, your body digests it easily.

Water-rich foods are essential due to their ability to clean the body and maintain health as well. They are digested with ease and the water in them helps to flush impurities out of the system. If you do not consume enough water-rich foods, you will have to drink a great deal of water to compensate.

Plants have the natural ability to distill water. Water held in the plant's living cells is organically purified and can be obtained by juicing or eating watery fruits and vegetables, or by drinking sweet coconut water. The highest quality water can be found in fresh sun-ripened, organically grown fruits and vegetables. This is some of the purest water on the planet because the plant has filtered it through its root system. Water from a fresh plant is called structured or charged water. When our bodies are energized with the high quality charged water in organic foods, it will function efficiently and maintain health. Denatured foods will always tend to clog the body and create

Ama - toxins in the system.

Remember you are Water-electrified charged water.

Tongue Cleaning

The cleaning of the tongue first thing in the morning is like brushing your teeth, only it's even more important. This is a very essential practice that is recommended in Ayurvedic. A scraper is used to free the tongue of its coating; the scraper is made from gold, silver, or a twig. It is used to stimulate all the pranic nadis that terminate in the tongue. Cleaning the tongue will give you a very fresh feeling, cleans off the accumulation of gunk on the tongue, serves as the best prevention against bad breath, protects teeth from bacteria, and makes food taste better. The bonus is that you do not have to use as much toothpaste, which simply kills the mouth and throat flora, allowing those substances to reach the stomach and intestine. The final step is to gargle with cool water. During the winter season, warm water would be preferable.

Why Clean the Tongue?

Tongue cleaning has been a recommended practice in Ayurveda for over 5000 years. Cleaning the tongue is just a basic part of oral hygiene that the West has over looked. If you look at it for a moment, it makes total sense that you would want to clean this part of your anatomy daily.

Detxification

The body also uses the tongue as one of its detoxification paths, something you can attest to the morning after you eat a pint of ice cream. If you use a tongue cleaner you can easily remove this "gunk."

Decrease Bad Breath and Infections

80% of bad breath starts in the mouth, mainly on the tongue. The tongue harbors countless bacteria that can colonize to cause sore throats, or worse. Because of this, the tongue is one of the main sources of bad breath and other infections in the mouth and throat.

Use of a tongue cleaner helps remove this bacteria and the phlegm that they live in. Brushing the tongue to get rid of them does not work because it tends to just move them around or embed them in your brush.

Increasing Your Attractiveness

According to Ayurveda, the number one anti-aphrodisiac (social/sexual turn-off) is bad breath.

Increase Your Sense of Taste

As you peel off layers of bacteria and phlegm from your taste buds, you will be able to taste your food with more acuity and pleasure.

Activate Your Digestion

Rubbing the tongue with a tongue cleaner activates digestion; therefore, you will digest your food better when you clean your tongue.

Decrease Plaque and Oral Debris

The tongue is the main source of plaque and oral debris, so keep it clean.

Cleansing of the Tongue

Mouth/Tongue/Throat Cleaning Regimes

An important morning ritual in Ayurvedic practices is mouth and tongue hygiene. In ancient Ayurvedic times, twigs from various trees were used to clean teeth. Today, we prefer to use toothpaste. A note of interest regarding toothpaste is:

Sweet toothpaste for Vata
Bitter toothpaste for Pitta
Tangy toothpaste for Kapha

Tongue Scraping

First begin with tongue scraping.

Gargling Treatments

It is advisable to sit upright and to clear the mind of hurried and stressful thoughts when doing gargling treatments. The purpose of gargling is to stimulate and sooth the sense organs, freshen the breath and invigorate the mind. It is recommended to do this treatment every morning after brushing and tongue scraping.

Benefits: Gargling helps with loss of taste, bad breath, dullness of senses, dryness of face, exhaustion, anorexia, impaired sight, sore throat and most Kapha related disorders. An additional benefit is the effect of drawing out excess doshas through the eyes, ears, nose and mouth. For severe conditions, increase the oral retention time to two minutes or until the eyes and nose begin to ooze.

For Vata disorders, use heat-producing unctuous fluids. Caraway seeds, ashwagandha, sesame oil, cinnamon or eucalyptus oil.

For Pitta disorders, use sweet, cooling, pungent, and salty fluids. Fennel seeds, peppermint, turmeric, shatavari, blackberry essential oil.

For Kapha disorders, use heat-producing and drying fluids. Cardamom, neem, black pepper, guggulu, eucalyptus essential oil.

Salt Water Gargle - All body types

1/2 cup water

1 tsp. Rock salt or sea salt

1/4 tsp. turmeric powder

Bring water to a boil; then dissolve the sea salt and powder in it. Remove from heat, cover, and steep for 5 minutes. Use when the temperature is comfortable enough to retain in the mouth.

Gargling Procedures:

1. Place your gargling solution and hand towel next to the sink.
2. Allow your mind to become peaceful by sitting in a comfortable position.

3. Bring yourself to an upright, seated position with your back comfortably erect.
4. Fill your mouth two-thirds full with the gargling solution. Retain for 60 seconds.
5. Release the fluid from your mouth, then refill the mouth with the same quality of fluid and retain it for one to two minutes. Then release again.
6. Pour another measure of decoction into the mouth. Lean the head into a comfortable backwards position and gargle the fluid in the throat. Then release from the mouth.

Acid/Alkaline Balance

The understanding of acid and alkaline balance is beneficial with tongue diagnosis because acidity is easy to identify as coating on the tongue. When the tongue is coated with a thick layer of slimy whitish or yellowish film, this means over acidic condition in the body. This is particularly true with the stomach. We can take this further by doing a salvia pH test to determine acidity of the digestive system. The more acidic the salvia test shows, the more toxins are in the system. It is an excellent indicator showing that the person needs to do some purification and rejuvenation practices.

The terms acid and alkaline, when used in reference to food, refer to the pH (acid or alkaline) of the ash that results when the foods are burned. As your digestive system is a kind of fire, the inference is that alkaline ash equals alkaline in digestion and in its effect on your body, with similar comments applying to acid ash food. This result in a classification of foods into the categories: acid or alkaline.

Most live food diets are predominantly alkaline forming foods, although many fermented foods such as raw sauerkraut, seed cheese, raw pickles, etc., are acid forming. Sprouting and soaking reportedly reduces the acidity of seeds and nuts.

The idea behind using acid / alkaline as a guide is to balance the pH of your system. Excess acidity is regarded as unhealthy. It is reported that your system "borrows" calcium from your central nervous system to compensate for excess acidity elsewhere. Excess alkalinity is also reportedly unhealthy even though less likely. The myelin sheath surrounding your nerves is rich in calcium.

Dr. Gabriel Cousens discusses the topic of acid/alkaline balance in his book Conscious Eating. He suggests collecting a 24-hour urine sample (all urine passed in 24 hour period) and testing it for pH using pH paper. This is a way of monitoring the pH of your body. The idea of this test has some intellectual appeal but the logistical aspects of collection are not so appealing.

Acid/alkaline balance is one of a number of food selection systems that one can use. A partial list of potentially relevant systems is as follows:

Balanced healthy eating:

- to obtain all the nutrients of the body on a cellular level
- balancing acid/alkaline (Western nutrition)
- balancing Yin-Yang (Traditional Chinese Medicine)
- balancing/controlling the Ayurvedic doshas- Vata (Air), Pitta (Fire), Kapha (Water)
- eating to get all six tastes (Ayurveda)

It would be nice if the above systems were consistent with each other but life is not that simple. What one can do is to choose/use a system for general guidance as you experiment to see which foods agree with you. The most important thing is how you personally react to a particular food not the general claims of a particular system. Over time, you will learn which foods are good for you and which don't agree with you.

Detoxification in Relationship to Acid-Alkaline Balance

According to Ayurvedic teachings, the purpose of the practitioner is to teach the patient how to take better care of him or herself; in other words, how to prevent an illness from occurring. The first step is for them to know a little about the foods they eat.

Alkaline Foods

Alkaline foods, such as fruits and vegetables, are great detoxifiers of the body. Alkaline constituents are also used to feed the body; they are truly the regenerators. Acidic foods slow, inhibit or stop the detoxification process. They are inflammatory and mucus forming, causing tissue failure to the body. Acids can become free radicals causing tissue damage unless linked to an antioxidant (alkaline) and removed. Examples of acid-forming foods are meats, dairy products, processed flour products and proteins in general.

Alkalization is the key to regeneration and getting healthy. Alkaline foods cool and soothe inflamed tissue, heal ulcerations and enhance cellular functions. A healthy diet consists of 80 percent alkaline-forming foods.

Acidic Foods

Acidic foods are high in sulfur, phosphorus and nitrogen. These include: all meats, eggs, grains, beans, nuts, seeds, pasteurized dairy products and cooked tomatoes. Most animal protein foods are irritants to the mucosa and cells of the body invoking an immune response. Foreign proteins cause mucus production thus creating congestive issues until the lungs, sinus cavities, ear canals, throat and other areas become saturated. The intestines can also become saturated in mucus, resulting in parasites and inflammation. This congestion and inflammation eventually leads to cellular death. The best example of this congestive process results from the consumption of dairy products. Much of the mucus and toxins resulting from dairy consumption is stored or filtered through the lymphatic system, especially in the lymph nodes. Is it any wonder that lymphatic cancers are on the rise in the U.S. today? Remember: What you don't eliminate, you accumulate!

The human body is biologically suited for predominately alkaline-forming foods.

10.4a Alkalizing Food Chart

ALKALIZING FOODS 75-80%		
VEGETABLES **Most Fresh Vegetables:** Asparagus Avocado Beets Broccoli Brussels sprouts Cabbage Carrot Cauliflower Celery Chard Collard Greens Cucumber Daikon Eggplant Garlic Horseradish Kale Kohlrabi Lemons Limes Lettuce Mushrooms Mustard Greens Dandelions Edible Flowers Onions Parsnips (high glycemic) Peas Peppers Pumpkin Rutabaga Spinach Squash Turnip Wild Greens Watercress Zucchini	**Sea Vegetables:** Arame Dulse Kelp Kombu Hiziki Nori Wakame **Fermented Foods:** Apple Cider Vinegar Kefir Kim Chee Miso Seed or Nut Cheese and Yogurt Sauerkraut Tamari Umeboshi Plums **FRUITS** All Berries Apple Apricot Avocado Banana (high glycemic) Cantaloupe Cherries Currants Dates/Figs Goji (Lycii) Berries Grapes Grapefruit Lime Honeydew Melon Nectarine Orange Lemon Peach Pear Pineapple	Plums Tangerine Tomato Tropical Fruits Watermelon **ALKALIZING PROTEINS** All Algaes Spirulina Chlorella Blue Green Sea Vegetables Hemp Seeds **Seeds & Nuts:** Almonds Chestnuts Coconut water Flax Macadamia nuts Pine nuts Poppy Pumpkin Sesame Sunflower Seed-Nut Cheese **Sprouted Grains & Grasses:** Amaranth Barley Buckwheat Kamut Millet Oat groats Spelt Sprouts: Most Seeds Alfalfa Red Clover Broccoli Mung

ALKALIZING FOODS 75-80%		
MISCELLANEOUS	**SWEETENERS**	**ORIENTAL MUSHROOMS**
Bee Pollen	Stevia	Maitake
Lecithin Granules	Carob raw	Shitake
Probiotic Cultures	Bee Pollen	Reishi
Green Juices	Honey, raw	**ALKALIZERS**
Veggies Juices	Agave nectar	Cold Showers
Fresh Fruit Juice	**SPICES/ SEASONINGS**	Love & Joy
Alkaline Antioxidant	Celtic Sea Salt	Hugs & Laughter
Energized Water	Cinnamon	Calming Exercises
Green Tea	Curry	Fresh Air & Pure Water
Herbal Tea	Chili Pepper	**ALKALIZING MINERALS**
Dandelion Tea	Ginger	Calcium
Ginseng Tea	Mustard	Potassium
Kombucha Tea	Most Herbs & Spices	Magnesium
		Sodium
		Iron

10.4b Acidifying Food Chart

ACIDIFYING FOODS 20-25%		
FATS & OILS	**GRAIN PRODUCTS**	**SWEETENERS**
Heated Oils:	**Processed Grain Products:**	Artificial sweeteners
Avocado	Biscuits	Sugar
Canola	Breads	Barley malt
Corn	Rice	Brown rice syrup
Hemp	Cakes	Molasses
Flax	Wheat Cakes	Sucanat
Lard	Corn flour	Pasteurized honey
Olive	Oats (rolled)	**NUTS & BUTTERS**
Safflower	Rice Product	Cashews
Sesame	Wheat Flour	Brazil Nuts
Sunflower	**DAIRY & EGGS**	Peanuts
FRUITS	Butter	Peanut Butter
Most Unripe or Processed Fruits:	Cow's Cheese	Pecans
Cranberries	Goat's Cheese	Pistachio
Unripe Bananas	Processed Cheese	Tahini
	Sheep's Cheese	Walnuts
	Milk	
	Eggs	

ACIDIFYING FOODS 20-25%		
ANIMAL PROTEIN	**MISCELLANEOUS**	**BEANS & LEGUMES**
All Meats:	Black tea	Black Beans
Beef	Caffeine	Chick Peas
Carp	Chocolate	Green Peas
Clams	Coffee	Kidney Beans
Fish	Distilled	Lentils
Lamb	Vinegar	Lima Beans
Liver	Ketchup	Pinto Beans
Lobster	Mayonnaise	Red Beans
Mussels	Peanuts	Soy Beans
Oyster	Soy sauce	Soy Milk
Pork	Bottled juices	White Beans
Rabbit	Canned foods	**ACIDIFERS**
Salmon	Processed foods	Lack of sleep
Shrimp	Microwaved foods	Overwork
Scallops	Tobacco	Tension
Tuna	Wheat germ	Anger
Turkey	White Vinegar	Jealousy
Venison	Yeasts	Resentment
PASTA (WHITE)	**DRUGS & CHEMICALS**	**ACIDITY REMEDIES:**
Noodles	Chemicals	Lemon Juice with 1 tsp.
Macaroni	Drugs	Cider Vinegar & Honey
Spaghetti	Herbicides	**ACIDIFYING MINERALS**
	Psychedelic	Sulfur
	Pesticides	Phosphorus
	ALCOHOL	Iodine
	Beer	Chlorine
	Liquor	
	Spirits	
	Wine	

Alkaline pH Testing

The pH of saliva indicates the state of the beginning part of digestion (mouth and stomach). The pH of urine indicates the state of the blood. This shows us what is occurring in the latter half of the digestive system, (liver, pancreas, small and large intestine).

When we eat acid forming foods such as grains, beans, nuts, meat, processed foods, frozen or cold foods, the body will need to rid itself of the acid buildup. This is reflected in the pH of your urine and saliva. A morning saliva and urine test result of

7.4 indicates a well functioning organism; if the results range from 5.8 to 6.8 a slightly acidic condition is indicated. This is something you would want to rectify. A test result of 5.8 or lower indicates a very acidic internal environment and something you would want to take immediate action to rectify. This can be done through an alkalizing diet, an increase in healthy water, exercises, meditation, etc.

The two most important things a person can do to alkalize is to drink more pure water and eat plenty of alkalizing fresh fruits and vegetables, leafy greens, soups and juices

Simple Saliva pH Testing

Follow These Three Simple Steps:

1) Wait for two hours after having anything in your mouth. The reason for this is that you are testing the saliva produced by the body, about six quarts each day, and not just the saliva and food in your mouth.
2) Swallow the saliva in your mouth and then suck new saliva from below your tongue (there are two saliva glands below the tongue). Repeat two more times.
3) Apply saliva to a piece of the pH paper, wait 20 to 30 seconds, and compare the resulting color to the pH color chart.

Check Your Results:

1) If your pH is 7.5, your body fluids are in the healthy range, meaning that, for the moment, you are not mineral deficient.
2) If your pH is between 6.0 and 6.5, you are becoming acidic and therefore prone to one or more of the 150 degenerative diseases.
3) If your pH is below 6.0, then you are highly acidic, indicating mineral deficiency.

Daily Cycle Test

This test will determine how your pH fluctuates during the day under different circumstances and food consumption habits.

10.5 Daily Cycle Test Chart

Day	Time	Consumption	Salvia pH	Urine pH	Feel
Day 1					
Day 2					
Day 3					
Day 4					
Day 5					
Day 6					
Day 7					

Using a copy of the Test Chart above, record your saliva and urine pH every time you go to the bathroom. When you wake up in the morning, record the time and your pH values and how you feel. When you eat breakfast, record the time. Now, the next time you urinate, record the time, your pH values and how you feel. Do this throughout the whole day, for at least seven days.

You will start to track what you eat, how that affects your pH levels, and how you feel during the process. It can be an invaluable tool to begin to make associations like; every time I eat a certain food my pH drops, or rises and I feel like... You will start to notice patterns that do or do not support you. Do this for a long enough period of time and you will start to see cause and effect. You are on the road to taking charge of your health.

Wake-Up Test

A simpler way of testing your pH is to do this wake-up test. Upon rising, check the level of your first urination and saliva (make sure you don't drink or brush you teeth before testing). First thing in the morning is the most reliable time to check your pH balance.

Fasting and Purification Practices

Fasting is considered to be an important medicine in Ayurveda, as long as it is not a long-term fast that would deplete the individual. During an illness, you should fast as long as you have no real desire for food. As long as you feel lighter, brighter and healthier without food, continue your fast. Fasting is one of the alternative procedures used instead of emesis therapy. Fasting is used as purification only if panchakarma cannot be done. If you have never fasted before and you decide to do a prolonged fast, you should get professional guidance and support.

Fasting is the first and best of all medicines. It is nature's ancient, universal "remedy" for numerous ailments. When possible, fast for 24-48 hours. A couple of ways to know that Ama is gone from the digestive system is your tongue, urine and feces become lighter and clearer.

The "missing link" in the Western dietary regime is fasting. To cleanse and detoxify is one of the essential components in the trilogy of healthy nutrition, balancing, maintaining and building/ toning are the others. Fasting is an important corrective and rejuvenative process in our cycle of nutrition. If we ate a balanced and well-combined diet, suited for our constitution, there would be less need for fasting and toning plans. The fasting regimes that would need to be practiced would be more preventative in nature. We would, in other words, be living in harmony and balance with the rhythms of the earth.

Dr. Gabriel Cousens, M.D., a California physician and spiritual teacher, author of Conscious Eating and Spiritual Nutrition and the Rainbow Diet, includes a whole chapter focusing on fasting in which he describes his concepts of fasting and his own 40-day fast.

> *"Fasting in a larger context, means to abstain from that which is toxic to mind, body, and soul. A way to understand this is that fasting is the elimination of physical, emotional, and mental toxins from our organism, rather than simply cutting down or stopping food intake. Fasting for spiritual purposes usually involves some degree of removal of oneself from worldly responsibilities. It can mean complete silence and social isolation during the fast which can be a great revival to those of us who*

have been putting our energy outward."

— Dr. Gabriel Cousens, 'Spiritual Nutrition and the Rainbow Diet'

Fasting Defined

The definition of fasting is "a complete and total abstinence from all food, including juices, for a short or long period of time, for any number of purposes." True fasting is the avoidance of anything by mouth. Continual eating without periods of fasting can cause internal toxemia or food poisoning. Fasting allows the eliminative organs to literally "catch up" on their work.

Fasting - Nourishing Our Spirit

Spiritual purification or fasting rejuvenates our mind and body but also our spirit. It allows our physical bodies to turn to the nutrition that is found in the essence of spirit or cosmic energy rather than biochemical energy. It enhances and accelerates the purification of the body; freeing up the energy and movement at all levels in the body, including the spiritualizing energy. One spiritualizing and positive effect of the fast is that the more we are attuned with God/Goddess, the easier it is for us to be motivated to live in a way that will continue to enhance spiritual development.

Paramahansa Yogananda suggested that fasting is a way to increase our natural resistance to disease, he made some of the following states from his 1947 lecture entitled Healing by God's Unlimited Power.

"Fasting is one of the great ways of approaching God: it releases the life- force from enslavement to food, showing you that it is God who really sustains the life in your body."

"Fasting is a natural method of healing. When animals or savages are sick, they fast. Judicious fasting can cure most diseases. Unless one has a weak heart, regular short fasts have been recommended by the yogis as an excellent health measure."

— Paramahanasa Yogananda

When fasting with a spiritual intent, one withdraws from everything that is toxic to the mind, body and spirit. This allows the mind to become freer to merge into higher states of spiritual communion. There are literally thousands of spiritual teachers through the centuries who have encouraged people to fast. Mahatma Gandhi told people to fast and purify their minds and bodies, and these people would find peace, joy and contentment.

> *"Fasting will bring spiritual rebirth... the light of the world will illuminate you when you fast and purify yourself."*
> — Mahatma Gandhi

> *"The greatest discovery by modern man is the power to rejuvenate himself physically, mentally, and spiritually with rational fasting."*
> — Dr. Paul Bragg, The Miracle of Fasting

CONSTITUTIONAL FASTING

Vata individuals should not fast on water or any other severely restricted diet for more than two or three days. Fasting for up to a week can cause metabolic disorders that can take months to bring back to balance. Vata people may fast once weekly or bi-monthly on liquids other than water alone. Some individuals like lemon juice and honey in pure water or juices.

Pitta individuals can fast on liquids like fruit or vegetable juices or broths, or on raw fruits and vegetables, but not on water alone. They should not skimp on quantity. Ideally its good for them to dilute fruit juices, like prune, grape or pomegranate, or cucumber juice, which is both astringent and bitter in taste, and should avoid strong sour tasting juices.

Kapha individuals can easily do prolonged water fasts if they so chose. Otherwise, they may use raw juices. For Kapha people to maintain a good strong digestion, it would be healthy for them to do weekly fasts. These types should avoid strong tasting sweet and sour juices.

Ten Physical Reasons for Fasting

1) Blood purification

2) Colds and flues

3) Stabilizing and losing weight

4) To prevent acute and chronic disorders

5) Revitalizing internal glands and hormones

6) To lower blood pressure and cholesterol levels

7) Improving digestion and bowel movements

8) Overcoming stress and to sleep more soundly

9) When physically exhausted

10) To break unhealthy habits such as sugar, alcohol, smoking, drugs, etc.

Five Psychological and Spiritual Reasons for Fasting

1) When mentally exhausted

2) To increase mental discipline and clarity

3) To improve one self-esteem and self-image

4) For spiritual development

5) To transform one's mental habits

Cycles of Fasting

The cycles of the weeks, months and seasons form the harmony and beat of daily life.

Daily Fasts (8-12 hours)

We should not consume any foods after sunset. Once we go to sleep, our body is in the state of rest, it is fasting from the day's activities; when we awake to begin a new day we break our fast by having breakfast.

Weekly Fasts (1-2 days)

The week is a musical octave of seven notes, with the eighth being the same note with which the week began. Within the span of seven days one completes a full cycle of existence. When we observe weekly fasts this help to cure chronic disorders of the digestive system, lessens the desire to eat and promotes good health and longevity. While fasting, the system becomes more sensitive to energy patterns and attuning to the energy and harmony with his or her individual cycles.

Moon Fasting (2-3 days)

There are monthly fasts for the beginning of the new moon or for the full moon. During the time of the eclipse, it is actually forbidden even to drink water. This allows the individual to become more sensitive to cosmic consciousness.

Seasonal or Equinox or Solstice Fasting (7-10 days)
The change of the seasons is when it is common for people to come down with an illness. By going on a seven-day fast you are allowing your inner being to come into tune with the outer rhythms of mother earth. These fasts are associated with various ceremonies of planting, harvesting, etc. and they also serve an important function for inner cleansing.

> *"Fasting renovates, revivifies, and purifies each and every one of the millions of cells that make up the human body."*
> — Dr. Paul Bragg

Juice Fasting

A mild and yet effective way to cleanse is through juice fasting. Fresh organic juices are easily assimilated and require minimum digestion while supplying many nutrients and stimulating our body to clear its wastes. Juice fasting is more commonly practiced today because of the business of today's lifestyles. It is a safer way to fast, especially if there is a need to continue working because it supports the body nutritionally while purifying the system; probably even producing a better detoxification and quicker recovery.

Precautions in Fasting

Fasting is most beneficial in acute diseases, but not in degenerative conditions.

Acute symptoms and diseases are quick in releasing body toxins. It is an indication that the body has enough reserve and vital power to discharge and eliminate the internal poisons and heal the organism. Those who need to fast are usually those who have been over-nourished rather than malnourished.

Chronic or degenerative diseases are conditions that are long standing, leaving a person with little vital healing power. Degenerative diseases, such as Parkinson's disease, cancer, tuberculosis, diabetes, rheumatoid arthritis, heart disease, anorexia nervosa or any other extreme malnutrition disorders, do not respond well to long fasts,

Living Water

Water and life are synonymous. Without water there is no life. Our planet would be similar Mars. Where there is pure living water organisms can thrive. Water vibrates within all life as the blood of Nature. From the vast oceans, rivers, lakes and waterfalls, to the life blood in our bodies and every cell that is alive within us. Water's pure essence is reality. On a symbolic level, we can think of water as the movement of consciousness of the Earth.

Water is the basic substance on which all life is based. The basic function of water is to bring active natural hydrogen into the cell, so the cell becomes hydrated and the DNA of the nucleus becomes hydrated. This has been one of the greatest secrets of water.

Drinking pure revitalizing water which is alive can actually make you feel thirstier. Understanding these basic water principles; that carbonated water, coffee, soft drinks, and all beverages that contain sugar or alcohol cause a dehydration to occur within the body. They are dehydrating us intercellularly, robbing the essential hydrogen from our cells.

Functions of Water

Water has numerous important functions. Besides its solvent effect, it also has an electrical and mineral content that supports and regulates all bodily systems. When the body is dehydrated the vital function of flushing out toxins is impaired and information transfer, an action that is completely dependant upon sufficient fluids in the system. Drinking energized, structured water which has not been heated to temperatures above 140 degrees, builds Ojas and prevents dehydration, and has the full presence of mineral salts in ionic form. Mineral salts that are in ionic form are much more easily absorbed by the body.

Water's Antioxidant Functions

One of the less known functions of water is its role as an antioxidant. When the water has a high-electron charge it brings electrons into the system so they are able to disrupt and destroy free radical activity.

Dehydration: One Cause of Aging

Babies are 90 – 95% water. It makes sense that the early part of our life is classified as the Kapha stage. The healthier the flow of water is in the body the healthier we are. One of the main factors in aging is dehydration. A drying up process occurs later in life. The latter stage of life is classified as the Vata stage. In other words the more we can slow down the drying up process, the more we slow the aging process.

Studies have shown that 75% of people are chronically dehydrated and that in 37% of North Americans the thirst mechanism has become so weak that the dehydration is mistaken for hunger. Metabolism will drop down as much as 3% when an individual is dehydrated. One glass of pure structured water can significantly reverse dehydration.

Structured Water

Structured water is water that is alive and has a high degree of energetic organism. As an example, there is more structured water in biological systems then in plain water that has become stagnant and denatured from its natural state. Fresh fruits and vegetables constitute the highest percentage of water approximately 80-90 percent compared to most foods which are half of this, especially processed foods. The more sunlight food is exposed to the more it becomes structured. The structured water of fresh picked food has the highest degree of enzymes, mineral content and other trace mineral and phytonutrients. This makes it easier to penetrate into the extracellular fluids and systems in the body. In other words vitamins arrive more efficiently at the correct reaction site. The more structured the water in any system, the more easily minerals and vitamins are absorbed into the cells, and the better the enzymes metabolize. Structured water is found in the cytoplasm of healthy tissue, so the nutrients which are formed with this water, tend to go from the digestive tract and bloodstream into the tissues.

Water Content in the Body

85% Brain
80% Blood & Liver

75% Muscles
70% Skin & Liver

Water makes up such a high percent of the body. Even the bones in your body are one-third water. To lose even a tenth of your body's water supply is considered dangerous, and to lose a fifth can be fatal. Losing lesser amounts disturbs body functions and impairs chemical and physical processes necessary to good health. An individual can do without food for five weeks or more, but without water he can survive for only a few days.

All life is based on water. Without water, protoplasm cannot exist, nor a plant, or an insect, or any animal. It must have fluid liquid. Human cells are exactly the same, they need liquid to survive; even oxygen needs a moist surface to be absorbed by your lungs.

Rasayana Therapy: The Essence and Delight

RASA: THE TASTES OF NATURE

The term rasa has numerous meanings and definitions in Sanskrit. According to Maya Tiwari in her wonderful book Diet for Natural Beauty she defines rasa as "the culmination of maturity." In other words, rasa is the beauty that is earned. It is the achievement of a calm and resolved being. It is the vital lymph fluid or plasma that nurtures the cells of the body. The Indian word for the life-giving fluid of the internal and external environment is Rasa. In Ayurveda, the term rasa refers to the complex chain of reactions that occur from the initial registration of a perception by a sense organ to the stimulation of the brain cells that excite the appetite. It means not only the lymph which bathes the cells of our bodies, but also the food-essence detected by our sense of taste and instinctively sought by our appetites to maintain the total environment within our bodies. Appetite is the total intelligence of the body acting in harmony with the external environment. Appetite, in this sense of the word, is the point of intersection of constriction, education, weather change, seasonal variation and the body's internal economy. It is a complex regulator of our behavior and not simply a process of eating. Rasa is not merely the taste of foods. Taste is a just a tiny aspect of the prodigious spectrum within which rasa operates. Nourishing substances are desired, ingested, digested, and its waste ejected. Rasa is present through all stages of the vital process of assimilation.

> *"We have reached a point where taste has been sacrificed for the sake of convenience and profit. Fewer and fewer people are aware of the great gulf dividing mass-produced from homemade food. And even when they are aware of it, they have no time to trouble themselves over it or else they feel the matter is too trivial."*
>
> *"Foregoing the simple, fundamental contact opportunities offered us in the taste of food is only a short step away from devaluing contact in general."*
>
> — Erving and Miriam Polster, American Psychotherapist

One of the main aspects of rasa is discrimination. Rasa is an intelligence to be learned; it's not just the throwing together of foods or herbs to simply stimulate the sense of sight and taste, irrespective of indigestion and digestion.

The proper "foreplay" of eating arises from:

1. An understanding and knowledge of nature, its environs and the body.
2. A deep regard for the universe and the bounty of its grains and greens.
3. The selection of seasonal and repertory produce.

> *"When food ceases to be medicine, medicine becomes impotent."*

How do we learn which foods are nourishing and which are potentially toxic? As was spoken of earlier, taste combined with constitutional wisdom is a primal indicator of what to eat and not eat.

Rasayana (rah-sigh-yah-na) is a Sanskrit term for procedures that rejuvenate the physiology. Rasa literally means, "sap" or "juice." Rasa represents tissue fluids, including lymph and blood plasma. Its accessory tissues are breast milk and menstrual blood and its waste product is mucus. Its primary function is nourishment.

Rasa has at least two dozen important meanings in Sanskrit; meanings as varied as taste, elixir, water, semen, plant sap, food juice, lymphatic fluid, plasma, essence, purified metallic oxide or mercury, and even gravy or sauce.

Taste is "Rasa." It means delight or essence, both of which promote healing. Another definition of Rasayana in Ayurveda is described as "That which destroys the old age and disease is called Rasayana." A channel extends from the mouth into the head and brings the essence (one meaning of taste) to the brain. This essence stimulates Prana, which in turn stimulate the Agni- digestive fires.

In Ayurvedic medicine there is a particular science called "Rasayana." "Ayana" means "pathway", "to circulate" or "to have a home." Rasayana is what enters "ayana" in the "essence." It is what infiltrates and rejuvenates the essence of our psycho-physiological being. Rasayana foods and herbs regenerate the mind and body, slowing down the aging process. They work on strengthening the quality of the body's organs and tissues. Rasayana nourishing medicines are specific and work on a subtle and more long-term basis than do most herbal nutritive tonics. Their healing quality sustains and maintains body function. The majority of Rasayana herbs are classified as sweet in the post-digestive stage, even though Rasayana tonics for a Kapha constitution will usually be warming and pungent. Rasayana herbs are determined by their taste, energy and their unique qualities.

THE AIM OF RASAYANA

The Rasayana or rejuvenation therapy aims at keeping the enzymes in the tissue cells in their normal functioning condition. These cells are to be revitalized and their composition has to be changed. The tranquility of the mind has to be promoted and the nerves, as well as the bones, are to be kept soft and smoothened. This prevents the process of aging and makes the individual free from any disease, even during an advanced age. The sharpness of hearing and vision continues; the glow in the face and the color of the skin remains as before. It is with this in mind that one may partake of rejuvenation therapy.

The universe's rasa is expressed through the six tastes: Sweet,

Sour, Salty, Pungent, Bitter and Astringent. Each taste is permeated with the universe's remembrance of its original seed from the beginning of time.

In Ayurveda Revisited, Dr. SharadiniA. Dahanukar and Dr. Urmila M. T Hatte in Bombay, India, gives experimental evidence that Rasayana's rejuvenative foods and herbs of Ayurveda harmonize the body's functions by modulating the neuroendocrine-immune function. This strengthens the individual's resistance. It seems logical to conclude that increased immuno-competence improves the quality of tissues so that they sustain effects of external and internal stress better. Perhaps Rasayana therapy may prove to be the most effective integrated treatment for immune system and emotional problems.

Rasa Dhatu

Rasa Dhatu mainly signifies blood plasma, lymph and chyle. It also refers to "taste" and "emotion." The fact that Rasa means, "taste" suggests that good quality Rasa Dhatu can be generated only when the ingested food possesses all the Six Tastes that the individual needs. These Tastes make sure that the three Doshas do their work well.

The deep meaning or function of Rasa Dhatu is to provide nourishment. When our body is hungry, every cell in our body is hungry. As soon as we see or smell the aroma of a food we like, our mouth begins to water, all of our cells perk up and come to life, both physically and emotionally. Once you bite into the food you receive the "sap' of Rasa Dhatu. This is the anticipation - the promise of good things to come. Rasa is not sufficient in itself to nourish the whole being of the individual. It is the zest for more, the wetting of the lips, the desire for more.

If your meal is not well-digested and assimilated, you will feel a lack of energy and vitality. The process of digestion after thorough chewing and swallowing and good assimilation of healthy Rasa will lead to great stamina.

Symptoms when Rasa is disturbed are numerous but we'll focus on one of the major ones, the "lack of taste." This has two meanings. First, at the physiological level, it indicates a lack of desire for food. This happens when Ama is generated in preference to Rasa Dhatu. For nutritional absorption to occur, the bodily systems must first clear the toxins and any obstructions of Ama. The second meaning at the psychological level", signifying a lack of curiosity or concern in living, lack of "flavor" for the things of life. The symptoms would be an inability to get excited regarding anything in life, often accompanied by bad moods and displeasure. The displeasure is Kapha related, and it's the waste product generated at the phase of exchange of food into Rasa. Wasteful exchange makes disproportionate Kapha that supports Ama production and produces this sluggishness.

Developing emotional and mental health is next to impossible as long as the body is filled with undigested Ama. Eating wholesome foods in such a way that Ama does not build, incorporating daily movement and breath practices and rejuvenation therapies when needed, will create an organism that is clean, vital, mentally and emotionally balanced, loving and peaceful.

Disease and Rasayana

- Rasayana increases tissue resistance to disease.
- Rasayana treats healthier tissues by providing a protective cover.
- Rasayana treatment delays the onset of diseases and reduces the severity and complications of them.
- During convalescence, Rasayana speeds up the process of recovery.

Rasayana treatment maintains the normal status of Agni promoting easy and speedy treatment of diseases takes place.

Aging and Rejuvenation

The following are the main causes of aging and premature aging:

1. Excessive use of food and drinks that have spicy, salty and sour tastes.
2. Intake of alkalis, for example certain preservatives, processed, baking soda etc.
3. Consumption of old food (canned foods).

4. Over intake of oily or fried food.
5. Excessive intake of non-vegetarian food.
6. Incompatible /antagonistic food
7. Untimely eating schedule.
8. Over eating.
9. Intake of food when suffering from indigestion.
10. Sleep during the daytime.
11. Excess consumption of alcohol and over indulgence in vices.
12. Overexertion.
13. Negative emotions like greediness, fear, anger, grief etc.

Knowingly or unknowingly most of us indulge in some of these activities that result in aging, even in the young or Middle Ages, with the following symptoms:

The person is subdued with malaise, depression, sleep, drowsiness, lassitude, lack of enthusiasm, dyspnoea, incompetence in physical and mental activities, loss of memory, intellect and luster, and gradually becomes ill and does not enjoy a normal life span.

The Principles of Rejuvenation Therapy

Briefly, it is the treatment for the nourishment of the body tissues. This therapy slows down the aging process by decreasing the degenerative process. The appropriate time for this therapy is between the ages of 16 - 80 year.

the Merits of Rejuvenation Therapy

The Rasayana Rejuvenation Therapy offers: prolonged life span, great memory, intelligence, perfect health, youthfulness, bright complexion and color, bold voice and magnanimity, physical endurance and strong sense organs, perfection in speech, sexual powers and brilliance. It is the best means of keeping the tissues in peak condition.

Who Will Benefit from Rasayana Rejuvenation Therapy

• Individuals with chronic diseases who are able to fully participate in the therapy.

- Individuals who are recovering from chronic diseases and are seeking to enhance or accelerate the recovery process, and who would like to develop and maintain new habits of a health lifestyle.
- Healthy individuals seeking optimum health or peak performance in whatever area of life they have chosen to pursue excellence.
- Spiritual practitioners who would like to purify and balance in order to deepen and broaden their spiritual practice.

Rasayana Rejuvenation: The Role of Rasayana Therapy

In Ayurveda, Rasayana is a well-developed ancient science. As stated earlier, Rasayana literally, means the "augmentation of rasa," the vital fluid produced by the digestion of food which sustains the body through the strengthening of the dhatus. It is the rasa flowing in the body, which sustains life; when it stops flowing, life comes to an end. Rasayana is, therefore, the medium through which the rasa is maintained, freshened and augmented. Rasayana is a part of Ayurveda and its aims are: to increase longevity to over 100 years, to increase the power of the brain, to improve health and make a person more active, to remove all morbidity from the body and to maintain the youth of the individual. Another connotation of rasa, which follows from the first, is that it is a medicine that will maintain the life and health of the individual. Medicines are categorized according to whether they promote general health and longevity, sexual vigor or fight disease.

The sages of old, who lived long, disease-free and vigorous lives, did so with the help of Rasayanas. Ancient Reishi masters supposedly gave the knowledge of these panaceas to the sages. The Rasayanas were based on such herbs as: Endri, Brahmi, Kakoti, Kshirpushpi, Shravani, Mahashravani, Shatavari, Vadarikanda, Jeevanti, Punarnava, Sthira, Vacha, Chhatra, Atichattra, Meda and countless others.

Rasayanas prepared from Amalaki, Haritaki, Triphala, Bhringaraja, Ashwagandha, Punarnava, Chitraka and many other herbs have been used from time immemorial and have been instrumental in giving long, disease-free and vigorous lives to their users.

TIME OF ADMINISTRATION

The sooner the therapy is administered to the individual the better it is. In more advanced age, its effect becomes limited. Before starting the therapy, the following two points are to be observed:

The body of the individual is cleaned of the dirt or the metabolic waste products through specialized therapies indicated in the Pancha Karma. If the Rasayana is taken after cleaning the toxins from the body, it gives the best results, though it can be also taken without it.

The person taking Rasayana is taught to think, speak and work in such a way that would be conducive to the development of a healthy society. In fact, these conducts are given much importance in Ayurveda and they themselves are considered to have rejuvenating effects on the human body.

METHOD OF TAKING RASAYANA

The Rasayana therapy can be taken in two different ways:

IN A COUNTRY RETREAT: A country setting is both calming and allows a person the opportunity to 'retreat' from daily life and focus on healing. Through a program that is geared to nourish the seven tissues, and specific to your constitution the practitioner draws on the healing aspects of foods, herbs, aromatherapy, body work, yoga, meditation and nature therapies, a person is guided back to health. Ideally it is a good practice to undergo panchakarma therapy before taking the rejuvenation.

AT HOME RETREAT: This method, while not ideal, will support those unable to go for a country retreat. This can be done while still participating in your normal workday. It is comprised of different types of Ayurvedic herbal preparations as recommended by a skilled practitioner.

11 The Six Healing Tastes

- The Healing Tastes Quotes
- The Essential Aspects of the Healing Tastes
- The Significance to Tastes and Digestion
- The Effect of Tastes on the Dosha
- The Six Tastes in Nature
- Tastes & Energy and Food
- The Six Tastes and their Values
- Adaptation of Seasonal and Daily Regime
- The Six Tastes and Constitution
- Tastes & Emotions
- The Six Tastes and the Mind
- Tastes, Intoxicants and the Mind
- A Happy Home Recipe

The Healing Tastes Quotes

Our entire psychology is connected with our nutrition.
Salt: basis for awakening consciousness;
Sour: refreshing, activating;
Sweet: general sense of well-being;
Bitter: resistance for the will.

— Albert Soesman, Our Twelve Senses

"You know exactly the mouthful you still need, and the next mouthful you don't need."

— Dr. F. W. Zeylmans van Emmichichoven(1893-1961), physian and psychiatrist

"We are always healed by means of fructification process."
"Our mouth is an inner room."

— Albert Soesman, Our Twelve Senses

The Essential Aspects of the Healing Tastes

The mouth is the beginning of the digestive tract. What you eat becomes a part of you. With smell it's different. It does not become a part of you. When we smell a flower, it is "in" us for only a moment. With taste it is not just a moment. Eating something has a long-standing effect on us. The effect is that what we take in is what we become.

No sense is as degenerated as the sense of taste. It started a long time ago in the Garden of Eden. Just imagine, the temptation in paradise taking place by means of smell or by means of, let's say, sight, such as a nice picture of the serpent. Impossible! The serpent had to intervene by means of the sense of taste for it is through taste that it laid hold of man.

If I ask you how something tastes, you may say "good" or "terrible." Yet, life is so much more than good or terrible. What we need to bring to our awareness, is that when you taste something, you take in a piece of the macrocosm and this substance becomes a part of your body - the instrument with which you have been given to enjoy this beautiful planet we live on.

What happens when you eat? Food is a primary aspect of your nourishment, a kind of fertilization process. What you actually do, is taste how the world will fertilize you and whether or not this agrees with you. The universe, or Earth, fertilizes you and then you fertilize the world around you. You taste the "moment of transition", in which the world starts to form you. 'Tasting" is living and living is "tasting."

Eating is a sacred affair, just as the formation of culture is a sacred matter. The first is the fertilization of a human being by the Earth, the second that of the world by human beings.

In early times, medicines were always discovered by means of taste. The first herb gatherers went off into nature and the taste of each plant told them whether it would have an effect on the liver, kidneys, heart or lungs. This kind of wisdom, by means of taste, can still be our teacher today.

Ancient writings of India, China, the Middle East and even in older Western healing systems such as the Four Humor classification of the Greeks, have documentation of classifying herbs and foods according to the properties and tastes of the natural elements. This empirical evidence of the ages has shown that each flavor has a specific pharmacological trait and specific pathological effect.

The Six Tastes

The six healing tastes are the missing key in the Western World. This holistic energetic system of tastes gives us a method to choose our food, spices and medicinal herbs systematically for our constitution.

The six tastes are:

Sweet or bland
Salty or moistening
Sour or acidic
Pungent or hot
Bitter or tart
Astringent or dry

Energetics

What is needed is a model of understanding the language of plants, a way of knowing the foods and herbs in all aspects of healing according to the plant's energy and how it matches the condition accordingly. Traditional healing systems used herbs and foods according to a system called energetics. Energetics look beyond the systems of the disease to alleviating the underlying imbalance that caused the disease. This cause will vary from individual to individual; therefore, all aspects of the individual are taken into account, their unique inborn constitution and not just the disease.

The tastes are the most important instrument used in understanding the "science of life," which is what Ayurveda means. The taste is for perceiving the healing quality of a food.

> *"We have reached the point where taste has been sacrificed for the sake of convenience and profit."*
>
> — American psychotherapist Erving and Miriam Polster

Each of your cells has a sense of taste and is affected by the taste of its nutrients. Since each cell in your body affects every other cell, and since all those cells affect your senses and your mind, the tastes in the food you eat exert a critical influence on your health. Taste predominates over all other physical influences.

One of the reasons for prescribing certain foods is to rebalance whatever taste is lacking in the body. The plant transmits that taste effect. In Ayurvedic healing, herbs and foods are classified according to their predominant taste, secondary aftertaste and potential taste.

The main taste acts on the plasma, whose function it is to provide nutrition to all cells of the body. The effect a food has on your body begins with the taste.

The second effect, which is experienced during digestion, is the food's energy. Heating herbs increase the body's ability to digest, freeing energy for other metabolic tasks. Cooling herbs require extra energy to digest. The stomach and the digestive organs obtain this energy from the rest of the body, which means reducing its other activities.

The aftertaste, or post-digestive effect, is that which occurs once digestion is complete and the nutrients are assimilated. The final effect or taste has either a heating or a cooling effect. When the tastes are used in the proper amounts, individually and collectively, they bring about balance of our bodily systems.

It is important for practitioners to taste and smell the actual herbs and foods themselves; developing their own sense of the gifts / properties and how the food relates to a person's physiology. It is just as important for the patient seeking healing to slow down and "smell the flowers" or "tastes the herbs" and then feel how they move within them. The determination of flavor is a very subjective experience, especially when one considers that the sense of smell is intimately linked to, and very much influences, our perception of taste, as does memory and emotions. In other words our tastes are our own.

Characteristic Qualities of the Six Tastes

Sweet Taste - sticks to the tongue, is tasty and creates desire for it.

Sour Taste - causes people to make a face, produces salvia.

Salty Taste - provides increased salivation and has additional healing effect.

Pungent Taste - produces a flow of tears, burns on the tongue and palate and has a strong heating effect.

Bitter Taste - improves mouth odor, is considered an appetite stimulant and a regulative for digestion.

Astringent Taste - has a tart taste, sticks to the palate and creates a roughened feeling.

Water Element: The Sense of Taste

According to Ayurvedic medicine, the sense of taste arises out of the presence of the water element. The capacity to taste is dependant on the liquidity that exists within the mouth in the form of salvia. If your tongue and mouth are completely dry, you will not be able to taste anything. Taste does not exist in a mouth totally devoid of wetness. Taste does not occur when water is the only liquid in the mouth, since pure water is experienced by the sense of taste as an absolute – totally devoid of taste.

The Water Element and then the Earth Element are the basis for taste. Together these two elements accommodate the possibility for taste and, in addition, provide the basis of most of our food. Ninety percent of our food and herbs have the tastes predominant in the Water and Earth principles.

Water, in the form of saliva, will act as a medium in which the sense of taste discerns the relative quality and quantity of solids dispersed within it. The body needs to know the percentage of solids to liquids. The sense of taste also gives information as to the composition of those substances.

Taste, in the strictest sense, detects substances that can dissolve in water. Since most of the body's tissues are water-based, compounds that can be tasted may be more simply and directly related to the body's biochemical balance. According to the traditional wisdom of India, taste is considered the most reliable index of the properties of food. The foundation of ancient Indian pharmacology and medical science is a highly systematized and refined science of taste, enumerating 64 basic taste qualities. Ayurvedic physicians who have studied and practiced taste pharmacology are part of an ancient science that has evolved over thousands of years. It is a complex science, and yet, can be incorporated into one's practice quite easily after some study and practical application. The properties and healing actions of about 80% of foods and herbs can be deduced according to their taste. Another 10% - 15% must be explained by what happens after digestion occurs. The other 5% - 10% can be explained by the plants energetic properties as either heating or cooling.

If we were to examine medicinal herbs the way the Traditional Asian herbalists of India and China did, we would consider an herb's taste because it affects Prana / Chi, which involves all body and mind functions. Studying the patient, we would pay close attention to which energy channels the herb / food affects and any other actions. The Asian healers see both the plant and the individual as energetic beings with internal organs that encompass pathways of energy called channels or nadis.

Within your own mouth, you have a laboratory where you can test any food or herb to see and know what its properties are. You do not have to be dependant on vast laboratories with high-tech auto-analyzers. To know the basic language or alphabet of the plants, all you need to be equipped with is your tongue and palate. With this sensitivity you can understand the universal language-properties of plants anywhere in the world.

> *"Everyone should have all six tastes at their main meals but in different proportions, depending upon what dosha they need to balance."*
>
> — Dr. Mary Jo Cravatta

The Significance of Taste to Digestion

As food moves through the three specific stages of metabolism, it takes on the taste associated with that particular region. The influence of the gastrointestinal tract will first cause the whole food mass to be converted to a predominantly sweet taste in the Kapha region, then to a sour taste in the Pitta region and finally to a pungent taste in the Vata region. These basic tastes will predominate regardless of the taste the food had at the time it was eaten. This is a universal phenomenon and is not just an incidence to human physiology.

One of the aspects of Ayurveda and the healing tastes is to ensure that all six tastes are part of each meal so as to experience all tastes in a way that maintains one's own constitutional balance. This is what creates health. This requires an artful intelligence, intuition and trial and error concerning what tastes of foods and spices are balancing and when to eat these foods.

The Ayurvedic texts describe the influence of tastes and their affect upon the human body.

11.1 Digestive Effect and Post-Digestive Effect

TASTE (RASA)	DIGESTIVE EFFECT (VIRYA)	POST-DIGESTIVE EFFECT (VIPAK)
Sweet	Cooling	Sweet
Sour	Heating	Sour
Salty	Heating	Sweet
Pungent	Heating	Pungent
Bitter	Cooling	Pungent
Astringent	Cooling	Pungent

11.2 Tastes, Substances, Energetics and Actions

TASTES	SUBSTANCES	ENERGETICS	ACTIONS
Sweet	Sugars, amino acids	Cooling	Tonic, Nutritive, Nervine, Expectorant
Sour	Organic acids	Heating	Carminative, Digestive Stimulant
Salty	Mineral salts	Heating	Demulcent, Increases Appetite
Pungent	Volatile oils	Heating	Diaphoretic, Stimulant, Carminative
Bitter	Alkaloids, glycosides	Cooling	Hepatic, Antibacterial, Alterative
Astringent	Tannins	Cooling	Vulnerary, Haemostatic, Antiseptic

11.3 Classification of Foods: by the Six Tastes, Their Qualities and Effects

The six major food qualities in Ayurveda are:
Heavy/light, oily/dry, and hot/cold

Taste	Quality	Effects
Sweet	oily, cold, heavy	**Positive:** promotes weight increase, vitalizes, aperient, diuretic action **Negative:** obesity, anorexia, goiter, diabetes, respiratory disorders **Herbs:** alfalfa, comfrey, hibiscus, licorice rt., marshmallow, psyllium seeds
Sour	Oily, hot, heavy	**Positive:** stimulates appetite and digestion, combats anorexia **Negative:** blood disorders, swellings, inflammation, nausea **Herbs:** hawthorn berries, rosehips, raspberry leaves
Salty	oily, hot, heavy	**Positive:** appetite stimulant & digestion, expectorant **Negative:** graying & falling hair, impotence, skin & stomach disorders **Herbs:** Irish moss, kelp and all seaweeds, sea salt, rock salt
Pungent	rough, hot, light	**Positive:** appetite stimulant, promotes weight loss, verifuge **Negative:** nausea, mental weakness-unconsciousness, impotence, thirst **Herbs:** angelica, basil, cinnamon, coriander, cumin, garlic, ginger rt.
Bitter	rough, cold, light	**Positive:** stimulates appetite, digestion, antitoxic, vermifuge, febifuge **Negative:** nervous disorders, consumption, mental weakness and nausea **Herbs:** gentian rt., wormwood, dandelion rt., pau d'arco, yellow dock
Astringent	rough, cold, light	**Positive:** astringes, anti-inflammatory, absorbs **Negative:** dry mouth, clogging through contraction of the canals **Herbs:** cranesbills, uva ursi, plantain, white oak bark, witch hazel

The Six Tastes and the Doshas

SWEET

- composed mainly of Earth and Water
- increases Kapha
- decreases Vata and Pitta
- attributes are cooling, heavy and unctuous
- promotes increase in all tissues

SALTY

- composed mainly of Water and Earth
- increases Kapha and Pitta
- decreases Vata
- attributes are heavy, heating and unctuous
- softens and loosens the tissues.

SOUR

- composed mainly of Earth and Fire
- increases Kapha and Pitta
- decreases Vata
- attributes are heating, heavy and unctuous
- improves appetite and digestion

PUNGENT

- composed mainly of Fire and Air
- increases Pitta and Vata
- decreases Kapha
- attributes are heating, light and dry

BITTER

- composed mainly of Air and Ether
- increases Vata
- decreases Pitta and Kapha
- attributes are cooling, light and dry

ASTRINGENT

- composed mainly of Air and Earth
- increases Vata
- decreases Pitta and Kapha
- attributes are cooling, light and dry

11.4 Effects of Tastes on the Doshas

	Vata	Pitta	Kapha
Sweet	+	-	-
Sour	+	+	-
Salty	+	+	-
Pungent	-	+	+
Bitter	-	-	+
Astringent	-	-	+

Each taste has definite effects in terms of the three doshas. The plus and minus symbols indicate increasing or diminishing effects of the particular dosha.

Taste reflects certain qualities in the food and its ability to modify the doshas. From this, one can know how the substance will influence the energetic balance of the body-mind. By studying the chart, we can see how a taste of the food or spice immediately affects the doshas. As knowledge and intuition increases, one can become aware of the dynamic balance of the elements in their body and which foods (tastes) should be eaten at that moment. The Ayurvedic pharmacology of taste is essentially a way of putting into proper terms the intuitive and experiential sense of what is the best and healthiest food to eat at any moment.

The Six Tastes and the Three Humors

VATA

- sweet, sour and salty
- heavy, oily and hot

PITTA

- heavy, oily, cold
- sweet, bitter and astringent

KAPHA

- hot, light, and dry

- pungent, bitter and astringent

Pungent herbs and foods act on the lungs and large intestines. They induce perspiration and are appropriate to use during the fall months due to their dispersing effect. Excessive and/or lack of pungent foods injure the lungs and large intestines. Excessive pungent foods injure the liver, knot the muscles, slow the pulse and injure the spirit. Pungent tastes are balanced by a moderate amount of bitter food.

Sweet herbs and foods act upon the stomach, spleen and pancreas. They neutralize toxins and are appropriate to use during the late summer due to their retarding effect. Excessive and/or lack of sweet foods injure the stomach, spleen and pancreas and excessive sweet food injures the kidneys, causes hair loss and aching bones. Sweet taste is balanced by moderate amounts of sour foods.

Bitter herbs and foods act upon the heart and small intestines. They reduce fever and induce diarrhea and are appropriate to use during the summer months due to their strengthening effect. Excessive and/or lack of bitter foods injure the heart and small intestines and excessive bitter food injure the lungs, whither the skin, body hair falls out, and stomach becomes congested. Bitter taste is balanced by moderate amounts of salty food.

Sour herbs and foods act upon the liver and gallbladder and stop diarrhea and perspiration. They are appropriate to use during the spring season due to their gathering (astringent) effect. Excessive and /or lack of sour foods injure the liver and gallbladder and excessive sour food injures the spleen and stomach, toughens and wrinkles the flesh, and the skin and lips become slack. Sour taste is balanced by a moderate amount of pungent food.

Salty herbs and foods act upon the kidneys and urinary bladder and soften hard mass and tissues. They are appropriate to use during the cold winter months due to their softening effect. Excessive and/or lack of salty foods injure the kidneys and bladder and excessive salty food injures the heart, causes high blood pressure, hardened pulse and weak bones. Salty taste is balanced by a moderate amount of sweet food.

The Chemical Compounds of Tastes

SWEET

The sweet tastes are stimulated by a host of simple sugars, among them sucrose, glucose, fructose, maltose and charose as well as by some unlikely chemicals such as the amino acid D-leucine, lead acetate (sugar of lead), nonnutritive saccharin, chloroform and beryllium choride. (The first name given to the element beryllium was glucinium, which means "sweet." The sweet constituents are also mucilage, fatty oils, and starches. Its medicinal actions are to support tissue growth and development. The sweet taste of foods and herbs helps with assimilation and provides nourishment through their demulcent, antispasmodic, nervine and nutritive action and also tonifies and balances the internal organs and tissues.

SOUR

The sour tastes are stimulated by such substances as hydrochloric acid, acetic acid, citric acid, malic acid, tartic acid, hydrogen ions (H+), tannins and ascorbic acid (Vitamin C). Its medicinal actions are carminative, digestive stimulant, nutritive, increases appetite and a refrigerant. It helps in absorption, binding and holding the tissues of the internal organs together.

SALTY

The salty tastes are stimulated by salts such as sodium chloride, ammonium chloride, magnesium chloride and sodium fluoride. Its medicinal actions are sedative, digestive, appetite enhancer, purgative, demulcent and laxative. It moistens and softens the internal organs and tissues.

PUNGENT

A pungent taste is found in chili peppers, garlic, onions, mustard or horseradish due to their volatile oils, phenols and alcohols. Its medicinal actions are as a stimulant, diaphoretic, expectorant, digestive aid and carminative. It disperses and causes movement of energy on the internal organs and tissues.

The potent capsaicinoids that impart the flaming bite of chili peppers and cayenne have almost no odor or flavor. They act directly on the pain receptors in the mouth and throat and will irritate other tissues as well. One drop of capsaicin in 100,000 drops of water will produce a persistent burning on the tongue. Capsaicin makes cold solutions appear less cool and warm solutions appear hotter. It also lessens the perception of bitter and sour tastes, while the piperine in black and white pepper affects the sweet and salty tastes. Curry will anesthetize the tongue.

BITTER

The bitter compounds are quite potent medicinally or can be classified as toxic in large amounts. These chemical constituents are alkaloids (over 4,000 alkaloids have been identified), terpenes, phenolics, or glycosides that are stored in plant tissues or exuded to deter the plant's enemies. The herbal actions that are usually found in bitter tasting foods and herbs are effective against bacteria, fungi and insects. It sedates, dries and hardens the internal organs and tissues.

The best-known strong bitter tasting drugs are caffeine, quinine, codeine, nicotine, morphine and strychnine. Digitalis is one common drug that comes from the beautiful foxglove plants. Many of these toxic bitters also have a strong addictive quality. Very bitter substances detected by the taste buds on the back of the tongue will evoke a gagging reflex with the adaptive significance of getting rid of a dangerous substance; that is why bitters need to be used in small amounts, for in large amounts they can disrupt normal biological function to the point of death.

ASTRINGENT

Tannins and acids stimulate the astringent tastes. It tightens and cools the internal organs and tissues. Its medicinal actions are vulnerary, haemostatic, febrifuge, sedative, anti-inflammatory, styptic and antiseptic.

The Six Tastes in Nature

The Fine Art of Tasting

We can sharpen their sense of taste. The taste buds need to be fresh, not fatigued. Tasting is a completely individual experience; each person will react differently to a particular taste…

nobody has the right to dictate how you should react to a taste sensation.

Sweet Taste

- **SIMPLE SUGARS**
  Fruit sugars, cane and beet sugar, honey, barley malt, rice syrup, maple sugar and syrup, dried fruits and fruit syrups, agave nectar, stevia, Yacon syrup, etc. These are derived from fruit, vegetable and sugar producing plants and herbs like stevia leaves. Other sweet herbs are licorice root, red dates, rehmannia and panax ginseng root.
- **STARCHES AND CARBOHYDRATES**
  Starches, as from grains, are more balanced, sometimes diuretic and sometimes heating but in most cases neutral. Vegetable starches like sweet potatoes and yams are similar.
- **LIPIDS/ OILS AND FATS**
  These are derived from seeds and nuts. They are in most cases heating.

Salty Taste

- **MINERAL SALTS**
  Sea salt, Celtic sea salt, rock salt, alkalis and laxative salts. Laxative salts draw fluids from the tissues and can aggravate Vata if used in excess.
- **SEA PRODUCTS/SODIUM RICH-FOODS**
  Sea vegetables, such as dulse, nori, arame, hiziki, kombu, kelp and bladderwrack, etc., and also certain natural products, such as tamari or natural soy sauce, Bragg's amimo acids, celery and celery seeds, irish moss and most naturally sodium rich foods, have a salty quality. These are less heating then the mineral salts and may combine other tastes.

Sour Taste

- **ACID FRUITS**
  Citrus fruit, sour plums, sour cherries, sour grapes, passion fruit, sour pineapple, sour apples, blackberry, strawberry, raspberry, hawthorn berries, raspberries, schisandra berries and most fruits.

- **ACID VEGETABLES**
  There are less acid vegetables then there are fruits, the main category is the nightshade family such as tomatoes, peppers, eggplant, potatoes and paprika. The oxalis family; like Swiss chard and spinach when eaten in excess. Also rhubarb stems can create acidity in the body.
- **FERMENTS**
  These are foods that have been naturally fermented, for example, sauerkraut from cabbage. Herbal medicinal wines are also in this category. The sour taste of herbs can be increased by preparing herbs through a fermentation process as in herbal wines and tinctures using an alcohol whose taste is sour in energy.
- **CARMINATIVE HERBS/ ANTI-OXIDANT HERBS**
  Sour herbs such as ginkgo, sheep sorrel and culinary seeds and spices.

Pungent Taste

- **ESSENTIAL OILS, AROMATICS, HERBS, SPICES**
  Most aromatic herbs and spices like garlic, horseradish, ginger root, turmeric, cayenne pepper, red and black pepper, mustard, rosemary, basil, prickly ash bark, turmeric, coriander seeds, cumin, chamomile, mints, and all culinary seeds and spices.
- **PUNGENT-BITTER ALKALOIDS, NARCOTICS, POISONS**
  Alkaloid herbs and beverages include black and green tea, coffee, stronger ones include ma huang, and even stronger ones like aconite, which is quite toxic. In small and appropriate doses these strong stimulating herbs can have a powerful cleansing effect, and yet in large doses are narcotic and paralyzing. They can be deranging to all constitutions.

Bitter Taste

- **SIMPLE BITTERS**
  Herbs such as goldenseal, gentian root, senna pods and leaves, yellow dock root, coptis; generally bitter in their properties. Herbs generally contain constituent principles like Bererine.

- **ASTRINGENT BITTERS**
  There are numerous astringent bitter foods such as endive, chicory, and romaine lettuce. Also leafy greens in general, tonic water, bitter cucumbers and burdock root. Other herbs include aloe vera, centaury, Herbs such as dandelion root, burdock root, black haw, uva ursi, and pippsessowa; combine some effects of pungent taste. Herbs generally contain constituents that have bitters and tannins.
- **BITTER AROMATICS**
  Herbs such as wormwood, mugwort, rue, tansy, fenugreek seeds, and vetivert. Combine some effects of pungent taste; may be anthelmintic, some are warming and others can be even toxic. Herbs generally contain constituents that have bitters and aromatics.

Astringent Taste

- **RESINS, SAPS, BARKS**
  White oak bark, witch hazel, horse chestnut are a few herbal barks. Numerous saps and resins (like coniferous or myrrh gum-like resins) combine the four tastes of astringent, bitter, pungent and even sweet. They have rejuvenative healing properties with some warming action. The majority of resins are astringent to aid in the healing of plants. Saps are astringent in most cases.
- **ASTRINGENT HERBS AND VEGETABLES**
  Fruits usually have a secondary astringent action especially if they are not quite ripe, huckleberry and blackberry are two examples that taste astringent. Vegetables that are starchy like potatoes may also have some secondary astringency, as well as beans, lentils, amaranth, apples, carrots pomegranate and the cabbage family.

  Most green herbs are astringent, like alfalfa, lettuce, dandelion leaves, plantain leaves, comfrey leaves and all lettuces. Grasses and trees are usually astringent. Other medicinal herbs are purple loosestrife, sumac, nettles, eyebright, ginkgo leaves, lotus seeds, plantain uva ursi white pond lily and lotus seeds. Herbs generally contain constituents that contain tannins.

Plant Constituents that are Warming in Nature

Aromatic Essential Oils
Acids
Resins, most of which are flammable
Lipids and fats
Salts and alkalis have a sharp acid caustic effect.

Plant Constituents that are Cooling in Nature

Most alkaloids
Sugars and starches
Bitter principles
Tannins
Proteins are fairly neutral

Tastes According to Degree of Potency

Smaller amounts of the elevated tastes will counteract or reverse large amounts of the lesser tastes. For example:

Sweet taste holds certain neutrality and can provide as a medium for the other tastes.

Salty cancels out all the other tastes.

Bitter rises above all other tastes.

A Taste Experiment

To check out the taste buds on your own tongue try this experiment. Take a bit of salt, lemon juice and ground coffee on the tip of the tongue (rinse with water in between). You will notice that the four main tastes can be quite clearly distinguished here. Try the sides of the tongue (use a small brush and a mirror): You will notice that this works quite well, too, especially with salt and sour. At the back of the tongue, a bitter taste is noticeable, and salt, sour and sweet are less noticeable.

The Six Tastes

Sweet - as in sugars and starches.

Salty - as in rock and sea salt or seaweed.

Sour - as in fermented food or acid fruit.

Pungent - as in hot spices like cayenne or ginger.

Bitter - as in bitter herbs like golden seal or gentian.

Astringent - as in herbs containing tannins, like alum or witch hazel.

11.5 TASTE, ENERGY AND FOOD

Taste (Rasa)	Energy	Food
Sweet	Cold	Fruits & complex carbohydrates
Sour	Acidic	Sour fruits & fermented foods
Salty	Hot	Sea vegetables
Pungent	Hot	Culinary seeds & spices
Bitter	Cold	Mild bitters & greens
Astringent	Constricting	Mild astringents & sprouts

Taste Relationship to the Five Elements

Sweet - of Earth and Water
Salty - of Water and Fire
Sour - of Earth and Fire
Pungent - of Fire and Air
Bitter - of Air and Ether
Astringent - of Earth and Air

Taste Relationship to the Three Humors

VATA:
Decreased by salty, then sour and sweet
Increased by bitter, then astringent and pungent
Balanced by sour, then pungent and sweet

PITTA:
Decreased by bitter, then astringent and sweet
Increased by sour, then pungent and salty
Balanced by bitter, then sweet and astringent

KAPHA:
Decreased by pungent, then bitter and astringent
Increased by sweet, then salty and sour

Balanced by pungent, then bitter and astringent

The Heating and Cooling Actions (Virya)

Heating - hottest being pungent, then sour and salty
Cooling - coldest being bitter, then astringent and sweet

The Post-Digestive Effect (Vipaka)

The post-digestive effect (vipaka) can result in three long-term post-digestive effects upon the digestive process:

- Sweet and salty have a sweet post-digestive effect increasing saliva and alkaline secretions in the stomach.
- Sour tastes have a sour post-digestive effect increasing acid and bile secretions in the small intestines.
- Pungent, bitter and astringent tastes have a pungent post-digestive effect involved in last stage in the colon.

11.6 Tastes and Digestive Phase

Taste Before Digestion	Taste After Digestion	Cures Bodily Energy
Sweet & Salty	Sweet	Vata & Pitta
Sour	Sour	Vata & Kapha
Pungent, Bitter, & Astringent	Pungent	Kapha & Pitta

The Special Action (Prabhava)

The special action is the effect that results from a specific action; this could be due to its chemical constituents or an effect on the mind or emotions.

Sweet - demulcent, expectorant, mildly laxative, it counters burning sensation, strengthening

Salty - softening, laxative, sedative, digestive stimulants, purgative, nervine

Sour - digestive stimulant, carminative, circulatory stimulant, heart tonic

Pungent - stimulant, carminative, diaphoretic, improves circulation, rubefacient, anti-spasmodic

Bitter - alterative, cleansing, and detoxifying antibiotic, antiseptic, hepatic, cholagogue

Astringent - hemostatic, vulnerary, expectorant, diuretic

Tastes and Organs

Excess Sweet - damages the spleen/pancreas and may cause hypoglycemia or even diabetes. Builds toxins and increases mucus.

Excess Salty - damages the kidneys and may cause edema, hypertension or kidney stones. Causes looseness of tissues.

Excess Sour - damages liver and gallbladder and may cause ulcers and disturbed blood chemistry. Causes acidity, burning sensations and bleeding.

Excess Pungent - damages, dries the lungs and may cause dry cough or bleeding from the lungs. Causes burning sensation, dryness and tissue depletion.

Excess Bitter - damages the heart and may cause anemia, low blood pressure or insomnia. Causes cold, vertigo and emaciation.

Excess Astringent - damages the colon and may cause gas, distention and constipation. Causes contractions, muscle tension, blood clotting, constipation and nerve pain.

Effects of Overuse

The appropriate balance of the six tastes is essential according to the constitutional balance of the individual. Health is maintained as long as you do not persist in over using one or more of the tastes. The harmful effects of overuse of particular tastes include:

SWEET

Obesity, respiratory congestion, blocked circulation, indigestion, gas, vomiting, lethargy, parasites, dropsy, diabetes, eye inflammation problems and all types of Kapha disturbances.

SALTY

Edema, joint and tissue disorders and inflammations, excessive bleeding, skin disorders, hives, hernias, early wrinkling of the skin, premature baldness, impotence and all types of Kapha disturbances.

SOUR

Heat and burning sensations, looseness of the body tissues, suppuration, itchiness, premature aging and all types of Pitta disturbances.

PUNGENT

Increased thirst, fever and excessive body heat, burning sensations, dryness of the mouth, debility, pain, tremors, faintness and dizziness, emaciation, drying of the sexual organs, loss of consciousness and all types of Pitta disturbances.

BITTER

Hurtful, colicky pain, numbness, emaciation, headache, joint stiffness, tremors, decreased sexual secretions and all types of Vata disturbances.

ASTRINGENT

Constipation, gas, emaciation, shivers, fits, distention, tingling numbness, dryness, thirst and all types of Vata disturbances.

The inability to experience taste at all or mistaking one taste for another is the first signs of disturbance in body tissues. This results from the overuse of one or more of the tastes. This dulling of the taste sense organ of the tongue and taste buds literally makes it impossible for the body to prepare for the incoming of nourishment physically, emotionally or mentally.

Constitutional Predominant Tastes

The relative intensity of the tastes in a food, spice or herb medicine determines the substance's effect on the three doshas.

Vata - salty is balancing because its qualities are heating, heavy and oily and it activates the digestive process. Sour comes next then sweet.

Pitta - bitter is balancing because its qualities are cooling, light and drying and it activates the liver. Sweet comes next and then astringent.

Kapha - pungent is balancing because its qualities are heating, light and drying and it flushes toxic secretions from the bowels, tissues and skin. Bitter comes next then astringent.

ACTIONS OF THE TASTES

Each taste has its specific therapeutic actions.

SWEET taste is building and strengthening to all body tissues. It's demulcent, expectorant and mildly laxative. It counters burning sensation.

SALTY taste is softening, laxative and sedative. It stimulates digestion. When used in small amounts it is purgative and in large amounts causes vomiting. It softens hard tumors and decongests hard masses. It relieves anxiety and calms the nervous system.

SOUR taste is stimulating, carminative, nourishing and thirst relieving. It promotes circulation, strengthens the heart and increases all tissues except for reproductive tissues.

PUNGENT taste is stimulating, carminative and diaphoretic. It promotes heat and digestion and counters cold sensations. It's excellent for improving circulation and resolves stagnant blood or blood clots. It improves all organic functions and metabolism. It also relieves muscle tension and nerve pain and clears the channels.

BITTER taste is alterative, cleansing and detoxifying. It's antibiotic, antiseptic and in small amounts is a digestive stimulant, it helps digest fat and sugar. It reduces all bodily tissues.

ASTRINGENT taste is expectorant and diuretic. It stops bleeding and other excess discharges (such as diarrhea and sweating) and tightens tissues and treats prolapses. It promotes the healing of skin and mucus membranes.

Heating and Cooling Effects (Virya)

The six tastes are classified as heating or cooling to various degrees. There are a few exceptions to the rule. One example, sweet and oily, as in nuts, is usually warming. They are still considered to increase Vata and decrease Pitta and Kapha. The variations of taste combinations may also show combinations of qualities.

HOTTEST - is pungent, followed by sour and then salty.

COLDEST - is bitter, followed by astringent and then sweet.

Heavy and Light Properties

The six tastes are also classified as heavy and light. Variations and exceptions exist. One example, which is both sweet and sour, is yogurt, which is heavy.

HEAVIEST - is sweet, followed by salty and astringent.

LIGHTEST - is bitter, followed by pungent and sour.

Moist and Dry Properties

They are also classified as moist or dry. Moist and dry properties also vary by the fluid content of the food or herb. Plums and apples, although they are both sweet, differ in that plums have more water than apples.

Long Term Effect:

WETTEST - is sweet, followed by salty and sour

DRIEST - is pungent, followed by bitter and astringent.

Intermediate Effect:

SOUR - is most thirst relieving

PUNGENT - is moistening to the skin by promoting sweating

SWEET - is emollient and thirst relieving

ASTRINGENT - dries out the skin and mouth

SALTY - aggravates thirst, promotes water retention

BITTER - promotes salivation, internally drying

Relationship Between Tastes

COUNTERACTING TASTES

Counteracting tastes tend to neutralize each other. Because their properties are opposite, one is used to treat an excess of the other.

Bitter / light—Sweet / heavy

Bitter reduces cravings for sweets and improves digestion of fats and sweets.

Pungent / expanding—Astringent / contracting

Pungent promotes excess discharges: sweating, bleeding and diarrhea. Astringent contracts the tissues and reduces the amount of fluid discharge.

Sour/acid—Salty/ alkaline

Sour increases acidity; Salty counters acidity and promotes alkalinity.

SYNERGISTIC COMBINATIONS

Tastes will reinforce the actions and energies they have in common.

Bitter and Astringent - Anti-Pitta- used for cooling, detoxifying and diuretic action.

Pungent and Astringent - Anti-Kapha- used for drying and expectorant action.

Pungent and Bitter - Anti- Kapha- used for detoxification action and cleansing Ama.

Pungent, Sour, and Salty - Anti-Vata- for stimulating digestion.

BALANCING

Some tastes help in relieving the side effects of the other.

Sweet and Pungent - sweet relieves heat, pungent relieves heaviness.

ANTAGONISTIC

Some tastes cause side effects if used together.

Sweet and salty aggravate each other, by opposite hot and cold properties.

11.7 The Six Tastes and Their Values

TASTE	NUTRITIONAL VALUE	MEDICAL VALUE	IN EXCESS CAUSES	ORGAN AFFECTED IN EXCESS
SWEET	Great	Little	Toxins	Pancreas, Spleen
SOUR	Moderate	Little	Acidity	Liver
SALTY	Some	Little	Looseness	Kidneys
PUNGENT	Some	Good	Burning	Lungs, Small Intestine
BITTER	Least	Great	Cold	Heart
ASTRINGENT	Small	Great	Contract	Colon

Post-Digestive Effect (Vipaka)

The long-term post-digestive effect of the six tastes is the long-term affect upon the digestive process. This is different from a secondary taste or aftertaste that is still felt in the mouth.

Sweet and salty tastes have a sweet post-digestive effect. They increase saliva and alkaline secretions of the stomach and assist in building all bodily tissues.

Sour tastes have a sour post-digestive effect. It increases acid and bile secretion in the digestive process, mainly in the small intestine. It strengthens and builds all body tissues except the reproductive system.

Pungent, bitter and astringent have a pungent post-digestive effect. They increase gas and are involved in the final stage of the digestive process. They have a long-term astringent or drying and contracting action on the tissues.

Determining The Taste and Energetics of Herbs and Food

11.8 The Anatomy of the Six Tastes

RASA	ELEMENTS	QUALITIES	VIRYA
Sweet	Earth/Water	Oily, cold, heavy	Cold
Sour	Earth/Fire	Oily, hot, heavy	Hot
Salty	Water/Fire	Oily, hot, heavy	Hot
Pungent	Fire/Air	Rough, hot, light	Hot
Bitter	Air/Space	Rough, cold, light	Cold
Astringent	Air/Earth	Rough, cold, light	Cold

11.9 The Six Tastes and the Five Elements Chart

Adopted from *Ayurveda & Aromatherapy*, by Dr. Light Millar and Dr. Bryan Millar, DC

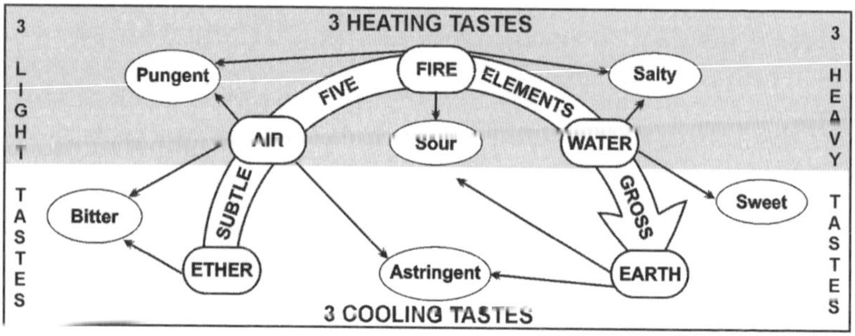

Adaptation of Seasonal and Daily Regime

We are always in a continuous flux with the ever-changing environmental conditions to maintain optimum health and vigor throughout the day and in all seasons of the year. The existence of the human body depends on the continuous interaction in a wholistic way between the internal environment and external factors. When this holistic interaction is in a state of equilibrium, the human being enjoys health. When this fails, either due to innate deficiency or hostile environmental factors, the balance is disturbed and leads to disease and disharmony. Environmental factors include the nature of the land, water and various atmospheric phenomena such as temperature, humidity, wind, rain, snow etc. All these factors are continuously changing.

Rhythms in Nature and the Variation of Doshas

There are three levels at which there are rhythmic variations of doshas. These are cycles that occur in nature, namely variations through the day during the course of twenty-four hours and variations through the seasons during a year. The other is the variation during the course of a human life span.

Daily Variation

There is a rhythmic variation in the predominance of the doshas during the course of the twenty-four hour day. There are six four-hour periods beginning at runrise. For example, if the sun rises at 6.00 A.M. on a particular day, then:

6 a.m. - 10 a.m. is Kapha period
10 a.m. - 2 p.m. is Pitta period and
2 p.m. - 6 p.m. is Vata period

Again in the evening and night
6 p.m. - 10 p.m.. is Kapha period
10 p.m.. - 2 a.m. is Pitta period and
2 a.m. - 6 a.m. is Vata period

The Ayurvedic advice for a healthy daily regimen is drawn up taking these rhythms into consideration. For example:

An important aspect of good health is to get up just before sunrise. This, as we can see, is the Vata period. Getting up at this time will help you to have more energy during the course of the day.

The Kapha period (6 a.m.- 10 a.m) is the time of the day to perform various daily practices, such as brushing your teeth and scraping your tongue, the use of eye ointments and nasal drops meant to control Kapha.

The Pitta period (10 a.m. - 2 p.m) is the time when we are advised to take the major meal of the day. This is the time when the digestive power is strong.

However, this is a variation of a relativity small magnitude. A more significant variation is the variation of dosha predominance in nature through the year with the changing seasons. This is taken up in detail later.

VARIATION DURING AN INDIVIDUAL'S LIFETIME

During the course of a human lifespan, the predominance of dosha varies as follows:

First 1/3 of life (birth to 30 years) Kapha period, this is the growing stage of life.

Second 1/3 of life (31 to 60 years) Pitta period, this is the ripening stage of life.

Last 1/3 of life (61 to end of life) Vata period, this is the maturing stage of life.

What this means is that Kapha disorders will usually manifest themselves with additional vigor in youth one may get relief from chronic Kapha conditions as one goes on to middle age. Similarly, chronic Vata disorders may manifest themselves with full vigor in old age.

The Tridoshas and the Seasons

The environmental condition in various seasons and also the food habits of the individual are the two important factors that affect the doshas. An individual may control his diet but cannot protect himself totally against the environmental factors. These factors cast their influence on the entire system and bring about changes in the equilibrium of the doshas.

If the qualities of these factors are opposite to those of the constitutional qualities, the individual enjoys perfect health. On the contrary, if the qualities of the constitution were similar, the result would be accumulation of doshas and change in the equilibrium culminating in diseases. For example, in winter, the cool and dry environment is beneficial for the Pitta constitution but is detrimental to individuals of Vata constitution.

Seasons

The calendar year has been divided into seasons. Each of these seasons is associated with the characteristic environmen-tal factors by which they are identified. Each has specific effects on the equilibrium of the doshas of an individual.

The Concept of the Cycle of the Sun

The seasons can be classified into two groups based on the movement of the sun. When the sun is in the Southern course and the seasons correspond to it are the rainy season, of late autumn and early winter. When the sun is in the Northern course and the seasons correspond to it are late winter, spring and Indian summer.

The Sanskrit meaning for the term Visarga is "sending forth," "shedding," or "giving away." In this period, the moon is predominant and endows to all living beings nourishment and thus increases their bodily strength. This period bestows strength and is soft in nature. Human beings are endowed with natural strength during this period, which begins with the rainy season and reaches its peak energy Ojas during early winter.

Adaana means, "taking away," "seizing" or "pulling out." In this period, the sun is powerful and saps the strength and energy (Ojas) from the living beings. This period starts with early winter and culminates with summer. During this period human beings begin to loose their natural strength and energy, which reaches the minimum during the summer season.

Relationship Between Seasons and the Tastes (Rasa)

Rasa is an important nutritional concept in Ayurveda. Rasa is not merely incidental in terms of rendering the food palatable but it is important in terms of nutrition as it relates to the changing seasons.

However, it is also observed that specific Rasas predominate in particular seasons and this has implications for how our food and regimen must change in various seasons. The predominance of a particular taste in a season can be illustrated from the following examples of summer and monsoon seasons. In the summer months, the sun's rays are hot and all the directions appear to be blazing. Due to this extreme heat, roughness quality increases in the atmosphere. These rough and penetrative qualities are predominant in Air and Fire Elements are also predominant in pungent taste. Thus, all living creatures on Earth experience the pungent quality thereby causing increased roughness and dryness creating a parched condition in the body. Similarly, to the rainy seasons that follow summer, the rain drops falling on the dry earth create warm vapors. This increases the Earth and Fire Elements in the atmosphere, which is also predominant in sour taste. Thus, the atmospheric quality becomes predominantly sour and permeates all living creatures. The table below illustrates this concept.

11.10 Relationship Between Seasons and the Tastes

Seasons	Predominant Element (in Nature)	Predominant Taste	Element in Rasa (Taste)
Late Winter	Air +Ether	Bitter	Air + Ether
Spring	Air + Earth	Astringent	Air + Earth
Summer	Ether + Fire	Pungent	Ether + Fire
Monsoon	Air + Fire	Sour	Air + Fire
Autumn	Water + Fire	Salt	Water + Fire
Early Winter	Earth + Water	Sweet	Earth + Water

11.10 Time Cycle Chart

Adapted from the chart of Dr. Vasant Lad, *Ayurveda: The Science of Self-Healing*

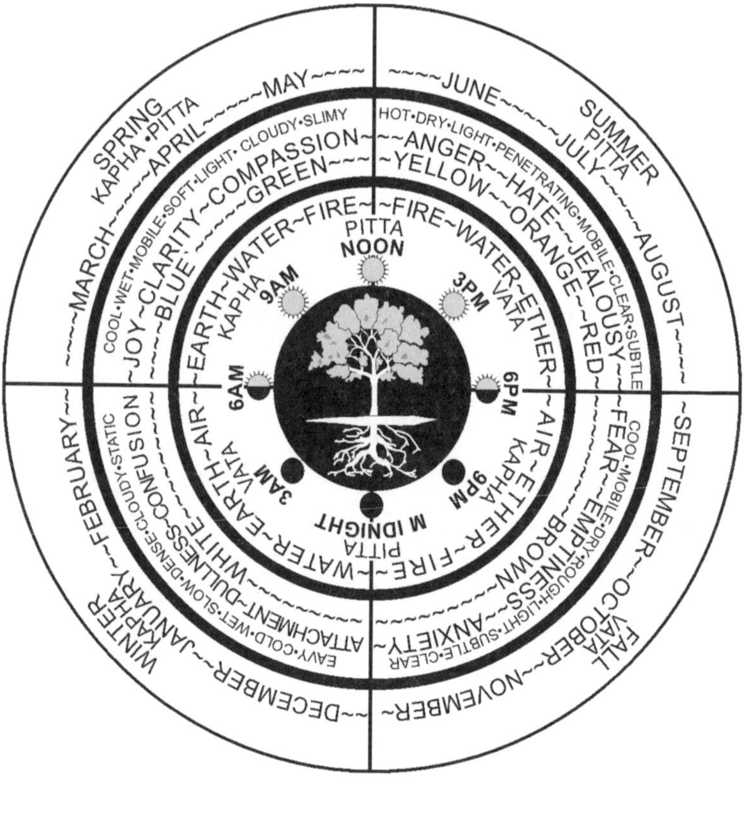

RASA (Initial taste)	VIRYA (Energy of Food)	VIPAKA (Post-digestive Taste)
Sweet	Cold	Sweet
Sour	Hot	Sour
Salty	Hot	Sweet
Pungent	Hot	Pungent
Bitter	Cold	Pungent
Astringent	Cold	Pungent

> *"The healing tastes are an essential component of the alphabet that forms the comprehensive language of nature. The tastes are a basic language saturating all of life, present in every structure of the cosmos"*
>
> — Walter Kacera

Dr. James Brooks, author of *Ayurvedic Secrets to Longevity and Total Health* suggested that Ayurvedic principles of six tastes can be used to analyze what is wrong with the Western diet and why we get into so many problems. Dr. Brooks notes that the average fast food diet includes only three tastes, sweet, salty and sour. (hamburger, french fries, coke and ketchup only have these three tastes. The meat, bread and coke are sweet; the fries are salty; the vinegar in the ketchup is sour).They are all Vata pacifying. Vata imbalance is very common in the Western society due to the fast pace of life and emotional instability such as anxiety, fear and feeling of emptiness. These tastes are attractive because Vata pacifiers give relief to these imbalances; however, when taken in excess they will induce further imbalance

The further problem is that fast food is not a healthy diet. It generally contains too much fat, is difficult to digest and does not contain the ingredients a body needs for health. Such a diet tends to imbalance Kapha, characterized by lethargy, overweight, depression, mental dullness and greediness.

Dr. Brooks also suggests that nutritional imbalance can lead to addictive behavior of all kinds. The mind / body system feels dissatisfied and is craving for something. The person does not know what is missing. This, left untreated, can result in addiction, and not necessarily just in food. Addiction may be in tobacco, alcohol, drugs, sex, excitement, shopping, over work, etc. The answer to this is to eat a balanced diet incorporating all the tastes. This will balance our Tridoshas and we will feel mentally and physically satisfied.

The Six Tastes and Constitutions

11.11a The Six Tastes and the Constitutions

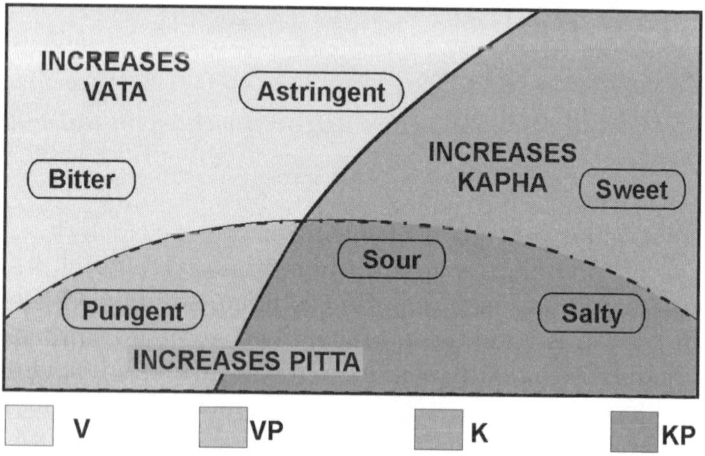

11.11b The Six Tastes and the Constitutions

Adopted from *Ayurveda & Aromatherapy*, by Dr. Light Millar and Dr. Bryan Millar, DC

Dosha	Tastes That Increases Dosha	Tastes That Decreases Dosha
Vata	• Pungent • Bitter • Astringent	• Sweet • Sour • Salty
Pitta	• Pungent • Sour • Salty	• Sweet • Bitter • Astringent
Kapha	• Sweet • Sour • Salty	• Pungent • Bitter • Astringent

The table above summarizes how the six tastes affect the Doshas and offers practical ways to balance an imbalanced diet. For example, a woman who a few days from menstruating may feel bloated from fluid retention. This may be accompanied by mood change and depression (we call this PMS). Ayurvedically speaking, this means that there is an excess of Kapha in the system prior to menstruation period.

Looking at the table above we can see that in order to reduce Kapha, we need to eat pungent foods such as onions, radishes, ginger, cumin etc., bitter foods such as green leafy vegetables, (such as spinach, bitter greens, turmeric) and astringent foods such as broccoli, cabbage, sprouted legumes, etc. Most people tend to go for the sweet foods (candy bar) or salty foods (potato chips, salted nuts, etc.). This will make things worse. Similarly, for a person who feels very irritated or annoyed (signs of Pitta imbalance), foods that are sweet, bitter or astringent will be helpful. Herbs can also be useful, along with foods to restore balance.

11.12 Effects of the Sweet Taste

Taste:	Sweet (Earth + Water)
Property	Cooling
Food Sources/ Examples	Basically all natural substances containing sugars, fruits with natural sugar such as peaches, sweet plums, grapes, melons, raisins, and dried fruits; honey, vegetables such as squash, pumpkins, sweet potatoes, most root vegetables, such as carrots, parsnips and beets; nut and seed milks, and sprouted whole grains, nuts, seeds and high-quality oils. Alkalizing protein-rich foods, organic-high-mineral-rich have a richer flavor and are classified as being sweeter in taste. Sweet applies not only to foods that are just sweet to the taste buds but includes carbohydrates, protein, and fats.
Herbs & Spices Sources/ Examples	Herbs and spices such as basil, licorice root, red cloves, peppermint, slippery Elm and fennel. Ayurveda recommends that you avoid highly processed sweets such as candy bars and sugar, which also contain additives, food coloring and preservatives.
Effect on Tridosha	• Decreases Vata • Decreases Pitta • Increases Kapha
Actions	Sweet is the taste of pleasure. It makes us feel comforted and contented. It is one of the most important healing tools for debilitating weaknesses in Ayurveda.

11.12 Effects of the Sweet Taste (cont'd)

Actions	It is nourishing, strengthening and promotes growth of all tissues so is good for growing children, the elderly and the weak or injured. Sweet increases Ojas, prolongs life, is good for hair, skin and complexion, and for healing broken bones. It adds wholesomeness to the body, increases Rasa, water and Ojas, relieves thirst, creates a burning sensation and nourishes and soothes the body.
If taken Moderately	• is nutritious and agreeable to the body • has a regenerating effect • increases seven bodily constituents • promotes overall body weight • is agreeable to the young, aged and the weak • soothes the throat • suppresses cough • promotes wound healing • acts as an anti-toxin • beneficial for clarity of sensory organs • beneficial for children and the elderly • excellent for people suffering from undernourishment • promotes longevity
If taken in excess	• increases fatty tissue and bodily phlegm • decreases digestive and bodily heat • increases need for sleep • increases mental sluggishness • promotes obesity, polyurea, goiter and boils • can lead to excessive growth of the glands (thyroid gland & pancreas)
Disorders	In excess, sweet taste promotes Kapha imbalances and disorders such as heaviness, laziness, dullness, colds, obesity, excessive sleeping, loss of appetite, cough, diabetes and abnormal growth of muscles

11.12 Effects of the Salty Taste

Taste:	Salty (saline) (Water + Fire)
Property	Heating
Food Sources/ Examples	Celery, Sea Vegetables and other sodium rich foods, miso, tamari, organic high mineral-rich foods
Herbs & Spices Source/ Examples	Sea Salt, Rock Salt, Celtic Salt, Himalayan Salt, Nori, Hiziki, Dulse, Kelp, Bladderwrack and all other edible sea vegetable
Effect on Tridosha	• Decreases Vata • Increases Pitta • Increases Kapha
Actions	A basic unit of electricity, natural Salt helps retain moisture in Vata, helps digestion, acts as an anti-spasmodic and laxative, promotes salivation, nullifies the effect of all other tastes, retains water, is heavy, unctuous and hot.
If taken Moderately	• opens all forms of blockages and induces perspiration • promotes bodily weight • develops appetite
If taken in Excess	• promotes loss of hair, premature graying and white hair • increases formation of wrinkles • reduces bodily bulk • decreases body strength • leads to diseases of the blood • can lead to bad teeth • leads to excessive thirst • promotes swelling and edema • gives rise to certain skin disorders • disturbs liver function • leads to Pitta diseases • can lead to hardening (also in emotional life)
Disorders	Excess salt can aggravate skin conditions, weaken the system, cause wrinkling of the skin and graying and failing out of hair, it promotes inflammatory skin diseases, gout, and other Pitta disorders, disturbs blood, causes fainting and heating of the body, causes peptic ulcer, rash, pimples and hypertension.

11.12 Effects of the Sour Taste

Taste:	Sour (Earth + Fire)
Property	Heating
Food Sources/ Examples	Cultured seed and nut foods, milks, yogurts and cheeses, naturally fermented vinegars, sour pickles, green grapes, sorrel, lemon and other citrus fruits, most berries and unripe fruits
Herb & Spice Sources/ Examples	Hibiscus, Rose Hips, Tamarind, Miso (fermented soybean paste) and in most most culinary seeds/spices such as: Caraway, Coriander, Cardamom, Cloves, Juniper Berries, etc.
Effect on Tridosha	• Decreases Vata • Increases Pitta • Increases Kapha
Actions	Creates a feeling of adventurousness, adds deliciousness to food, stimulates appetite and sharpens the mind, strengthens the sense organs, causes secretions and salivation, is light, hot and unctuous, good for the heart, digestion and assimilation, helps dispel gas.
If taken Moderately	• promotes bodily heat • develops appetite • quenches thirst • increases metabolism and decomposition of food • sets blocked energy back into motion • has an invigorating effect • helps clear the senses • controls diarrhea • acts as a digestive • develops the sense of touch • opens blocked wind element energies
If taken in Excess	• disturbs liver function • promotes laziness • impairs vision, blurry vision & flickering in front of eyes • creates clouding of the senses and feelings of dizziness • leads to pimples and itching of the skin • weakens immune system • increases the blood • allows the body to become limp and wilted • can lead to nervousness and aggression
Disorders	Increases thirst, sensitiveness of teeth, closure of eyes, liquefaction of Kapha, toxification of blood, edema, ulceration, heartburn and acidity, weakness and giddiness; may also cause itching and irritation, thirst, and blood toxicity.

11.12 Effects of the Pungent Taste

Taste:	Pungent (Fire + Air)
Property	Heating
Food Sourc-es/ Examples	Onion and Garlic Family, Radish-Cabbage Sulfur Family
Herb & Spice Sources/ Examples	Primarily in Spices: Chili, Ginger, Garlic, Asafetida, Cayenne Pepper, Black Pepper, Horseradish, Mustard, Cloves
Effect on Tridosha	• Increases Vata • Increases Pitta • Decreases Kapha
Actions	Stimulates appetite and improves digestion, like Salty and Sour, Pungent improves the taste of food, gives mental clarity, helps restore Kapha disorders such as obesity, sluggish digestion and excess water in the body, improves circulation, is germicidal, stops itching, facilitates sweating and elimination of Ama (toxic accumulations), keeps the mouth clean, purifies the blood, cures skin disease, helps to eliminate blood clots, and cleanses the body. Its light, hot and unctuous.
If taken Moderately	• increases digestive heat & provides heat to the stomach • develops appetite • heals throat disorders • helps expand arteries and veins • opens the bodily channels • has a drying effect • dries up fat and rotting tissues • beneficial against swelling • purgative effect and intestinal cleansing
If taken in Excess	• lessens semen production • weakens and stiffens the body • promotes shivering and fainting • pain in the waist region • consumes bodily strength • creates a drying effect on skin and mucous membranes • intensifies skin irritations and burns • dries up blood, fat and rotting tissues • can lead to slight sense of coldness and shivering • can promote aggressions and desires • can lead to loss of consciousness
Disorders	Too much pungent taste can cause weakness, feeling of weari-ness, impurities, burning sensations in the body, increases heat, sweating, can cause a peptic ulcer, dizziness and unconscious-ness

11.12 Effects of the Bitter Taste

Taste:	Bitter (Air + Ether)
Property	Cooling
Food Sources/ Examples	Fresh Greens such as Romaine Lettuce, Radicchio, Spinach Chard and Bitter Melon
Herb & Spice Sources/ Examples	Wild Lettuce, Chicory, Dandelion, Holy Thistle, Yellow Dock, Turkey Rhubarb Rt., Turmeric Root, Fenugreek, Gentian Root, Goldenseal
Effect on Tridosha	• Increases Vata • Decreases Pitta • Decreases Kapha
Actions	Considered to be one of the most healing tastes for many kinds of imbalances in the mind-body. Bitter foods and herbs are drying and cooling and create lightness, promotes other tastes, acts as an, anti-bacterial, anti-toxic agent and germicidal, is an antidote for fainting, itching and burning sensations in the body, relieves thirst, good for reducing fever, promotes digestion, cleansing to the blood and helps remove Ama in system.
If taken Moderately	• develops appetite • regulates the digestion • beneficial against diseases in the chest area • quenches thirst and has a drying effect • excellent for treating food poisoning • controls fainting and infections • dries fat, grease, marrow, urine and feces • beneficial against anorexia • intensifies mental alertness
If taken in Excess	• weakens the seven bodily constituents • disturbs digestion • consumes the bodily constituents which can result in emaciation, dizziness, tiredness, certain deficiencies, etc.
Disorders	Too much bitterness can cause dehydration. It can also increase roughness, emaciation and dryness, reduces bone marrow and semen, can cause dizziness and eventual unconsciousness.

11.12 Effects of the Astringent Taste

Taste:	Astringent (Air+ Earth)
Property	Cooling
Food Source/ Examples	Most Greens and Sprouts, Okra, Parsley, Cranberries, Wild Apples and Berries, Acorns, Pomegranate, Unripe Banana, Beans, Legumes
Herb & Spice Sources/ Examples	Various Tree Barks, Myrrh, Sandalwood, Plantain Leaves, Turmeric, Mace, Witch Hazel, Meadowsweet, Parsley, Saffron, and Alum.
Effect on Tridosha	• Increases Vata • Decreases Pitta • Decreases Kapha
Actions	Astringent foods and herbs squeeze out water. They are drying and firming, Astringent taste stops diarrhea, reduces sweating, slows or stops bleeding causing constriction of blood vessels and coagulation of blood; anti-inflammatory promotes healing, has a sedative action, is constipative, dry, rough and cold.
If taken Moderately	• heals wounds • beneficial against diarrhea • slows down the digestive fire • promotes luster to fats and complexion
If taken in Excess	• disturbs digestion • promotes swelling of abdomen • blocks bodily channels • promotes constipation • promotes general weakening of the body • generally dries up fluids • lets the nutrients and bodily constituents dry out • constricts arteries and veins • promotes coronary heart ailments and diseases
Disorders	Excess astringent is weakening and causes premature aging. Its drying effect causes constipation and retention of gas. It promotes dry mouth and Vata disorders such as paralysis and spasms and obstructs speech. Too much astringent taste can adversely affect the heart.

11.13 Ayurvedic Taste Chart

The Knowledge for attaining Long Life

Ayurvedic Food Preparation & Food Combining

Taste	Elements	State Gunas	Virya Essence Hot/Cold	Vipaka Effect	Vata Dosha	Pitta Dosha	Kapha Dosha	State of energy Guna
Sweet	Earth / Water	Heavy, Cold, Unctuous	Cold	Sweet, Heavy	Balances	Balances	Increases	Sattvic
Sour	Earth /Fire	Light, Hot, Unctuous	Hot	Sour, Light	Balances	Increases	Increases	Rajasic Tamasic
Salty	Water /Fire	Heavy, Hot, Unctuous	Hot	Sweet, Heavy	Balances	Increases	Increases	Rajasic Tamasic
Pungent	Air /Fire	Light, Hot, Dry	Hot	Pungent, Light	Increases	Increases	Balances	Rajasic Tamasic
Bitter	Air /Space	Light, Cold, Dry	Cold	Pungent, Light	Increases	Balances	Balances	Rajasic Tamasic
Astringent	Air /Earth	Light, Cold, Dry	Cold	Pungent, Light	Increases	Balances	Balances	Rajasic Tamasic

11.14 Positive Effects Due to Balanced Taste

Taste (Rasa)	Physical Effect	Mental Effect
Sweet VP-	Builds and strengthens tissues, complexion, bones, life sap	Pleasure, contentment
Sour VK-	Digestive aid, relieves thirst, maintains acidity, aids in circulation, and elimination of urine and feces, strengthens heart, dispels gas, nourishes, supports all bodily tissues except the reproductive system	Clears mind and wakens senses
Salty V-	Sedative, emetic, laxative, purgative, softening, lubricates tissues, softening hard tumors, decongests hard phlegm, maintains mineral balance, improves taste, holds water, aids digestion, promotes sweating, decongests hard phlegm	Calms nerves and stops anxiety

11.14 Positive Effects Due to Balanced Taste (cont'd)

Taste (Rasa)	Physical Effect	Mental Effect
Pungent VK-	Promotes sweat, breaks up stagnant blood or clots and other hard masses, clears nadis, relieves muscle tension and nerve disorders and pains, digestive aid, dispels gas, counters fat and grease, improves taste, metabolism and organic functions, removes edema, heals throat disturbances, allergic rashes, skin diseases	Opens senses, clarity to mind
Bitter PK-	Digestive aid, digests fats and sugars, reduces fat, tissue and water in excess, cleanses, detoxifies, heals anorexia, thirst, skin diseases, fever, burning, bacteria and parasites, cleanses breast milk	Clears emotions and senses
Astringent PK-	Dries moisture and fat, tightens tissues, stops bleeding and cleanses the blood, reduces sweat and diarrhea, acts as an expectorant and diuretic	Removes lethargy and cools fire emotions and minds

11.15 Negative Effects Due to Escess Taste

Taste (Rasa)	Physical Effect	Mental Effect
Sweet K+	Excess fat diseases; obesity, diabetes, indigestion, neck gland enlargement, malignant tumors	Vata-anxiety Kapha-lethargy
Sour P+	Thirst, loss of strength, fever, blindness, itching, pallor, anemia, herpes, small pox, flabbiness	Irritation, Anxiety, Giddiness
Salty PK+	Hypertension, skin diseases, thirst, baldness, herpes, abscesses, gray hair, skin disorders, wrinkles, loss of strength	Lethargy, Resentment, Unease
Pungent P+	Depletion of reproductive fluid and strength, thirst, tremors, fainting, waist/ back pain	Anger, Impatience
Bitter V+	Vata disorders, tissue depletion	Anxiety, Fear, Insomnia
Astringent VK+	Constipation, emaciation, thirst, heart pain, blocked channels, loss of virility	Fear, Worry, Trepidation, Insomnia

11.16 Effects of Overuse

Sweet	Obesity, diabetes, dropsy, parasites, obstruction circulation, eye inflammation, indigestion, vomiting, flatulence, respiratory congestion, lethargy and other Kapha-type disturbances
Sour	Burning sensations, itches, giddiness, looseness of body tissues, suppuration and premature aging
Salty	Edema, joint diseases, skin disorders including herpes and hives, easy bleeding, impotence, early baldness, early wrinkling of the skin
Pungent	Burning sensations, fevers, increased thirst, emaciation, dryness of the mouth, debility, drying of sexual secretions, loss of consciousness
Bitter	Tremors, numbness, headaches, stiffness, emaciation, cutting or breaking or colicky pain, giddiness, decreased sexual secretions
Astringent	Stiffness, emaciation, constipation, distention, thirst, dryness of the body, tingling, numbness, fits, tremors, decreased sexual secretions

11.17 Taste Chart

	Sweet (Earth & Water)	**Sour** (Earth & Fire)	**Salty** (Water & Fire)	**Pungent** (Fire & Air)	**Bitter** (Air & Ether)	**Astringent** (Air & Earth)
Related Organs	Stomach, Spleen, Pancreas	Liver, Gall Bladder	Kidneys, Adrenals, Bladder	Lungs, Large Intestines	Heart, Small Intestines	Skin, Colon
Action	Tissue Growth & Development	Maintains Acidity Counters Thirst	Mineral Balance & Holding Water	Metabolism, Improving Appetite & Digestion	Detoxifying, but also Depleting	Maintains Firmness of Tissues
Excess	Builds Toxins	Causes Acidity	Causes Looseness	Causes Burning	Causes Coldness	Causes Contraction
Organ Damage	Spleen-Pancreas	Liver	Kidneys	Lungs	Heart	Colon
Complementary Tastes	Sweet helps alleviate burning sensation of Pungent taste	Sour reduces thirst (created by Salt)	Salt aids in stimulating slow digestion of excess Sweets	Pungent aids in the digestion of Sweet	Bitter counters the cravings for Sweet	Astringent stops sweating caused by Pungent

11.17 Taste Chart (cont'd)

	Sweet (Earth & Water)	**Sour** (Earth & Fire)	**Salty** (Water & Fire)	**Pungent** (Fire & Air)	**Bitter** (Air & Ether)	**Astringent** (Air & Earth)
Examples of Above	As in taking honey with cloves	As in taking fermented foods or pickles	As in the use of sea salt & plants from the sea	As the use of spices with sweets	As in taking Digestive Bitters	As in taking Tannin-rich herbs
Pure (aggravating) **Versus Complex** (pacifying)	Sugar vs. Complex Carbohydrate	Alcohol vs. Sour & fermented foods	Table salt vs. Seaweed	Hot peppers (cayenne) vs. mild spices (cardamom & cinnamon)	Pure bitters (goldenseal root) vs. mild bitters (aloe vera, leafy dark greens)	Pure astringents (strong tannins) mild astringents (alfalfa, red raspberry)
Constituents	Sugars, Mucilage, Fatty Oils, Sucrose, Starch	Acid, Tannins, Ascorbic Acid	Sodium, Trace minerals	Volatile oils, Phenols, Alcohols	Alkaloids, Derivatives (aloe vera)	Tannins, Acids
Actions	Tonifies	Absorbs & Binds	Moistens & Softens	Disperses & Causes Movement	Sedates, Dries & Hardens	Tightens Cools
Herbal Actions	Demulcent Tonic Nutritive Nervine Antispasmodic Expectorant Aperient	Carminative Nutritive Refrigerant Digestive & Appetite Stimulant	Demulcent Sedative Digestive Purgative Laxative Increases Appetite	Stimulant Diaphoretic Carminative Vermifuge Digestive Expectorant	Detoxifies Hepatic Chologogue Antibacterial Antiviral Antipyretic	Haematogenic Antiseptic Vulnerary Febrifuge Sedative Anti-inflammatory Styptic
Excess Taste Balanced By...	Excess Sweet is balanced by Sour	Excess Sour is balanced by Pungent	Excess Salty is balanced by Sweet	Excess Pungent is balanced by Bitter	Excess Bitter is balanced by Salty	Excess Astringent is balanced by Pungent

Tastes and Emotions

The tastes have a profound effect, not just on the tongue, but also on our whole organism including our emotional-psychological realm. The tastes are even more important to the emotions and mind then they are to the body, due to the mind's craving for sensory stimulation. The most vital aspect of the numerous factors that influence the dilation and constriction of the sensory pathways are, in all probability, taste and emotions. The Sanskrit word "rasa" means, among several other things, "tastes" and "emotions." If we look at the meaning of rasa, we would come to the conclusion that tastes and emotions are actually one and the same force on different realms of reality. Emotion is to the mind is what taste is to the body. For example, a particular taste, when ingested, tends to create in the mind its corresponding emotion, and so the same would be true that a particular emotion that emerges in the mind would produce in the body its equivalent taste

HOT AND COLD TASTES AND EMOTIONS

The six tastes are the flavors of our various emotions and each of the six tastes corresponds to particular emotions according to their heating and cooling properties. In health, as in physics, heat expands and cold contracts. Heat expands physical and mental pathways and cold contracts them. At all times, your body and emotions are working to maintain a state of balance. Depending upon its needs at the time, it will select a certain taste that will provide a warming or cooling action.

COLD EMOTIONS - Inner Contractive Expressions

satisfaction, inner peace and contentment
fear, grief and unhappiness

Sweet, bitter and astringent are cooling tastes; their related emotions are cold and contracting. They diminish an individual's craving to experience or take in other aspects of life. Fear is the most controlling of all constricting emotions, constricting all senses.

HOT EMOTION - Outer Expansive Expressions

passion, love, outer peace and joy
anger, hatred and envy

Sour, salty and pungent are hot tastes and their related emotions are hot and expansive. They enhance an individual's craving to take in food and experience other aspects of life. Love is the most powerful of all expansive emotions, expanding all senses.

Light and Heavy Tastes and Emotions

LIGHT EMOTIONS - Upward Energy

Bitter, pungent and astringent tastes increase Vata and decrease Kapha. Their light properties make it challenging for you to self-identify with your physical body, and decreases your desire to stay attached with your body even if it wishes to.

HEAVY EMOTIONS - Downward Energy

Sweet, sour and salty tastes increase Kapha and decrease Vata. Their heavy properties make for both the ability to self-identify with the physical body and your wishes and interest in doing just that.

The Trials of Life Are Also Expressed in Terms of Taste

Emotional expressions commonly used are:

SWEET

Positive - "isn't she sweet," "hi honey," "you are the sweetest little thing," "hey sugar," "life is sweet," and "sweet taste of success."

Negative - "she was a little too sweet for me."

SALTY

Positive - "an old salt," and "he's the salt of the earth."

Negative - "that old salty dog."

SOUR

Positive - "that's so refreshing."

Negative - "you have a sour expression on your face," "it left a sour taste in my mouth," and "she's such a sour puss."

PUNGENT

Positive - "wow she's hot," wow he's full of fire," and "all fired up and ready to go."

Negative -"boy is he steaming," "he's going to blow," "pungent language," "a sharp retort," and "he's got a hot tongue."

BITTER

Positive - "it was almost bitter-sweet."

Negative - "man is he ever bitter," and "he's still bitter after all these years."

ASTRINGENT

Positive - "he has such a wonderful dry sense of humor."

Negative - "a dried up old bag," and "shrivel up like a prune."

All these emotional expressions convey an individual's emotional tastes, or frame of mind. As with all forms of health, our mental attitude plays a crucial role in sustaining and healing.

Emotions affect us energetically much the same way as diet and herbs. They do this by increasing the therapeutic or disease causing effects of the tastes (experience) that correspond to them. In general, psychological factors can prevail over physical factors. Anger or hatred can actually cause as much injury to the liver as alcohol can. A healthy diet and herbs are not sufficient if the taste of the emotions or mind has not altered.

The Predominate Attitudes and Emotions Related With the Tastes Are:

SWEET

Decreases the fears of Vata.
Increases complacency of Kapha.
Decreases the anger of Pitta.

Mental effects are contentment and pleasure.
Supplies the short-term illusion of mental and physical satiation.
Sweet emotions will increase Kapha and may cause stagnation, harmonizes the mind and promotes a sense of contentment, satisfaction or satiation.
Represents love and attachment.

Negative effects due to an excess of sweet: in Vata: anxiety; Kapha: lethargy.
An overindulgence of sweet leads to its negative aspects: greed and complacency.

SALTY

Decreases the fears of Vata.
Increases the fireness of Pitta.
Increases hedonism of Kapha.

Mental effects are it stops anxiety and calms the nerves.
Reinforces the tendency toward complacency and sense indulgence.
Salty emotions will increase Kapha make us try to hold more weight of emotions.
Represents envy and resentment.

Negative effects due to an excess of salty: anger, impatience and lethargy.
An overindulgence in zest leads to hedonism, craving for indulgence in all sensory pleasures.

SOUR

Decreases distracted energy of Vata.
Increases the anger of Pitta.
Decreases the clutching of Kapha.

Mental effects are it wakens the mind and senses.
Sour leads to envy or jealousy about what is lacking in life.
It enhances the mind's yearning for assessing objects with a view to determine their desirability as ownerships. Creates a desire to search outside oneself for things to possess.
Sour emotions will cause hyperacidity or heartburn.
Awakens the mind and senses.
Represents abundance and greed.

Negative effects due to excess of sour: impatience, giddiness, hot temper and anger.
An overindulgence in evaluation leads to jealousy or greed, which may manifest as depreciation of the object most wanted.

PUNGENT

Increases depletion of Vata.
Increases heated emotions of Pitta.
Decreases self-satisfaction of Kapha.

Mental effects are it opens the mind and senses.
Brings about an extroverted energy and a desire for external stimuli.

Pungent - extroversion brings out the tendency to excitement and stimulation, and in particular the craving for intensity. Pungent emotions will make us hyperactive and hot blooded. Represents passion, and anger.

Negative effects due to an excess of pungent: anger and impatience.
An overindulgence of excitement and stimulation leads to impatience, irritability and anger.

BITTER

Increases insecurity and disturbs the mind of Vata.
Decreases anger of Pitta.
Decreases complacency of Kapha.

Mental effects are it clears the senses and emotions.
Creates a dissatisfaction, criticism and grief.
Bitter emotions will have a depleting and reducing effect.
Clears and cleanses the mind and emotions.
Represents grief and sorrow.

Negative emotions due to an excess of bitter: insomnia, dissatisfaction, fear and anxiety.
An overindulgence of disappointment leads to frustration, which confirms your body to grief/bitterness.

ASTRINGENT

Increases fears of Vata.
Decreases self-aggrandizement of Pitta.
Decreases self-satisfaction of Kapha.

Mental effects are it removes lethargy and cools fiery minds.
Causes mental contraction that brings out fear and anxiety
Astringent introversion drags the mind away from excitement and stimulation.
Astringent emotions will cause muscle tension and constipation.
Represents fear and fright.

Negative emotions due to excess of astringent: worry, anxiety and insomnia.
An overindulgence of excessive introversion leads to insecurity and fear.

An excess of any of the six tastes will lead any constitution to eventually develop these emotional symptoms.

We need to be careful not to let the sense of taste become distorted. Our emotional body has a taste for certain emotions which can easily develop into an addiction and obsession and become as habituated to them as the physical body does for food.

Sweet emotions will increase Kapha and phlegm and cause stagnation.

Salty emotions will increase Kapha and make us try to hold more heaviness and weight.

Sour emotions will increase Pitta symptoms of heartburn or hyperacidity.

Pungent emotions will increase Pitta and cause hyperactivity and make us hot.

Bitter emotions will increase Vata and cause a plummeting and exhausting effect.

Astringent emotions will increase Vata and cause muscle contraction and constipation.

11.18 Tastes and Emotions

Taste (Rasa)	Emotion	Deranges
Sweet	Desire	Kapha
Sour	Envy	Pitta
Salty	Greed	Kapha
Pungent	Anger	Pitta
Bitter	Grief	Vata
Astringent	Fear	Vata

Tastes: Gifts of the Universe

Sweet taste brings us virility, goodness, abundance, wealth and love.

Salty taste brings us the ability to penetrate and fortify the subtlest cell of the body.

Sour taste brings us courage, exuberance and cheerfulness.

Pungent taste brings us invigoration and stimulation to awaken and pursue our life's desire.

Bitter taste brings us support in flushing out negative forces stored within us.

Astringent taste brings us the ability to discard damaged tissue cells and toxicity.

The Six Tastes and the Mind

To understand Ayurvedic psychology, it is essential to understand the effects of the six tastes on the mind.

SWEET TASTE

The sweet taste has a nutritive, calming and grounding purpose for soothing the mind and nerves along with its rejuvenative effects. Individuals, who are suffering from depression, SAD, or any other psychological depression, are best to avoid using an excessive amount of sweet tonic nervines since these slow and consolidate our inner reserves.

The most important tonic nervines to use that are sweet are: licorice root, brown or black sesame seeds, lotus seeds, bala and shatavari and ashwagandha. These tonic nervines are composed of the Water and Earth Elements are not excessively sweet in taste.

SALTY TASTE

The salty taste has a sedative and grounding effect for most Vata conditions such as nervous debility, hyperacidity or a general weakness. Individuals who have a Kapha condition are best to avoid using an excessive amount of strong salty tasting herbal preparations.

The most important relaxing nervine herbs and minerals that are salty include: bladderwrack, kelp, nori, sea salt, black salt, pure rock salt, Himalayan salt and red coral powder. These nervine herbs and minerals are composed of the Water and Fire Elements.

SOUR TASTE

The sour taste does not have much nervine property, but it is a mild stimulant and can help counter general depression, lightheadedness and nausea. The sour taste needs to be used in moderation by Pitta individuals due to its heating effect.

The most important nervines that are sour are: tamarind, lime, amalaki and red wine. To extract the sour alkaloids substances from the herbs use alcohol or vinegar as the base of your tincture or herbal extract. These nerviness are composed of the Fire and Earth Elements.

PUNGENT TASTE

The pungent taste has a stimulating effect on the mind and promotes circulation in the brain. It aids in developing discernment, intelligibility and reasoning ability. It's beneficial for those complaining of blockages, lack of motivation, dreariness, hopelessness and depression. The pungent taste needs to be used with care if the individual is a Pitta constitution due to its high heating effect. Anyone who is prone to having a temper, restlessness, hyperactivity or insomnia should use pungent tasting herbs in small proportions.

The most important nervines that are pungent awaken us and help us get focused; on the other hand, they can also irritate the nerves.

Pungent nervine stimulant alkaloids are: damiana, ephedra, black or green tea and coffee.

Pungent nervine stimulants include: rosemary, camphor, hyssop, thyme and the mints.

Pungent nervine relaxants include: valerian root, lady's slipper, and nutmeg.

These nervines are composed of the Fire and Air Elements.

BITTER TASTE

The bitter taste expands and opens the mind and enhances the functional capacity and sensitivity of perception. The usefulness of bitter tasting herbs is that they help clam, cool and expand the effect of the mind. Individuals who have symptoms of toxicity, excess heat, or a heaviness or dullness of the mind, would get relief by using nervine bitters. On the other hand, those suffering from ungroundedness, hyperactivity and nervous exhaustion are best to avoid this category of herbs or use them for only a short time period and in small dosages.

The most important nervines that are bitter are: chamomile,

wood betony, skullcap, passionflower and hops. These nerviness are composed of the Air and Ether Elements.

ASTRINGENT TASTE

The astringent taste can be useful for minor spasms and to speed up healing of nerve tissue damage but it is not usually used for nerve system complaints.

The most important nervines that are astringent are: frankincense, bayberry, myrrh and nutmeg. These nerviness are composed of the Air and Earth Elements.

Cognitive Memory Through the Tastes

> *"The taste of things remain poised a long time, like souls, ready to remind us...."*
>
> -Marcel Proust

Rooted in the cognitive memory, the sense of taste is our primary receptor for accessing memory. Through the six tastes we can gain access to the memories held in the universe. Taste holds the memories from the beginning of time.

Sweet taste triggers the rapture of all the memories of the sweet taste held within the universe.

Sour taste is the universe's essential taste for healthy inquiry.

Pungent taste connects us to the vast memories of the universe's passion and stimulation.

Bitter taste sends a jolting signal to the system that cautions it to remain light.

Astringent taste stimulates the system into aliveness.

Salty taste cleanses bodily tissues and gives fresh potential for retrieving wisdom from the universe.

In eating, we are assimilating Spirit by churning the essences of the universe within our body, enabling us to recall our cognitive memories. Through the six tastes, the universe's rasa is expressed. Each of the six tastes is imbued with the cosmic memory of its original seed from the onset of creation.

Sweet taste brings us lavish love, virility, abundant wealth and goodness.

Sour taste imparts activity, courage and vivacity.

Salty taste brings fortification and the ability to penetrate the most subtle cell of the body.

Pungent taste provides stimulation and awakens our interest in pursuing life's challenges.

Bitter taste gives us the ability to look deeply into our cognitive memories and extract negativity.

Astringent taste discards damaged cells and toxicity, while restoring intelligence of mind and body.

Tastes, Intoxicants and Addictions

The sensory pathway and organ of the tongue can suffer from an excess of either contraction or expansion. If the sense of taste is underused, the tongue's pathway contracts eventually diminishing the mind's capacity to take pleasure along that pathway. Overuse of the sense of taste expands or overdilates its pathway, enervating that sense so that the mind can no longer obtain pleasure from its use. An over contracted pathway is an obstruction to air's unobstructed movement. An over expanded pathway provides too much air or ether to move properly through. Under use, overuse, misuse and abuse of the sense of taste are regarded in Ayurveda as one of the main causes of disease.

Each taste has the potential to be an intoxicant, which can then lead to self-abuse. We can see this very easily when we look around our modern world. Sweet (sugar) is the world's number one addictive drug, used to bring on the feeling of happiness and satisfaction. Sugary substances can be bought in just about any store in any country. Salt is right up there with sweet, providing the feeling of profligacy and self-indulgence. In some parts of the world, individuals may intoxicate themselves with the envy of sour or the tetchiness of pungent, and others may even set off the extreme by means of bitter and astringent for self-satisfaction. The food and herbs we eat affect the consciousness of our physical, emotional and mental body.

Our emotional body has taste or desire for certain emotions and easily becomes addicted or accustomed to them, much the same way as the physical body does to food. Awareness needs to be applied not to let the sense of taste become deranged or perverted.

Vata people often become addicted to sugar because they love to eat sugary foods that provide that instant satisfaction and temporary control of the mental state of being erratic. They can easily develop hypoglycemia due to this tendency.

Pitta people may become habituated to hot spices or meats that inflame, making them more obsessive, intense, goal-oriented and driven.

Kapha people may find themselves addicted to heavy, oily and fatty foods that reinforce their natural complacency.

All addictions must be broken to achieve optimal health. The key is to break the addictive habit gradually so as not to create even more stress than the individual is already experiencing.

It can be said that all addictions are basically an origin of a sweet taste imbalance; for sweet is the taste that creates and provides satisfaction. The terms "sweet," "sugar," and "satisfaction," are all tied together. For example, if an individual looks for satisfaction from sweet foods instead of a sweet life, the chances of an addiction developing are most likely. Anyone who consumes refined sugars, as found in alcohol and junk foods instead of fresh, natural sugar found in foods directly from Mother Nature's Garden, will exhaust their body. This may take a few years, but the refined sugar will deplete the pancreas and blood sugar levels will be thrown off, eventually leading to the digestive system being unable to digest properly. To break the vicious cycle of sugar consumption, the first thing is to start feeding your body natural complex carbohydrates and natural sugars as found in organic fruits, vegetables and seeds. This will satisfy your regular daily sweet fix. The difference being you will have eliminated the yo-yo effect of the blood sugar extremes. A sweet addiction is a sign of a Vata imbalance.

An alcohol dependency leads to all three Doshas becoming imbalanced. Vata is imbalanced by the obstruction of nerve energy. Pitta is imbalanced by its heating effect. Kapha is imbalanced by its effect on the brain and stomach. The late stages of alcoholism are mainly Vata symptoms, which reflect a deep physical and mental disturbance. The first objective in treating an alcoholic is to nourish and support the Vata (nerves) and then treat the Pitta and Kapha imbalances.

Taste Protocals for Alcoholics

Sweet - use whole grains, natural fruits, particularly those for Vata, for soothing the nerves.

Salty - use sea vegetables for their stabilizing effect and to balance depleted minerals.

Sour - use fermented foods and lemons for digestion and to improve mental perception.

Pungent - use warming spices to offset the dependency on the heat that alcohol provides.

Bitter - use herbal bitters and greens to detoxify the liver and keep things moving.

Astringent - use dark leafy greens to rejuvenate and discard damaged tissues.

A popular saying of Dr. Vasant Lad is "Bitter is Better." It is one of the most neglected tastes today, which means one of the most important herbs we need. In the right dosage in our foods or formulas, it aids in balancing all other tastes in our body. The way that bitter action works is by dilating pathways that are too constricted and constricting those that are too dilated. An example of being too constricted, such as in Kapha complacency, is it helps to open up and get energy moving. With Pitta and anger, it constricts by cooling down the energy. If your over-indulgences are interrupted, bitterness sets in. Bitterness is an emotion that will appear when desires are unfulfilled. Too many disappointments will end up with an excess of bitterness in your emotional and physical body. Just as dissatisfaction ignites bitterness, bitter's opposite, the sweet taste, eradicates frustration and disappointment. Our physical and emotional bodies return to balance and satisfaction once a sweet experience is taken in.

Salty is called "all tastes" due to its abilities to enhance all the different tastes in a food and, because of this, the individual's appetite to eat more food increases. When it is used in small doses it promotes good digestion, but when used in large amounts it weakens the body and mind. Self-gratification is one of the symptoms that manifests from an excessive use of salty substances. When powerfully impelled by the salty taste to gratify yourself, you will go toward worldly pursuits. That is one reason why salt is not recommended for those choosing a celibate lifestyle. In the appropriate amounts, salt increases the mind's desire for intensity of experience; overuse makes the mind uninspired, weak and lifeless. Like all other tastes, addictions and intoxicants, the salty taste also posses a possibility for abuse.

What Does the Universe Taste Likc?

According to Ayurveda, the entire universe has a taste (energetic quality). The more intimately we know the quality of the different tastes, the more intimately we know our universe. No machine can ever discover this for us.

11.19 A Happy Home Rcipe

4 Cups of Love	5 Spoons of Hope
3 Cups of Forgiveness	2 Spoons of Tenderness
2 Cups of Loyalty	4 Liters of Faith
1 Cup of Friendship	1 Barrel of Laughter

Take love and loyalty mix it thoroughly with faith. Blend it with tenderness, kindness and understanding. Add friendship and hope, sprinkle abundantly with laughter. Bake it with sunshine, serve daily with generous helpings.

Recipe for Life

"The priest cooked food of the four kinds and the six different flavors, in accordance with sacred prescription."

"All the world seeks food. It is the life source of all beings. Clarity, longevity, intelligence, happiness, contentment, strength and knowledge are All rooted in food." -Charaka

"A healing diet gladdens the heart, nourishes the body, and revives memory."

— Sushruta Samhita

"The right balance of tastes for our constitution, we would seldom, if ever, get ill."

12 The Sattvic Diet

- Food, Prana and Consciousness
- The Optimal Sattvic Diet
- Original Nourishment
- A Sattvic Live-Food Approach
- Nature's Foods vs. Denatured Foods
- The Seven Keys for Determining the Quality of Food
- Peace through a Sattvic Diet
- Relationship of Sattvic, Rajasic and Tamasic Foods
- Food Plan for Vata, Pitta, Kapha
- Vegetarian Facts

"When food is pure, the mind is pure this creates an oasis for awakening and provides an awakening that affects every level of our health."

— As it says in the Upanishads

Food, Prana and Consciousness

"When we look at nutrition from a purely scientific point of view, there is no place for consciousness. And yet, consciousness could be one of the crucial determinants of food itself."

— Deepak Chopra, M.D.

We cannot ignore the role of food on our consciousness. A Sattvic diet is a conscious diet, a diet of compassion, which has the greatest potential for healing and maintaining health. In Ayurveda, our focus is on the refinement and fine-tuning of the physical body as an aid to purifying the mind. Prana provides the energy that's required for this inner transformation. Prana essentially organizes the mind resulting in less distorted thoughts.

Sattvic means "pure essence." This is the purest diet for a spiritual and healthy life. It nourishes the body and maintains a peaceful state. According to Ayurveda, this is the best diet for physical strength, a good mind, good health and longevity. It calms and purifies the mind, enabling it to function at its maximum potential. A Sattvic diet thus leads to true health; a peaceful mind in control of a fit body, with a balanced flow of energy between them.

To live a purely Sattvic way, means acting with care and concern for our planet and the creatures that we share this beautiful planet with. It means making food choices that both support all life and the life of the earth.

Planetary Consciousness

We are living during challenging as well as exciting times on our planet. It is also a time when there is a great need for spiritual awakening both for healing the planet and healing ourselves. Choosing to eat foods that have their full life-potential and are low on the food chain is the diet that's best for preserving life on Earth, both animal and human life, and uses the least amount of resources for the survival of all creatures. It's no mistake that there is an increase of interest in a healthier and a more conscious way of eating, because it is time for all of us to embrace a lifestyle that supports all life. A Sattvic diet supports the awakening of consciousness that we may live more creative, peaceful and joyful lives. At the end of this chapter is an information list that outlines the effects of our food choices on individual health and the planet.

Vegetarianism

Eating vegetarian is one of the core ways of purifying the mind. When Ramana Maharshi, the most famous self-realized sage of modern India was asked what the most important aid to a spiritual way of life is, he replied "a pure vegetarian diet." He quoted the ancient *Chandogya Upanishad D II 26.2* that says *"when food is pure, the mind is pure, when the mind is pure, concentration is steady, and when concentration is achieved one can loosen all the knots of the heart that bind us."*

There are some people that say that animal food is part of their natural diet and so should not interfere with the unfoldment of their higher nature. As Sri Yukteswar, the guru of Paramahansa Yogananda, states in his *Holy Science, "Can flesh be considered the natural food of man, when both his eyes and his nose are so much against it, unless deceived by flavors of spices, salt and sugar. On the other hand, how delighted do we find the fragrance of fruits, the very sight of which often makes the mouth water?"*

Animal foods create a tamasic effect on the physical body and mind. It blocks the channels of the subtle body, the 72,000 nadis. Even Western historians such as Herodotus have suggested that not only violence and crime, but also religious intolerance is more common among people who consume meat. Numerous spiritual teachings support this. The *Manusmirti (5.49)*, an ancient law code of Hindu society states, *"Having well considered the origin of flesh foods, and the cruelty of fettering and slaying of sentient beings, a person should abstain from eating flesh."* It also states *(6.60), "By not killing any living being one becomes fit for liberation."* The *Yajur Veda (12.32)* states, *"You must not use your God-given body for killing God's creatures whether a human, animal, or whatever."*

Environmental Destruction

The consumption of meat is a destructive act and, sadly, one of the main causes of environmental degradation and devastation. Animal livestock uses approximately half of the water consumption in the United States. A diet that centers on meat creates a need for about 4,500 gallons per day, per meat-eater, as compared to 300 gallons per day for a vegan (a diet of no flesh or dairy). An animal based diet requires approximately eighteen times more energy to sustain than a plant-based diet. The destruction of the rainforest for grazing land, and the resultant greenhouse effect is one more case of the harmful effects of a flesh-centered diet on our environment. Our land, water, atmosphere and animal and human populations are not safe from the exhaustion of resources that results from the meat-centered diet. We simply cannot get away from the fact that raising animals for meat and dairy at this point in history has an overwhelming and destructive effect on our entire ecosystem, the ecosystem that is our home.

> *"Animal products are at the top of the food chain having about 15 times more pesticides and herbicides than fruits and veg-*

etables. Dairy products have about 5 times more pesticides and herbicides than vegetarian foods. A vegetarian mother has 1% the amount of pesticides in her breast milk as a meat-eating mother."

— Dr. Gabriel Cousens, Conscious Eating

Vegetarian Diet & Health

Ayurveda teaches that a vegetarian diet is not only essential for a healthy life, but is also the basis for living peacefully and spiritually supportive. Not only do vegetarians live longer but have, according to numerous studies, more endurance than meat-eaters. They are less subject to health problems such as: heart disease, hypertension, cancer, kidney disease and osteoporosis. People who consume meat are also at a higher risk of various viral, bacterial, fungal and parasitical infections. Toxoplasmosis is one of these and now there is also the possibility of Mad Cow Disease.

The ill-effects of a meat centered diet is clarified by the enlightened being Swami Prakashanada Saraswati in 1987 when he said, *"Every animal that is slaughtered for human consumption brings the pain of death into your body. Think about it. The animal is killed with violence. That violence causes the animal to experience very intense pain as it dies. That pain remains in the meat even after you've prepared and cooked it. When you eat the meat, then you eat pain. That pain becomes lodged in your body, heart, and mind. That violence and pain which you consume will also eat you. It consumes you so that you must experience the same pain in your life also."*

Dairy Products

Traditionally, a Sattvic diet in Ayurveda includes dairy products. This, however, depends upon the health and quality of the milk. It is difficult, these days, to get high quality dairy products that can be truly called Sattvic foods because of the conditions cows are raised in. Ayurveda recognizes and teaches that poor quality dairy products from unhealthily raised cows increases mucous, toxins and Ama in the system and turns milk into a poison rather than the elixir it was originally meant to be.

So many problems plague the meat and dairy industry, such as the possibility of contacting Mad Cow Disease and the high amounts of pesticides, herbicides, hormones and antibiotics in meat and dairy products. Industry is adding chemicals and genetically engineered substances that we don't yet know the long-term effect of. This type of milk and its byproducts is a deteriorated food overflowing with fear, the pain of enslavement. There is very little true nourishment or Prana left in it. It is a new day. What our grandparents thrived on no longer works for us. Lifestyle is different, environment is different and food is different. What is the diet of the Now?

The Optimal Sattvic Diet

Once we understand the necessity for a vegetarian diet, the question arises: "What kind of vegetarian food is best for our constitution?" The equivalent of a traditional Sattvic diet today consists of organic, whole, natural fruits, vegetables, nuts, seeds and grains. A modern Sattvic diet emphasizes foods grown organically and in harmony with nature and prepared with an attitude of love. Such foods carry the highest Prana and consciousness. A modern Sattvic diet does not include junk food, excessively spicy or salty foods, fried food, white flour, white sugar, and other forms of food that unnaturally stimulate your blood sugar or your mind. It avoids meat, fish and alcohol, garlic and onions (garlic and onions can be used as medicines) and eggs. It is careful about, but not necessarily exclusive of, dairy (as per the comments above). It does not include genetically engineered foods, irradiated foods, microwaved foods or day-old foods. The most Sattvic food is natural, organic food, home prepared with love and consciousness or food from organic restaurants based on such ideas.

Originally Sattvic foods, like all foods at the time, were organically-grown without any herbicides, pesticides, chemical fertilizer, hormones, genetic modification, irradiation to prevent spoilage and there were no microwave ovens to sap the food. In addition all means were prepared with unrefined and in their whole form. The modern denaturing and processing of food through monoculture and chemical treatment deranges their Pranic life-force. This unnatural way of growing and preparing food is making the food unable to contain their Sattvic essence and in addition is much of the cause creating the health problems of today.

Because of its focus on spiritual growth, the Sattvic diet is more disciplined than a regular vegetarian diet. It is generally lighter and includes spiritual fasting and the taking of living foods (roots, leafy vegetables and fruit). In the Vedas, live (uncooked) foods are called specifically the "food of the Rishis" or the "food of the yogis." Live foods are rich in Prana, which brings the Prana force not only into the body but also into the mind helping to purify the 72,000 nadis. Fresh Sattvic foods are the most powerful foods for enhancing the flow of energy and cleansing the nadis. A Sattvic diet helps us become superconductors of Prana. As the Prana in our body increases, these nadis naturally open, affording us deeper perceptions of truth, reality and universality.

Sattvic foods are full of life and create a peaceful disposition. Sattvic foods are living foods. Living foods are pure foods. The living-foods approach to dietary health incorporates the finest organic fruits, vegetables, grains, nuts and seeds. To ensure that the essence and total nutritional value of the foods are maintained, we recommend that you do not heat foods at a temperature higher than 118 degrees Fahrenheit, 44 C. When food is prepared in this way, the integrity of the food is maintained, vital minerals, overheating or processing does not destroy vitamins and enzymes, and we are guaranteed that we are receiving the absolute highest content from our foods. Other reasons for eating living foods are, we not only avoid loss of nutrients but we also avoid loss of taste. Our taste buds have been conditioned by cultural food habits, but the cleaner our body becomes and the more we incorporate a high level of wellness foods, the more we want to experience the pure tastes of the foods we are eating. An Ayurvedic living foods dietary lifestyle calms and clarifies the mind, soothes and balances the emotions and brings energy and strength to the body.

This we know, fresh organic fruits, vegetables, soaked and sprouted nuts, seeds and grains include everything needed to fulfill our nutritional needs. These foods are rich in life giving enzymes, vitamins and minerals. Plant foods are easier to digest, contain more electrified water, are sun-enzyme charged, contain more trace minerals, and are not laden with chemicals, hormones and medications. Our human physiology is adapted to thrive on a plant-based diet. It is a more Sattvic and most certainly a more peaceful way to live.

The Sattvic diet, as a Prana-rich approach to eating, differs slightly from the Ayurvedic approach that aims only at balancing the doshas and which covers the doshic effects of animal foods for those who choose to eat them. Note the book written by Dr. David Frawley *Yoga and Ayurveda* for a discussion of these differences between the yogic (Pranic) and Ayurvedic (doshic) diets. As Dr. Frawley states in his book *'Ayurveda and the Mind' "Ayurveda emphasizes a Sattvic diet for healthful living, particularly for keeping our minds happy and at peace. Sattvic diet was originally devised for the practice of Yoga and the development of higher consciousness"*. The Sattvic diet assists us to expand the highest attributes of peace, love, compassion and equanimity. It emphasizes increasing Prana and the subtle elements of Air and Ether that help open the mind and heart and make them more sensitive. The nature of the mind itself is Air and Ether and therefore the Sattvic diet works directly to expand the Sattvic mind and consciousness. A diet rich in Prana also lessens the heaviness in the body and eliminates excess weight and impurities that are usually heavy in nature. Following a spiritual lifestyle will support the achievement of a Sattvic diet. By cultivating peace, forgiveness and compassion, and avoiding stress, emotional agitation and conflict we help to stabilize ourselves in Sattva.

The consciousness of our bodies and minds are both the cause and result of the diet that we eat. Eating, as our most basic and habitual activity, defines not only our physical body but also our emotional state and our human interactions, which usually center around the dinner table. As we progress spiritually, we gain an increased sensitivity, not only to the sacred, but also to the food that is sacred. We require food that has both high Prana and love as its main ingredients. That is why eating together in a spiritual circumstance is one of the most transformative and spiritual actions that we can do.

A Sattvic approach to both eating and lifestyle is one way to regenerate the current environment and our bodily internal environment.

Fine-Tuning the Diet

A Sattvic diet, using mainly live foods, if not done thoughtfully, can imbalance Vata, the biological air-humor that has the tendency to get too airy or move too much out of the body. The aim is to keep Vata in balance while eating a Sattvic Prana-rich diet.

Most of the difficulty experienced when transitioning to a living-foods diet is caused by a lack of nutritional understanding and constitutional understanding. Once a person has the supporting knowledge, integrating a Prana rich living-foods lifestyle will be easy.

Original Nourishment

> *"See I give you every seed-bearing plant that is upon all the earth and every tree that has seed –bearing fruit; they shall be yours for food."*
>
> — Genesis 1:29

Nourishment comes to us directly from the life-giving elements of Air, Fire, Water, Earth and Ether. We experience these elements through the qualities of Prana, Tejas and Ojas. Without these three qualities, there would be no life. Let us look more closely at the source, or origin, of these qualities, and therefore the source of our nourishment.

Mother Nature has gifted us with all that we need to live in vibrant health within her abundant garden. Nature has provided for us the ultimate cuisine to ensure a long and good life. Each food and herb has been created to perfection, exquisitely designed to match our bodily needs. Nothing was forgotten. It is when we tamper with the original creation that we open the doorway for dis-ease to enter. The elements, in all their brilliance, have provided humans with fresh, whole, sun-ripened, enzyme-rich, organic, plant-based foods. It is these foods that come to us from the source, and it is these foods that "source" us.

The evolution of each species was centered on the elements available to ensure the survival of that species. Us humans have lost touch and, therefore, lost trust in nature's ways. Why do we think that we can take the gifts of nature and improve upon them? Why do we feel we need to alter them? If these gifts of nature are not broken, why fix them? When we see the abundance that nature offers us, do we really think that we can make it better without compromising health and well being?

Edwin Flatte, writes in The *Natural Nutrition Guide, "All fruits and vegetables in their natural state contain millions of living cells as well as vital enzymes. When food is subjected to intense heat for more then a few seconds, these enzymes and cells are devitalized."*

When the enzymes in fruits and vegetables are killed, our own body must be called upon to compensate by supplying the missing elements. This is an extraordinary drain on the body's reserves.

Foods ripened by Nature and cooked by the sun provide us ultimate nourishment. When we process or cook foods at high temperatures, we are changing and destroying some of the electrical energy - the life-giving properties of Prana, Tejas and Ojas.

A Life-Giving Approach to Eating

- Fresh, sun-ripened, organic plant foods contain enzymes that are the catalysts that regulate the digestive process in the body.
- Heating (or freezing) food degrades or destroys nutrients and enzymes in food.
- Foods without enzymes cause toxicity and obesity in the body.
- Nature's Prana, Tejas and Ojas rich foods have much higher nutrient values than foods which have been adulterated.
- Food that has been either frozen or heated over 118° F (44 degrees C) have lost most of it live-giving nutrients.

Nature's Foods vs Denatured Foods

Foods release their energy or Prana in the colon. This can provide long-term tissue building energy; however, when foods are cooked above 118 degrees F., much of the life-force of the food has been destroyed before it reaches the colon or, for that matter, even before the taste buds have a chance to taste them. The energies and materials that sustain life cannot be released from complex carbohydrates without the assistance of enzymes, which are destroyed in high temperatures. As well, nutrients are not properly digested or assimilated without enzymes. This leads to a build up of Ama, or toxins. Even though Ayurvedic food preparation uses certain herbs and spices to help stimulate the body to produce its own digestive enzymes, this can never replace the real thing.

There is a common misconception that processing or cooking foods at high temperatures makes them more digestible. While this is true in a few isolated incidences, on the whole it is utterly false. Heating at a high temperature can make a bad food safe to eat, but it never improves it or makes it a better food. It is more difficult for the digestive system to break down foods that are heated at high temperatures. The main reason is that, during the heating process, foods lose the nutrients that support the natural decomposing process and thus the supporting digestion.

When we experience discomfort, perhaps a stomachache, when eating live foods, this is not the result of the live food but because the digestive system or Agni (digestive fire) is deficient. Studies have shown that eighty percent of enzyme reserves are depleted by the time an individual is 30 years old. By the age of 50, half of the population has insufficient hydrochloric acid in the stomach, and 15 percent by the early age of 20. Many also have insufficient pancreatic and liver digestive juices; this is all because of improper eating habits. The shortage of any one of these will result in digestive disturbances. The whole subject of digestion is probably the most overlooked phase of human health care.

Nature Knows

All the species on this planet have been provided with foods that sustain them, without the necessity to transform the foods before consumption. All creatures have a natural, unadulterated diet, and my belief is that humans are no exception. We can find everything that we need for vital health from the trees and the plants, without needing to transform, denature or alter it in any way. Denatured or processed foods only seem to be more digestible and taste better because that is what we have been taught. If you give a baby the choice between whole, live foods and cooked food, they will choose the live foods. Their body knows. Of the 23 million creatures on this planet, we are the only ones who do to our foods what we do. Doesn't it make sense that nature would also provide her human children with foods that do not have to be cooked, microwaved or processed, in essence, de-natured, before consumption?

Nature gave us the sense of taste so we can decide what is healthy and delicious to eat and what is not. If it doesn't taste good in its fresh, whole, natural state, you may wish to reconsider your food choices. There is the power in nature. Let us tap into this power by making food choices that do not alter the power. **When you eat Alive, you feel Alive!**

A Sattvic Live-Food Approach

Remember, our body becomes what we eat. If we eat foods that are full of life-force, rich in enzymes, minerals and vitamins, this is what our body becomes. The healthier our body is the easier it is to experience the natural attunement with our true spiritual nature. Sattvic means "peaceful with essence," that which possesses the same nature as truth or reality. It is the cosmic force of balance and contentment. A Sattvic diet and lifestyle supports a spiritual life. Sattvic plant foods are those that are fresh and sweet, whole, sun-ripened, enzyme-rich, moist and organic.

Life-Force of Living Foods

Living-Foods are the wholeness of life. They are a gift of Mother Nature. Living-Foods literally mean wholeness. Modern day science seems to miss this picture, since the wholeness of living foods is really non-reproducible by scientific means, which tends to fragment nutrition.

The true purpose of a high quality diet is to assist in the expansion of our consciousness by providing a body which is free of Ama. It also helps purify the koshas, calm the mind, clear the nadis and supports the movement of prana. If we look at nutrition in its highest degree, we are following the example of the ancient rishi (sages) of India. They clearly understood that live-foods have the highest prana (life-force) and that prana helps to expand consciousness. This way of eating supports our spiritual growth and was the food of the rishi masters.

Dr. David Frawley, a Vedic and Ayurvedic scholar, states in his excellent book *'Yoga & Ayurveda'* that the traditional Yogic texts emphasized a way of eating that was a living-foods diet and primarily plant-based and high in prana. Also included, was an emphasis on wildcrafted foods and high-soma herbs and foods as well.

Denatured-Foods vs Living-Foods

Denatured foods cannot create true health because they are missing vital elements needed by the body for optimal functioning, like enzymes, oxygen, hormones, phytochemicals, bio-electrical energy and life-force. When foods are heated above 118° F, they begin to lose all of these. Over heating a food depletes it of its vital energy. Yes, some of the vitamins, minerals, carbohydrates, fats and proteins are still there, but in a greatly altered state – not at all what nature provided and therefore less able to be assimilated and with much less vitality.

Life force means "the energy that is able to create life." The sprouting ability of live foods demonstrates the presence of the life-force within them. Through observation, you can easily demonstrate for yourself what you are losing by eating denatured foods. A food that cannot create life cannot give our body the life-force energy needed for a long and healthy life.

Heating foods to high temperatures disrupts its molecular structure and kills all the enzymes as well. Enzymes are the indispensable catalysts that enable the body to utilize vitamins and minerals. Enzymes are extremely heat-sensitive and thus do not survive in high temperatures. As well, the vitamins and phytochemicals are injured and greatly diminished and left in an altered molecular state. The minerals are made less soluble. The fats have turned from life enhancing fatty acids to trans-fatty acids, which create damaging free radicals in the body. Trans-fatty acids also interfere with respiration of the cells. The proteins (including vegetable proteins) become denatured; they then coagulate (like the white of an egg) and are very difficult to digest. Some researchers report that un-metabolized protein particles in the bloodstream are a possible cause of allergies.

When you eat enzymeless foods, you put a heavy burden on your body that then has to produce the enzymes missing in the food. One of the reasons you feel lethargic or sleepy after a denatured meal is because the body is diverting its energy to replacing the enzymes that were not supplied. By comparison, a life-giving meal leaves you feeling light and full of energy. You can judge this for yourself. Fresh sun-ripened foods digest in 1/3 to 1/2 the time of denatured foods. The stress of creating and restoring enzymes, meal after meal, day after day, year after year, significantly contributes to a speeding up of the aging process. This is one of the main ways your body becomes low in Agni.

Ingesting denatured food also causes the body to produce a surge of white blood cells (leukocytosis). These cells normally defend against disease, infection and injury to the body, but their production is a routine effect of ingesting denatured foods (as if the body considers such food a threat or danger). Because leukocytes carry a variety of enzymes, there is another possible explanation for the increase in white blood cells. The leukocytes may be delivering the missing enzymes so that digestion can proceed unhindered. Leukocytosis does not occur when raw foods, cold or heated at low temperatures, are eaten. According to Viktoras Kulvinskas, *in any pathological condition, including the intoxification of the digestive system with foods cooked at high temperatures or other toxic materials, these white cells increase from 5 or 6 thousand per cubic millimeter to 7, 8 or 9 thousand per cu.m.m.* Leukocytosis also occurs when additives, pesticides and chemically based supplements are ingested; and, of course, producing these cells creates an additional stress upon the body.

Contrary to general belief, or misbelief, a major proportion of food enzymes are not denatured by stomach acid and can actually remain active throughout the digestive tract. Well over 50% of enzymes reach the colon unaltered. During this stage, they have the capacity to bring about changes in the intestinal environment by binding any free radical damage. This reduces the potential for fermentation and putrefaction and provides support in creating an environment in which healthy lactic-acid forming bacteria can thrive.

Nature's Antioxidants

What are antioxidants and how do they support body function? Antioxidants are substances that retard or prevent deterioration, damage or destruction by oxidation. There is a whole family of antioxidant enzymes that are in our healthy tissue as well as iron-containing transferring - a blood constituent which prevents the production of oxidative damaging molecules. In addition to these, nature provides us with antioxidant foods such as fresh orange and dark green fruit and vegetables as well as seeds, nuts, and sprouted whole grains, which are packed full of antioxidant nutrients that have the power to boost the body's natural antioxidant capacity.

12.1 Nine Antioxidants found in Food

Anthocyanidins	Found in all berries and grapes, most concentration found in the skin
Beta-carotene	Found in all yellowish-orange fruits and vegetables such as peaches, apricots, squash, pumpkin and carrots
Bioflavonoids	Found in all citrus fruits, most concentration is found in the white rind, also found in buckwheat, onions and garlic
Curcumin	Found in yellowish orange colored spices such as turmeric and mustard and some yellow foods like corn-on-the cob and yellow peppers
Lutein	Found in the carotene family and other dark-green vegetables such as spinach
Lycopene	Found in tomatoes
Proanthocyanidins	Found in green tea and grape seeds
Pycnogenal	Found in a large variety of fresh fruits and vegetables, most concentration found in Pinus maritma, a coast pine tree
Zeanzanthin	Found in most of the brassica or cabbage family and also spinach, peas and corn-on-the cob

Free Radicals

A free radical is a highly reactive molecule made inside the body. Free radicals are one electron molecule short (electrons are usually paired), so they grab an electron from another molecule, disturbing the chemical balance by making this molecule one electron short, thus setting up a chain reaction. Free radicals are produced constantly in the body as a part of normal functions. They need to be dealt with immediately because they can damage D.N.A. resulting in premature aging. Free radicals are produced whenever anything is burned or combustion occurs, so they will arise from tobacco smoke, exhaustion fumes, microwave radiation, fried, barbecued foods or foods heated to a high temperature. Natural oxidation processes occurring in the cells will produce their own free radicals. The body is designed to handle these easily if the body is in a natural state of balance.

It is when free radicals are present in excess that cellular damage occurs. This is because essential fatty acids and proteins in cell membranes become unstable and their traffic-directing effect of balancing the flow of nutrients in and out of the cells becomes ineffective. When the cell membrane is oxidized, it is either hardened so that nutrients cannot get to the cell, or it may be punctured so that the cell collapses as the cell fluid drains out. It is this that begins the aging process.

Cell Damage

The D.N.A. is damaged when the free radicals have gone into the genetic material of the cells. This causes inappropriate cell division and other changes that may lead to the progression of tumors and cancers. When free radicals are destroying more cells then we can create, they are then capable of causing inflammation and arterial damage, triggering cancer and speeding up the aging process.

With each passing year, there is more research affirming that oxidation damage is one of the main causes behind the aging phenomena and certain diseases. One of the best ways to reduce the amount of free radical damage is to eat fresh foods, such as fruits, vegetables and sprouted whole grains, nuts and seeds. A person enjoying the Sattvic diet and lifestyle will exhibit a tongue that is full of integrity and health.

Living on Nature's Foods

Nature has provided us with foods that are full of oxygen, especially green leafy vegetables, which contain an abundance of chlorophyll. The chemical structure of chlorophyll is almost identical to the hemoglobin in our red blood cells. The only difference is that the hemoglobin molecule has iron in its nucleus and the chlorophyll molecule has magnesium. Chlorophyll detoxifies the bloodstream better than anything else you could eat. When you eat fresh green chlorophyll foods, you oxygenate the blood. The bloodstream, through its capillary system, then delivers this oxygen to every cell in the body.

Soaked and sprouted grains, seeds and nuts contain vital elements that nourish our glands, nerves and brain. The hormones needed by the body are created out of the natural fat and other essential principles found in seeds. Reflect for a moment on how few seeds are found in the standard diet. The plant breeders are hybridizing almost all of the seeds out of our foods. Now we can get seedless watermelons, seedless grapes, seedless citrus, etc. Most people do not realize the importance of seeds and will disregard them rather than eat them. The seed is the beginning of life. It holds the "essence."

When you eat cooked starch, the body absorbs more than it needs. Getting rid of the excess starch then becomes another burden to the body. Those who favor cooking foods at high temperatures often make the point that since the body cannot absorb raw starch, that this is a sign the food should be cooked. Another way to look at this is that the body absorbs just enough of the raw starch for its needs and then passes out the rest. (When pig farmers feed their pigs raw potatoes, the pigs stay slender. Since farmers sell their pigs by the pound, they have learned to feed them cooked potatoes, which fatten them up.)

Cellulose, the woody, fibrous part of food, was previously believed to be unnecessary to the body. Because the body did not absorb it, it wasn't deemed important. Now we know that this fiber is what keeps things moving through our body so that we don't become constipated. Nature is justified once again. Natural whole foods high in fiber have the ability to act as a broom that sweeps the intestinal tract and keeps it clean. However, denatured fiber has lost the ability to do this for us. Colonics (a form of bowel cleansing) serve their purpose, but they are a poor substitute for what nature's foods have provided.

Foods high in nature's life-giving elements nourish and improve the body's internal environment. These foods enable the body to remove impurities. If there is a foreign substance in the body, the body will do everything in its power to remove it. Our natural body only knows how to use natural ingredients that have not been denatured.

Eating denatured food prevents the immune system from working on what is really vital. We exhaust and dissipate the body's strength by using the immune system to combat the effects of denatured and processed foods, chemically based supplements, pesticides, herbicides, fungicides, hormones (in meats, poultry, fish and dairy) and numerous other toxins we ingest, breathe in or absorb through our skin. What we really need is the immune system to support us, as when a disease or infection develops or an injury occurs. Yet, oftentimes, it is exhausted and lacks the strength to defend us properly.

Each cell of the body is like a tiny battery. To recharge a battery it requires the right electrical frequency. The same is true of our cells. The frequency that resonates, and therefore recharges, our cells can only come from a food that holds that similar frequency. Living foods do. Studies have been done with Kirlian photography showing the electrical discharges that naturally emanate from all living foods as luminescent, aura-like flares surrounding the subject, glowing brightly and radiant. The reverse is true of Kirlian pictures of cooked or processed foods. There is almost a total absence of life-force present.

The following is a passage from an article written by Dr. Gabriel Cousens, M.D., entitled *Living Foods: The Next Evolutionary Step* in which he states his view on the energetics of living food.

"Harry Oldfield and Roger Coghill in their book The Dark Side of the Brain discovered (with Kirlian photography research), that live foods are rich in Prana, Teja and Oja were surrounded by a considerably stronger bioluminescent field than processed foods. This field is related with greater cell bioelectricity and life force. Nobel laureate Szent-Gyorgyi described the essential life process as a little electric current sent to us by the sunshine. Live food is filled with these live electrons from the sun because the living food has not had its electron patterns (energized by the forces of nature) disrupted by cooking or processing in any way. I agree with Dr. Johanna Budwig, who holds degrees in medicine, physics, pharmacy, and biochemistry, that electron-rich live foods act as high powered electron donors and as solar resonant fields in the body to attract, store and conduct the sun's energy in our bodies. She feels, as I do, that the photons of sunlight are attracted by like electrons resonating in our own system, especially in the double bonded electron clouds found in our lipid systems, such as in flax oil."

"People who eat refined, cooked, highly processed foods diminish the amount of solar electrons energizing their bioelectric system. In fact, according to Dr. Budwig, processed foods may even act as insulators to the healthy flow of electricity in our bodies. The more we absorb solar electrons through live foods, the better we are able to resonate, attract, and absorb electrons in direct resonance from the sun and other star systems."

Eating healthy means giving yourself nature's best. Foods that have been unadulterated are easily assimilated and used for regeneration and rejuvenation. Life comes from life. The more you include nature's bountiful fresh organic foods in your diet, the more you will know what is means to be vibrantly healthy.

Without good health, the richest person in the world is poor. Without sufficient digestive fire-enzymes, the best food in the world is poorly digested.

12.2 The 10 Keys for Determining the Quality of Food

1. WHOLE: Whole foods are a complete food, packed in their own wrapping, complete with all their fiber, macronutrients, minerals, vitamins, phytonutrients and all the nutrients that science has yet to discover. Whole foods are always fresher and tastier.
2. FRESH: When a food is eaten fresh, it still contains all its life-force. Fresh means it is at its fullest potential with its rich array of nutrients, aroma, taste and color. Fresh is always the most nutritious. Fresh foods have ripened to perfection.
3. SUN-RIPENED: Means the sun has completed its cooking process for us. It tells us that the food is ripened to perfection and been imbued with the vital forces of the sun. When a food has fully ripened, the nutrient content of the food is now available for easier assimilation. Foods at the ripest stage have the greatest enzymes available. This is their peak stage. Foods that have been ripened by the sun have the greatest enzyme content.
4. ENZYME-RICH: Foods with the greatest enzyme content are those that are fresh and have naturally ripened on the vine. They have the most Agni potential and are the easiest to assimilate. They aid in the digestive process, creating

less work for our bodies, as compared to eating a processed food. Enzyme-rich foods have a wonderful scent and mouth-watering flavor. They have more nutrients and less calories then processed enzyme deficient foods. Most enzyme-rich foods are high on the alkaline pH scale.

5. ALKALIZING: Any food that is alkalizing will have more of a cleansing and purification effect on both the body and mind. They give the body a refreshing feeling. When a food is whole and fresh it will be much more alkalizing then a processed food. Our body needs high-alkaline fuel to work at its peak. Our body thrives in an alkaline environment. Mineral dense foods are organic foods.
6. ORGANIC: Since the beginning of time foods have been organic, with the exception of the last 60 years with the introduction of herbicides, pesticides, fungicides, insecticides, plant hormones, chemical fertilizers, irradiation and biotechnology. This new way of growing food has created serious human and environmental health challenges. Organically-grown food is much more nutritious, tastes better, is more easily assimilated by the body and has a vibration that is more attuned to the human body. The richer the soil is on minerals, the better it will taste with less concentrated sugars.
7. LOW-GLYCEMIC: Minimize high-sugar foods in your diet. Low-glycemic foods balance blood sugar levels. They also support a calm disposition and a balanced energy level. It is also much easier to meditate and have peace of mind. Foods with less sugar concentration are foods with high mineralization.
8. HIGH-MINERALIZED: Foods that are mineral-rich and packed full of trace minerals support the body and mind to function at its peak. This is due to all the physical body organs and glands have the nutrients they need to do their job. Mineral-rich foods hold more fluids and structured water.
9. WELL HYDRATED: Foods that well hydrated are high in hydrogen offered by structured water keep the body lubricated to run smoothly. Pick foods that are fresh and juicy. Pick foods that are fresh and juicy as they are more Sattvic.
10. SATTVIC: Choosing foods that are Sattvic in nature helps to create a peaceful body, mind and heart. By purchasing

Sattvic foods you are support in creating a more peaceful world. Foods in their pure form are the most Sattivic.

As you are making these conscious food choices to pick foods that are in season and appropriate according to your genetic constitutional blueprint.

Feel Alive!

Try it for yourself. For the next month create a diet that is 80% fresh, organic fruits, vegetables, seeds and nuts, sprouted whole grains, sea vegetables and algaes. Even better, if you really want to feel the difference, avoid all cooked food for one month. However, if this is a little too extreme for you right now, just do 80% and see what happens. You may well feel a remarkable increase in vitality, energy level, clarity of mind and peace of heart. Then go back to the way you used to eat (although you will likely not want to), evaluate and see the difference. Everyone can do something for one month, particularly if it can transform your life in a positive way. You are the scientist of your own life. Through curiosity and experimentation you will discover what is best, healthiest, most natural and joyful for yourself.

Peace through a Sattvic Diet

A Life Enhancing Diet to Balance the Mind

"Food is a dynamic force which interacts with the human on the physical body level, the mind emotional level, and also the energetic and spiritual level. The study of nutrition is the study of the interaction with and assimilation of the dynamic forces of food by the dynamic forces of our total being."

— Gabriel Cousens, M.D., 'Spiritual Nutrition and The Rainbow Diet

The Three Gunas

In the unmanifested Universe, energy has three qualities known as Gunas that exist together in equilibrium: Sattva (purity) Rajas (activity, passion, the process of change) and Tamas (darkness, inertia).Once energy takes form, one quality of the three predominates. Thus, on an apple tree some of the fruit is ripening (rajasic) some is ripe (sattva) and some overripe (tamasic).But no matter which quality prevails, an Element of each of the other two will always be present as well. An apple may be ripe, but part will be rotting even if the naked eye cannot see it, and part will be in the process of changing from one state to the other. The three gunas encompass all existence, all actions. If a man commits a robbery, the action is basically rajasic, but the decision to rob and the motive may be predominantly tamasic, rajasic or sattvic, according to the situation. In all people, one of the three gunas has superior strength and is reflected in all they do and think. Only in enlightenment are the gunas completely transcended.

Ancient Rishis have said you take on the karma of the animal you eat. When you eat meat you are ingesting all the stress hormones released when that animal was killed. The hormones released at death are present in the flesh when you eat it. At a cellular level, your body is getting the message that you are dying.

One goal and effect of Ayurveda and following a spiritual path is to raise our vibrational levels. Meat has a very low vibration. On a continuum of lower vibrations, fish, chicken, lamb, beef and finally pork have increasingly lower vibrations and their energy is very dark, dense and congested. Through the centuries it has been observed that vegetarians have a more refined Etheric body and brighter aura. A vegetarian, whose etheric body is brighter and healthier will generally heal at a much faster rate than those who are not vegetarian.

Ayurvedic Principles

Everything on earth has a primary quality (guna). Anything we hear, smell, see, taste or touch may be classified into the categories of sattvic, rajasic or tamasic.

Balancing the Emotional Body With Food

In Ayurveda, a dietary system was developed by the ancient masters and sages to support the development of the mind and help an individual on a spiritual path. The diet was complimented with yoga and meditation practices.

Sattvic foods all have one thing in common: they are high in Prana, the universal life force. More specifically, sattvic foods are natural, organically grown and as unrefined as possible. As was mentioned, modern food processing methods take the Prana out of many foods and make them heavy, impotent and lifeless - or simply "dead food."

Mind balance in Ayurveda means modifying the mind from tamasic or rajasic to a sattvic state. Choosing foods and activities that are sattvic in nature, in preference to those that are rajasic or tamasic, does that. With consistent and dedicated attention to diet, environment and sensory experiences, total mind balance can be achieved.

It often takes discipline and effort to become sattvic, but the peace of mind, health, strength and immunity that is obtained from this state of mind makes it worthwhile. However, some rajas and tamas qualities are still required. Rajas for action and motivation to achieve our goals and tamas for inaction such as sleep or relaxation.

There are three types of foods categorized by their primal essence or nature:

Tamasic Foods

Tamas energy is heavy, dark and dull. A tamasic diet benefits neither the mind nor the body. Prana, or energy, is withdrawn, powers of reasoning become clouded and a sense of inertia sets in. The body's resistance to disease is destroyed and the mind is filled with dark emotions such as jealousy and greed.

Tamasic foods include: meat, poultry, fish, eggs, onions, garlic, fermented foods such as vinegars, left over foods, contaminated or overripe foods, alcohol, tobacco and other intoxicants including drugs. Foods that are over-processed, no longer fresh and/or difficult to digest are Tamasic. Foods that are prepared unconsciously or while the preparer is in a negative mood are also considered tamasic as is overeating. If you are interested in vital health and spiritual growth, it is best to avoid tamasic foods, it is the unhealthiest food of all.

Rajasic Foods

Rajas signifies the "can do" kind of energy. It is the energy we need to accomplish, create and achieve. It represents worldly power and the sex drive. To include some rajasic foods is good for "householders" who aspire to maintain a meditative mind but need to live and work in the world as well. It has been recommended by the ancient Rishis teachers that a combination of sattvic and rajasic foods are beneficial for those who practice demanding disciplines such as endurance athletics, martial arts and Kundalini Yoga.

Foods that are very hot, bitter, sour, dry or salty are rajasic. Too much rjasic food will over stimulate the body and excite strong emotional qualities and passions, making the mind restless and uncontrollable. Rajasic foods include hot substances such as sharp spices or strong herbs, stimulants like coffee and tea, meat of animals and fish, eggs, salt and chocolate. Many of the ground foods are rajasic. Eating in a hurry is also considered rajasic.

Sattvic Foods

Sattvic foods are light, soothing and easily digested. Sattvic signifies etheric qualities and includes foods such as fruits and vegetables, especially sun foods and ground foods. Many sattvic foods are sun foods that grow one meter or more above the ground. They draw energy from the earth and are high in nutrients. They have a quickening and lightening effect on the body's nervous and digestive systems. Sattvic foods include sprouted whole grains, fresh fruit, land and sea vegetables, pure fruit juices, nut and seed milk and cheese, legumes, nuts, seeds, sprouted seeds, honey and herb teas. Sattvic foods are those foods which do not agitate your stomach at all. According to the diet, the best foods are those that are fresh, have a balance of all the six tastes and are consumed in moderate portions.

Becoming Sattvic

One should focus on work, self-improvement and intellectual or spiritual pursuits. Maintaining a positive nature, demonstrating generosity, kindness, openness, fairness (equality) and forgiveness increase the sattva guna. In addition, spiritual inclination, faith and belief in God, engaging in selfless service or charitable activities help one to become sattvic.

Spiritual Nutrition: Feeding the Body-Nourishing the Spirit

To truly be healthy, we need to be fed and be nourished on all levels. The tongue is not just a diagnosis of the physical body, but also on the deeper, emotional and spiritual levels. I do not believe that we can be healthy if we ignore these other levels. By choosing sattvic foods and bringing sacredness to our meal times we nourish our spirit.

> *"Nature's life-giving foods are God's gift to us to support us in taking the next evolutionary step on this planet into our destiny as peaceful, free, and joyous spiritual human beings."*
> — Gabriel Cousens, M.D., 'Spiritual Nutrition and The Rainbow Diet'

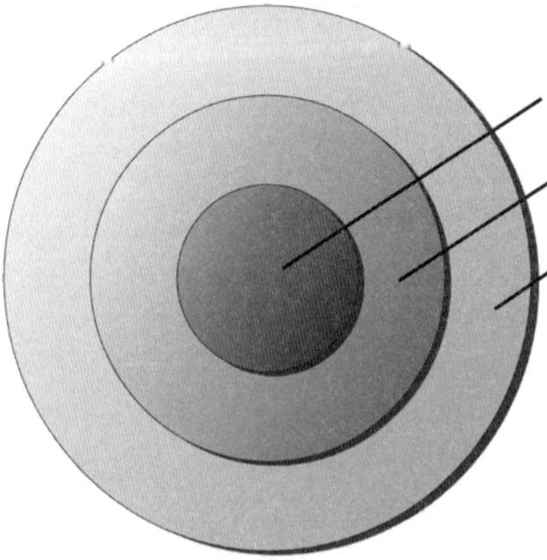

12.3 Nature's Sattvic Food

Nature's Sattvic Foods				
Fruits	Apples Apricots Bananas Cantaloupe Cherries Cranberry Grapefruits	Grapes Guava Kiwi Loquat Lychee Mango Melons	Honeydew Peaches Pears Prunes Tangerines Pomegranate Papaya	Nectarines Oranges Pineapples Plums Persimmons Watermelon
Vegetables	Artichokes Beets Daikon Fennel Shallots Lettuce Asparagus Shitake Mushrooms	Spinach Squash Eggplant Corn Green Beans Celery Chard	Watercress Leeks Carrots Sprouts Endive Yams Peas Parsnips	Cabbage Family: Bok Choy Broccoli Brussels Sprouts Cabbage Turnips Mustard Greens Radishes Cauliflower Kale

Nature's Sattvic Foods	
Sprouted Whole Grains	Amaranth, Buckwheat, Bulgur, Millet, Quinoa, Rye Rice: Basmati, Brown, Wild
Beans & Legumes	Adzuki, Garbanzo, Kidney, Lentils, Lima, Mung, Navy, Pinto, Split Peas
Nuts, seeds & Oils	Olive, Sesame, Sunflower, Hemp, Brazil Nuts, Pumpkin Seeds, Walnuts, Flax, Olive
Spices	Asafoetida (hing), Basil, Black Pepper, Cardamom, Cinnamon, Cloves Coriander, Cumin, Fennel seed, Fenugreek, Ginger, Horseradish, Nutmeg, Parsley, Turmeric
Sweeteners	Yacon root syrup, Raw carob, Mesquite meal, Raw Cacao, Dark Agave nectar, Cane juice, Raw Honey, Stevia, Fruit Juices, Dried Fruits, Maple Syrup, Most Berries & Fruit
Nut & Seed Milks, Cheeses & Yogurt	Almond or other nut or seed milk, Coconuts, Pecans

12.4 Relationship to Sattvic, Rajasic and Tamasic Foods

Foods	Sattvic	Rajasic	Tamasic
Fruits	Sweet Fruits: coconut, dates, figs, peaches, pears, mango, pomegranate	Sour Fruits: citrus, apples, guava, tamarind, apple	Fruit is overall sattvic, some oily fruits can be classified as tamasic
Vegetables	Sweet Vegetables: yams and sweet potatoes, asparagus, sprouts, leafy greens, lettuce, pumpkin, squash, zucchini	Nightshade Family: potatoes, peppers, eggplants, Cabbage Family: broccoli, Brussels sprouts, collards, cauliflower, broccoli, kohlrabi, daikon, radish, kale Onion Family: garlic, leeks, etc. Fermented Foods: pickles, sauerkraut, Kim chi	mushrooms, bland or dull tasting foods, also old and aged foods

12.5 A Food Plan to Balance Vata Dosha

Foods	Sattvic	Rajasic	Tamasic
Nuts and Seeds	Sweet Tasting: almonds, sesame seeds, fresh cashews, the fresher the sweeter they will be, also when soaked become more sattvic	nut and seed oils, also mustard seed oil, and buckwheat which is actually a seed	rancid nuts, peanuts, and dark bitter tasting nuts and seeds
Whole Grains	sprouted whole grains that are sweet in taste, quinoa, barley, blue corn, basmati rice	most grains that have processed, millet, corn and buckwheat	all grains that have been milled, baked or cooked, wheat, brown rice
Beans and Legumes	sprouted mung beans, red and yellow lentils	adzuki beans, brown lentils, and small amouns of black, pinto, pink beans	large amounts of black, pinto and pink beans
Herbs and Spices	Most Culinary Seeds and Mild Spices: fennel, dill, cumin, coriander, cardamom, saffron, turmeric	Hot Spices: curry, chili, cayenne and black pepper	most herbs that don't have much flavor
Drinks and Juices	sweet tasting spices and root herbs	coffee, black and green tea	most alcohol and drugs
Sweets	fresh sugarcane juice, raw honey, stevia leaves, fruits, berries, agave syrup, Yacon necter	processed sugar, artificial sweeteners, all cooked honey and sweeteners	molasses, soft drinks, processed or cooked foods that become sweet
Mental State	consciousness, meditation, spiritual practices and chanting	thinking, concentration, excessive travel and movement	unconsciousness, excessive sleep, laziness, coma
Emotions	love, compassion, forgiveness	anger, anxiety, jealousy, envy	attachment, depression, loneliness, drowsiness

These guidelines can be used for Vata mind-body constitutions, to maintain dosha balance, and to restore balance when necessary, regardless of the basic constitution. Vata influences the movement of thoughts, feelings, Prana flows, nerve impulses, and fluids in the body.

Favor:

Warm food, moderately heavy textures, added oils and fats.

Salt, Sour, and Sweet tastes; soothing and satisfying foods.

All soothing foods are good for settling disturbed Vata. Use foods such as: warm soaked nut and seed milks, warm soups, stews, sprouted warm whole grain cereals, sprouted breads. Since Vata is a cold dry dosha, warm, nourishing foods such as these are good for stabilizing Vata. On the other hand cold foods such as cold foods, iced drinks, hard to digest cabbage family use in moderation for persons with Vata imbalance.

Breakfast is highly recommended. Use sprouted whole grains such as Amaranth, Kamut, Oatgroats and Kamut, or any other breakfast that is warm, soothing, milky, and sweet.

Take a warm herbal tea with snacks in the late afternoon.

Use spicy foods such as spicy Mexican or Indian foods with plenty of high quality cold-pressed oils.

Use warm moist foods such as sprouted whole grains, bowl of warm oat groat gruel or cup of warm vegetable soup.

Warm nut and seed milk is good. You can add a little stevia to it if you prefer.

Prefer fresh nuts that are heavy and oily as opposed to dry salty snacks.

All sweet fruits are okay for Vata.

Take warm water instead of ice water and cold drinks.

Summary: Breakfast is usually desirable. Warming foods and Sweet and Sour tastes. Warm water, herbal teas and fresh juices. Raw nuts and nut butters. Spices: cinnamon, cardamom, cumin, ginger, cloves in moderation.

Avoid:

Avoid unripe fruits as they are Astringent.
Reduce dry foods and Bitter tastes.
Avoid drinks with high caffeine as it disturbs Vata.
Avoid eating candies as it disturbs Vata.

12.6 Nutritional Protocol for Vata

Nutritional Protocol for Vata			
Nourishing Elements	Fire, Water, Earth		
Nourishing Attributes	Moist, Heavy, Smooth, Warm		
Nourishing Tastes	Sweet, Salty, Sour		
Essential Minerals	Calcium, Copper, Iron, Magnesium, Zinc		
Fruits	_Sweet Fruits:_ Apricots, Avocados, Bananas, Berries, Cherries, Coconut, Fresh figs, Papaya, Peaches, Plums	_Sour Fruits:_ Grapefruit, Lemons, Grapes, Mangos, Sweet melons, Sour oranges, Pine-apples	_All Berries:_ Blackberries, Blueberries, Cranberries, Currants Black & Red, Goji (Lycii) berries, Goose berries, Huckle berries, Mulberries, Raspberries, Strawberries
Vegetables	_Warm vegetables:_ Asparagus, Beets, Carrots, Garlic, Green beans, Onions, dried Pars-nips, Peas, Pump-kin, Squash, Sweet potato, Tomatoes *Leafy greens in moderation	_Sea Vegetables:_ All sea veg-etables are excellent for Vata individuals	_*Cabbage (Sulfur) Fam-ily:_ (Best when Marinated, Fermented, Blended, Dried or Spiced) Arugula, Broccoli, Brussel sprouts, Bok choy, All Cabbage Family Sprouts, Cabbage, Cauliflower, Chinese Cab-bage, Collards, All Cresses, Diakon radish, Flowering Cabbage, Horseradish, Kale, Kohlrabi, Maca, All Mustards, Mustard, Mustard greens, Rappani, Radish, Rutabaga, Savoy Cabbage, Turnip, Watercress

Nutritional Protocol for Vata			
Nuts, Seeds & Oils	*All Nuts should be soaked:* Almonds, Brazil nuts, Cashews, Coconuts, Filberts, Hazelnuts, Macadamia nuts, Pecans, Pistachios, Pine nuts, Walnuts	*All Seeds should be soaked:* Chia seeds, Flax seeds, Hemp seeds, Golden flax seeds, Poppy Seeds, Pumpkin seeds, Sesame seeds, Sunflower seeds, Sunflower, Tahini	*Note*: are acceptable in small amounts.
Sprouted Whole Grains	Amaranth, Kamut, Oatgroats, Quinoa	Rice Brown, Spelt, Wild Rice	
Culinary Spices	Sweet and/or Warming herbs and spices, such as: Allspice, Anise, Asafoetida, Basil, Bay leaf, Black pepper (use sparingly)	Caraway, Cardamom, Cilantro (green coriander), Clove, Cumin, Cinnamon, Fennel, Fenugreek, Ginger, Juniper berries, Licorice root	Mace, Marjoram, Mustard, Nutmeg, Orange peel, Oregano, Sage, Tarragon, Thyme
Herbal Teas	Sweet & Nourishing Teas: Ajwan (Celery Seeds), Chamomile, Comfrey, Elderberry, Eucalyptus,	Fenugreek, Licorice Rt., Marshmallow, Lemon grass, Lavender, Hawthorn	Juniper berry, Oatstraw, Raspberry lf., Rosehip, Saffron, Sarsaparilla, Sassafras
Whole Food Supplements	Bee Pollen, Royal Jelly, Spirulina, Blue Green Algae	Nutritional Yeast, Aloe Vera Gel, Green Kamut, Green Chlorella	
Exercise	30 minutes 3 times per week Gentle movement Yoga	Walking Chi Gong Deep Breathing	
Avoid or Reduce	*Elements:* Air & Ether *Attributes:* Dry, Cold, Light, Mobile, Erratic *Tastes:* Bitter, Astringent, Pungent		

Vata dosha is aggravated and increased during autumn and early winter. During these seasons all mind-body types can include some of the above foods and decrease others.

Mental and emotional peace and constructive lifestyle routines are important to re-establishing and maintaining balance.

If your basic constitution is mixed (Vata-Pitta or Vata-Kapha), include portions of the second influential dosha.

General Tips on Health and Wellness for Vata Types

The Vata individuals find it very difficult to maintain regular habits, that is, to eat and sleep at regular times. But this is the most important thing for them to do. When Vata is out of balance this may feel almost impossible, but an effort to establish a regular routine is very important for all people with a Vata body type. Rest sufficiently, and choose foods, behaviors, personal relationships, and environmental circumstances, which can be instrumental in balancing Vata characteristics. It is also important to regulate mental and physical impulses and to modify mental attitudes, emotional states, and behaviors in supportive ways.

Sweet, Sour, and Salty tastes decrease Vata influences, so include these tastes if Vata influences need to be diminished. Nut and seeds milks, sprouted whole grains such as kamut, wheat, oat groats, wild rice and some fruits and berries can provide Sweet and Sour tastes.

Regular exercise should be relaxed and moderate. A regular movement practice in a meditative mood is good, as are also yoga, chi gong, tai chi, walking, and swimming. Avoid strenuous, competitive, frantic activities.

When possible, associate with people who are calmly purposeful. Meditate every day for deep relaxation.

12.7 A Food ood Plan to Balance Pitta Dosha

These guidelines can be used for Pitta mind-body constitutions, to maintain dosha balance and to restore balance if necessary regardless of the basic constitution. Pitta influences digestion and metabolism, body temperature, and biological transformations.

Favor:

- Use Bitter, Sweet, and Astringent tastes
- When practical, use less oils and added fatty foods. Consume food with moderately heavy textures.

- Take cool, refreshing food in summer. Salads are good, so is soaked nut and seeds milks.
- Herb tea is good. Prefer mint, licorice root or other Pitta pacifying teas.
- Breakfast: Cooling sprouted whole grain cereals sprinkled with cinnamon, and apple tea is a good breakfast for Pitta.
- The vegetarian foods are the best for Pitta. Consume abundant amounts of soaked nut and seed milks, sprouted whole grains and fresh vegetables.
- Eat carbohydrates foods such as root vegetables, sprouted whole grains and legumes.
- Cool or warm but do not steam hot cooked foods.

Avoid:

- Reduce the consumption of salt, oil, and spices, all of which are heating to the body.
- Avoid the tendency to overeat under stress.
- Avoid oily, hot, salty, and heavy foods such as fried food.
- Avoid consuming red meat tends to heat the body from the fat.
- Coffee is also Pitta aggravating due to the acid in coffee, as is also orange juice and doughnuts.
- Avoid processed and fast foods, as they tend to be heavy on salt and sour tastes. Japanese and Chinese foods are good choices. Avoid highly spicy food such as is found in Mexican restaurants.
- Avoid pickles, yogurt, sour cream, and cheese. Avoid vinegar in salad dressing; use lemon juice instead. Alcoholic and fermented foods should be avoided. Their Sour Rasa aggravates Pitta.
- Avoid the use of too much Salt, overuse of Sour and Pungent food and overeating.

Summary: Avoid egg yolks, hot spices, and hot drinks. Use honey in moderation. Cool foods and juices are better. Add Sweet, Bitter, and Astringent tastes. Reduce use of Sour tastes. Spices: black pepper, coriander, and cardamom.

12.8 Nutritional Protocal for Pitta

Nutritional Protocol for Pitta			
Nourishing Elements	Water, Air, Earth, Ether		
Nourishing Attributes	Cool, Substantial, Aromatic, Calming		
Nourishing Tastes	Sweet, Bitter, Astringent		
Essential Minerals	Copper, Iron, Magnesium, Potassium		
Macro-nutrients	Carbohydrate 60-70%	Protein 20%	Fat 10-15%
Fruits	*Sweet Fruits:* Apples, Avocados, Cherries, Coconut, Figs, Dark grapes, Mangoes, Melons	Oranges, Pears, Pineapples, Plums, Prunes, Raisins	*Note:* Fruits should be sweet and ripe.
Vegetables	*Cooling Sweet & Bitter Vegetables:* Asparagus, Beets, Beet greens, Bitter melon, Broccoli, Brussels sprouts, Cabbage, Carrots, Cauliflower, Celery, Chard, Cucumber, Dandelion greens, Endive Green beans, Green (sweet) peppers, Jerusalem artichokes	Kale, Leafy green vegetables, Lettuce, Mushrooms, Okra, Parsley, Peas, Sprouts, Squash, Sweet potatoes, Tomatoes, Turnips, Watercress, Zucchini	*Sea Vegetables:* Arami, Dulse, Kelp, Kombu, Hijiki, Nori
Nuts, Seeds & Oils	*All Nuts & Seeds should be soaked:* Almond	Coconut, Olive, Hemp seeds	Pumpkin seeds, Sesame seeds, Sunflower seeds
Sprouted Whole Grains	Barley, Buckwheat, Corn, Kamut, Millet	Spelt, Oat Groats, Wheat, Brown Basmati Rice, Wild Rice	
Beans & Legumes	All Beans & Legumes Soaked & Sprouted	Aduki beans, Chick-peas	Green peas, Mung beans

Nutritional Protocol for Pitta			
Culinary Spices	*Herbs and spices, such as:* Basil, Cardamom, Cinnamon, Cilantro (green coriander), Cinnamon, Coriander seed, Cumin, Dill, Fennel	Marjoram, Miso, Saffron, Tarragon, Thyme, Turmeric, Savory, Vanilla, Plus small amounts of cumin and black pepper	*Note:* Spices are generally avoided as too heating. In small amounts, the following Sweet and Astringent spices are good.
Herbal Teas	*Cooling & Refreshing Teas:* Alfalfa, Burdock, Blackberry, Catnip, Chamomile, Chicory, Cornsilk	Dandelion, Elderflower, Fennel, Hibiscus Hops, Honeysuckle, Lemon balm, Licorice root, Lemon grass	Mint, Nettle, Oatstraw, Peppermint, Red clover, Sarsaparilla, Spearmint, Violet, Wintergreen
Whole Food Supplements	Aloe Vera Gel, Spirulina, Blue Green Algae	Green Kamut, Green Chlorella, Kamut Grass	Nutritional Yeast, Wheat Grass
Exercise	40 Minutes 4 times per week Outdoor Activities Gardening	Walking Hiking Yoga Swimming Water skiing	Snow skiing Running Biking Tennis Calming Exercises Meditation
Avoid or Reduce	*Elements:* Fire *Attributes:* Hot, Oily, Light, Intense, Fluid, Fetid *Tastes:* Sour, Pungent, Salty		

Pitta dosha is aggravated and increased during summer. During hot, dry seasons, all mind-body types can choose some of the above foods and decrease others.

Mental and emotional peace and positive lifestyle routines are important to re-establish and maintaining balance.

If your basic constitution is mixed (Pitta-Vata or Pitta-Kapha), to maintain balance, include smaller portions for the second dosha.

General Tips on Health and Wellness For Pitta Persons Pitta constitutions will be disturbed by alcohol and cigarettes, as well as by overwork, overexertion, and overheating. When out of balance, they are vulnerable to feeling such negative emotions as aggression, hatred, intolerance, and resentment. Therefore it is very essential for Pitta people to remain cool (literally and figuratively) and to lead a wholesome and modest lifestyle. Choose foods, attitude, behaviors, personal relationships, and environmental conditions, which can be helpful in balancing Pitta character.

Because Sweet, Bitter, and Astringent tastes decrease Pitta influences, include these in your food plan if Pitta characteristics are too pronounced. Complex carbohydrates, soaked nut and seed milks, and some fruits are Sweet; some green, leafy vegetables are Bitter; beans and some green vegetables are Astringent.

Do things that cool the mind, emotions, and body. Avoid conflicts. Cultivate the virtues of honesty, morality, kindness, generosity, and self-control.

12.9 A Food Plan to Balance Kapha Dosha

These guidelines can be used for Kapha mind-body constitutions, to maintain dosha balance, and to restore balance if necessary, regardless of the basic constitution. Kapha influences the heavy, moist aspects of the body.

Food to Eat to Balance Kapha:

- Warm, light food.
- Dry food, prepared without much water, minimum of oil and sweeteners.
- Stimulating foods with Pungent, Bitter, and Astringent tastes.
- Light meals are to be favored such as light breakfast and dinner.
- Eat lightly warmed foods or fresh fruits and vegetables. Eat spicy, Bitter and Astringent foods. Watch out for eating too much food, a typical Kapha tendency.
- Select warming food and dry food preparation methods (dehydrated foods, gently warmed, and fresh).
- As an appetizer eat Bitter or Pungent foods instead of Salty or Sour. Foods such as romaine lettuce and endive are good to stimulate your appetite.

- Take ginger tea or a pinch or ginger to stimulate appetite. Other preferred spices are cumin, fenugreek, sesame seed and turmeric.
- Any food that is spicy is good for Kapha individuals such as very hot Mexican or Indian food, especially in winter.
- Foods that are good for Kapha breakfast are warmed-spiced cider, soaked buckwheat gruel with freshly made apple butter, and Bitter cocoa made with nut or seed milk and a touch of stevia or honey.
- To pep you up in the morning, use stevia or unpasteurized honey, warm water, lemon juice and ginger. Try warm ginger tea. Try skipping a meal or two and take a spoonful of honey in warm water to keep you going.
- Eat fresh raw fruits, vegetables and salads.
- Eat salad with minimum salad dressing. Take a glass of warm water instead of ice water. Eat salad instead of soup especially in hot weather.

Avoid:

- Don't overindulge on dairy foods.
- Avoid deep fried foods.
- Avoid cold food whenever feasible
- Avoid cold foods and juice , and sugary foods
- Kapha individuals need to watch the consumption of too much sweet foods or fatty foods. Keep an eye on the salt consumption also, which tend to result in fluid retention in Kapha individuals.
- Kapha individuals have a sweet tooth. So, cutting down on sugar is difficult for many of them. Cutting sugar is recommended. Take honey instead. Avoid taking more than a spoonful of honey a day.
- Avoid fast food restaurant foods, especially oily, Salty, Sweet or deep-fried foods – these are all Kapha aggravating.

Summary: Breakfast is usually not necessary. Avoid sugar, fats, dairy products, and salt. Oils only in small amounts. Choose foods that are light and dry. The main meal should be at the middle of the day, and only a light, dry meal in the evening.

Avoid cold foods and drinks. Reduce use of Sweet, Sour, and Salty tastes. Pungent, Astringent, and Bitter tastes are best. All spices are good.

12.10 Nutritional Protocol for Kapha

Nutritional Protocol for Kapha			
Nourishing Elements	Fire, Air, Ether		
Nourishing Attributes	Dry, Warm, Light, Unclogging		
Nourishing Tastes	Pungent, Bitter, Astringent		
Essential Minerals	Carbon, Chlorine, Hydrogen, Iron, Magnesium, Sulfur		
Macro-nutrients	Carbohydrates 70-80%	Protein 10 %	Fats 10%
Fruits	*Sour Fruits:* Apples, Apricots, Cherries, Dates, Figs, Mangoes, Papaya, Peaches, Pears, Pineapples, Prunes, Pomegranates	*All Berries:* Blackberries, Blueberries, Cranberries, Currants Black & Red, Goji (Lycii) berries, Goose berries, Huckle berries, Mulberries, Raspberries, Strawberries	*Citrus:* Grapefruit, Lemons, Limes Dried fruits: in general are good for Kapha. (Apricots, figs, prunes, raisins)
Vegetables	*Pungent and Bitter foods such as:* Asparagus, Beets, Broccoli, Brussels sprouts, Cabbage, Carrots, Cauliflower, Celery	Eggplant, Garlic, Leafy green vegetables, Lettuce, Mushrooms, Okra, Onions, Peas, Peppers, Potatoes, Radishes, Spinach, Sprouts, Tomatoes	Cabbage (Sulfur) Family, Arugula, Bok choy, Broccoli, Brussels sprouts, Cabbage, Cauliflower, Chinese Cabbage, Collards, Diakon Radish, Kale, Kohlrabi, Horseradish, Maca, Mustard greens, Rapini, Rutabaga, Turnips, Watercress

Nutritional Protocol for Kapha			
Nuts, Seeds & Oils	*All Nuts & Seeds should be soaked:* Almonds, Cashews, Chia seeds, Sunflower, Pecans, Filberts	Flax seeds, Hazelnuts, Sesame seeds, Sunflower seeds, Poppy seeds, Pumpkin seeds	*Note:* (Oils in small quantities)
Sprouted Whole Grains	*Soaked & Sprouted Whole Grains:* Barley, Buckwheat, Corn, Millet	Oats Groats, Quinoa, Spelt	Rye, Brown Basmati Rice, Wild Rice, Wheat
Beans & Legumes	All soaked and sprouted legumes are acceptable except kidney beans and tofu.		
Culinary Spices	Sweet and/or Warming herbs and spices, such as: Allspice, Anise, Asafoetida, Basil, Bay leaf, Black pepper (use sparingly), Caraway, Cardamom, Cilantro (green coriander)	Cinnamon, Clove, Cress, Cumin, Fennel, Ginger, Juniper berries, Licorice root, Mace, Maca, Marjoram, Mustard	Nutmeg, Oregano, Parsley, Rosemary, Sage, Savory, Tarragon, Thyme
Herbal Teas	Green &/ or Warming Teas: Ajwan, Alfalfa, Blackberry, Borage, Burdock, Catnip, Chamomile	Chicory, Clove, Chrysanthemum, Cinnamon, Cornsilk, Dandelion, Elderflower, Eucalyptus, Fennel, Fenugreek	Ginger, Juniper berry, Oatstraw, Nettle, Orange peel, Raspberry, Red clover, Sage, Sassafras
Sweeteners	Raw, unheated honey, maple syrup		
Whole Food Supplements	Bee Pollen, Royal Jelly, Spirulina, Blue Green Algae	Nutritional Yeast, Aloe Vera Gel, Green Kamut, Green Chlorella	
Exercise	*40-60 minutes daily* Outdoor Activities Gardening Walking Hiking Running	Biking Tennis Mountain climbing Deep Breathing Aerobic Weight Lifting Stair Climbers	
Avoid or Reduce	*Elements:* Water, Earth *Attributes:* Wet, Cold, Heavy, Condensed *Tastes:* Sweet, Sour, Salty		

Kapha dosha is aggravated and increased in the spring of the year. During this season, eat less and choose drier, fibrous foods. During wet, cold seasons, all mind-body types can choose some of the above foods and decrease others.

If you're basic constitution is mixed (Kapha-Pitta or Kapha-Vata), include smaller portions for the second dosha.

General Tips for Health and Wellness for Kapha Types Kapha's are prone to lethargy, sluggishness, depression, and being overweight. Kapha people need activity and stimulation. Daily exercise is more important for them than for any other dosha type. Getting out of the house and seeking new experiences is also valuable. Be receptive to useful change, renounce impediments to progress, be intentional in implementing life-enhancing actions, and choose foods, mental attitudes, behaviors, exercise routines, and relationships and environmental circumstances which can be instrumental in balancing Kapha characteristics.

Pungent, Bitter, and Astringent tastes decrease Kapha influences. Black pepper, ginger, cumin, chili, and some other spices provide the pungent taste; some green leafy vegetables provide Bitter; and some green vegetables and beans provide the astringent taste. Note that the taste that decreases a dosha usually increases one or both of the other two.

Meditation can be more intensive for Kapha constitutions than for Vata or Pitta constitutions. Take time every day.

12.11 The Six Tastes Percentage Chart

Dr. Michael Tierra- *Planetary Herbalism* page 74-77 1988

Vata	Pitta	Kapha
93% Sweet	90% Sweet	80 % Sweet
2 % Salty	1 % Salty	1% Salty
5% Sour	1% Sour	1% Sour
1% Pungent	1% Pungent	2% Pungent
1% Bitter	3% Bitter	2 % Bitter
1% Astringent	7% Astringent	14 % Astringent

12.11 The Six Tastes Percentage Chart

Dr. Michael Tierra- *Herb Course* page 23-24

Vata Building Diet	Pitta Cooling Diet	Kapha Dry Diet
90% Sweet	85% Sweet	75% Sweet
2% Salty	1% Salty	1% Salty
4% Sour	1% Sour	1% Sour
2% Pungent	1% Pungent	4% Pungent
1% Bitter	2% Bitter	4% Bitter
1% Astringent	10% Astringent	15% Astringent

The Deeper Meaning of Sweet Taste

In chart 12.11 The Six Tastes, the percentages for sweet vary from 75 % to 93%. While these may seem high, keep in mind that these percentages can easily be achieved with foods that are not necessarily high in sugar.

What we are referring to here is the subtle essence of the sweet taste, not sugar or high-glycemic foods. Low-glycemic sweet tasting foods have a minimal affect on blood sugar levels, unlike the high-glycemic foods. A high-glycemic index food is one that converts rapidly to sugar in the blood. This includes not only refined sugars, but all fruits that have a high amount of sugar content or are classified as a high glycemic such as cooked starches and flour products. This also includes most of processed sweeteners that are on the market today. The most common high-glycemic foods are processed and refined grain products, potatoes and of course white sugar. High sugary foods have become a norm in our modern fast paced world. Even many fruits especially the sweet tropical fruits because of hybridization are now high in sugars. Certain vegetables become more high-glycemic when cooked such as: beets, parsnips and the winter squashes.

Benefits of Low-Glycemic Foods

Most diseases, bacteria, virus and parasites thrive on high-glycemic foods. There are numerous disorders that occur from consuming high-glycemic foods over the long term. The one we hear the most about is diabetes. According to the Center for Disease Control and Prevention, there are 17 million diabetes cases in the U.S., 5-10 percent of these are Type I. This has been a 33 percent increase in diabetes in the last decade. Eating a low-glycemic diet will not only satisfy the natural desire for the sweet taste, it helps create and maintain a biological terrain for preventing disease. Most berries are an excellent choice. Avoiding, or at least reducing high glycemic fruits, refined sugars and carbohydrates and cooked starchy vegetables will be a positive step towards health. The deeper meaning of the sweet taste is foods that nourish and build the body and help build the Ojas.

This is partial list of potential problems that can occur as a result of consuming a high-glycemic diet:

- Asthma
- Atherosclerosis
- Acidic stomach
- Alcohol
- Candida
- Cardiovascular Disease
- Cancer (certain types)
- Emphysema
- Elevated Triglycerides
- Elevated Uric Acid
- Fatigue
- Food allergies
- Glucose Intolerance
- High cholesterol
- Hypertension
- Kidney damage
- Impaired structure of DNA
- Lowered enzyme ability to function
- Mellitus (NIDDM)
- Multiple sclerosis
- Obesity

- Osteoporosis
- Tooth decay
- Weakened eyesight

The healthiest of all low-glycemic foods are leafy green vegetables, all berries and non-sweet fruiting-vegetables such as cucumber, zucchini, tomatoes, peppers, etc., nuts and seeds that have not been roasted, cooked or gone rancid. Nutrient rich foods such as sea vegetables, algaes, bee pollen, have an alkalizing effect, are high in minerals and have higher water content.

The current state health of an individual is the determining factor of how moderate or how high they can go in the glycemic range before their internal terrain is thrown off balance. We are looking at this from a constitutional perspective as well as the present state of their inner terrain.

Stevia seems to be one of our better herbs to use as a natural sweetener since it has no calories or carbohydrates, and according to a study in Brazil (J. Medical Biological Res 1986; 19(6)): 771-4), the active constituent 'stevioside' does not raise blood sugar glucose. The study actually showed that it lowered blood glucose. Fresh coconut is another food that can be used as a healthy choice in sweetening up foods. Coconut is a wonderful Sattvic food.

12.12 Vata Menu Plan

	Spring/ Summer	Fall/ Winter
Waking (1/2 hour before meal)	warm tea (adaptogen herbs, culinary spices such as fennel, cardamom, etc.)	soaked almonds blended and made into warm drink with fresh ginger, turmeric and honey
Breakfast	sweet fruit or sprouted grains, seet-sour berries	sweet fruit salad, berries or soaked grain dish with a spicy seed milk such as cinnamon
Snack	sweet treat such as fruit with warming spices and herbs, berries or fruit	tahini or almond butter, in season fresh peaches or apricots
Lunch	sprouted wild rice or soaked buckwheat groats with yellowish-orange sweet root vegetables	fresh kale or collard salad marinated with lemon, hemp seed oil, tamari and warming spices, eaten with sprouted grain and flax seed crackers

	Spring/ Summer	Fall/ Winter
Snack	sesame seed fennel treat	apple sauce with cinnamon, nutmeg and sweetened with honey, spicy herbal tea
Dinner	spaghetti squash with tomato-basil sauce and pungent spring salad	stir-not-fry root vegetable dish spiced with warming seeds and nuts
Snack	carob brownie	pumpkin pudding, culinary seed tea
Bedtime	warm nervine tea with ginger and honey	warm spicy toddy with vanilla and carob meal

12.13 Pitta Menu Plan

	Spring/ Summer	Fall/ Winter
Waking	warm tea (herb tea, tur-meric, fennel)	soaked almonds blended and made into warm drink, turmeric and honey
Breakfast	sprouted grain dish with coriander coconut milk	soaked grain dish with a seed milk flavored with coriander
Snack	sweet or bitter fruit in season	apple or pear
Lunch	sprouted barley or kamut grains with cabbage or broccoli, bitter green salad with sprouts and a refreshing salad dressing	fresh kale or collard salad marinated with lemon, sunflower seed oil, tamari and cooling herbs, eaten with sprouted grains and herbed flax seed crackers
Snack	sunflower seeds, fennel, lemon grass tea	apple sauce with cinnamon, nutmeg and sweetened with stevia, mint tea
Dinner	cauliflower and Jerusalem artichoke dish with a spicy cilantro sauce	sprouted garbanzo beans blended with sesame seed and sunflower seed butters spread over sprouted grain and flax seed caraway crackers
Snack	coconut macaroons with red clover tea	pumpkin pudding, catnip tea

12.14 Kapha Menu Plan

	Spring/ Summer	Fall/ Winter
Breakfast	ginger and licorice root tea	grain dish with a cup of ginger tea
Snack	sour treat such as a bowl of cranberries with warming spices and herbs	fresh peaches or apricots, in season, with a warming spicy sauce
Lunch	sprouted barley with sauce, fresh celery soup and a fresh spring salad	soaked buckwheat and fresh Brussels sprouts salad marinated with sesame seed oil or mustard seed oil, and black pepper and other warming spices, eaten with sprouted grain and flax seed crackers
Snack	raspberries, lemon grass tea	pumpkin seeds, cup of saffron herbal tea
Dinner	root vegetable and burdock stir-not-fry dish with curry and cumin sauce and a dark green salad	stir-not-fry root vegetable dish spiced with warming seeds and nuts
Snack	cranberry dessert	sour apple and chamomile tea

The Significance of Dietary Therapy in Ayurveda

In Ayurvedic dietetics, it is not only what is eaten that is important, but also the manner in which it is eaten.

The major considerations that are applied in Ayurvedic are as follows:

1. The quantity of food
2. The quality of food
3. Preparation of food
4. Combination of food
5. Spicing of food
6. Right attitude in eating
7. Right time for eating
8. Regime for eating

Dietary variations by external factors
1. Seasons
2. Climate
3. Age and sex
4. Diet and Ama

Ten Factors That Reduce the Quality of Food

1. Over-cooked, burned or overcooked food.
2. Canned or junk food.
3. Artificially prepared food.
4. Spoiled or rancid food.
5. Additives, preservatives and artificial coloring.
6. Frozen food.
7. Freeze dried food.
8. Fast foods.
9. Animal products.
10. Refined or processed foods.

12.15 The Elemental Relationships

Guna	Sattva		Rajas		Tamas
Element	Ether	Air	Fire	Water	Earth
Attribute	Clarity	Mobility & Subtlety	Energy	Mobility with Inertia	Inertia
State of Matter	Ethereal	Gaseous	Radiant	Liquid	Solid
Physical Quality	Special Relationship	Movement	Electricity	Cohesion	Weight
Plant Part	Fruit	Leaves	Flowers	Stems and Branches	Roots
Senses	Hearing	Touch	Sight	Taste	Smell
Sense Organs	Ear	Skin	Eyes	Tongue	Nose
Action	Speech	Holding	Walking	Procreation	Excretion
Organ of Action	Vocal chords, Mouth	Hands	Feet	Genitals	Anus

Vegetarian Facts

Is a human being a carnivore, herbivore, or vegetarian? 20 Reasons we are more similar to anthropoids then carnivores in body physiology.

12.16

				Higher Primates	
		Carnivores	**Herbivores**	**Anthropoids**	**Humans**
1.	**Primary Diet**	Lives on flesh-foods	Lives on grass, herbs & plants	Diet is veg-etarian	Diet is veg-etarian
2.	**Blood**	Acidic	Alkaline	Alkaline	Alkaline
3.	**Teeth**	Teeth are long, sharp, and pointed. Sharp canine teeth.	Front and canine teeth may be sharp or pointed. Back teeth are flattened for grinding.	All teeth are flattened. Dullest canine teeth of all primates.	All teeth are flattened. Dullest canine teeth of all primates.
4.	**Molars**	Pointed molars	Molar teeth in folds	Well-developed incision teeth	Well-developed incision teeth
5.	**Dental Formation**	5to8/1/6/1/5to 8 (upper) 5to8/1/6/1/5to 8 (lower)	6/0/0/0/6 (up-per) 6/1/6/1/6 (lower)	5/1/4/1/5 (up-per) 5/1/4/1/5 (lower)	5/1/4/1/5 (up-per) 5/1/4/1/5 (lower)
6.	**Salivary Glands**	Small	Well-developed	Well-developed	Well-developed
7.	**Reaction of salvia & urine**	Acid	Alkaline	Alkaline	Alkaline
8.	**Tongue**	Rasping	Smooth	Smooth	Smooth
9.	**Jaw**	Jaw ca move up & down (vertically) To facilitate tear-ing & biting	Jaw can move both up and down (vertical-ly) To facilitate grinding of vegetables	Jaw can move both up and down (verti-cally) To facili-tate grinding of vegetables	Jaw can move both up and down (verti-cally) To facili-tate grinding of vegetables

				Higher Primates	
		Carnivores	**Herbivores**	**Anthropoids**	**Humans**
10.	**Drinks**	Drinks by lifting it into the throat with tongue	Drinks water by suction	Drinks water by suction	Drinks water by suction
11.	**Stomach**	Simple & roundish	Ruminant: four compartment	Stomach with duodenum (as second stomach)	Stomach with duodenum (as second stomach)
12.	**Intestinal Tract**	Tract 3 times length of the body	Tract varies by species; usually 10 times length of body	Tract 12 times the length of the body	Tract 12 times the length of the body
13.	**Colon**	Smooth	Smooth & convoluted	Colon is convoluted	Colon is convoluted
14.	**Hands**	Four-footed	Four-footed	Two hands and two feet.	Two hands and two feet.
15.	**Nails**	Have paws & claws	Hooved (cloven)	Flat nails	Flat nails
16.	**Walking**	Go on all fours	Go on all fours	Upright or semi-upright	Upright or semi-upright
17.	**Tails**	Have tails	Have tails	No tails	No tails
18.	**Vision**	Stereoscopic vision	Stereoscopic vision	Forward vision	Forward vision
19.	**Pores**	Skin with pores	Skin with pores	Millions of pores	Millions of pores
20.	**Placenta**	Zonary	Non-deciduate	Discoidal	Discoidal

The human being is the most herbivores of the herbivores; actually a frugivore.

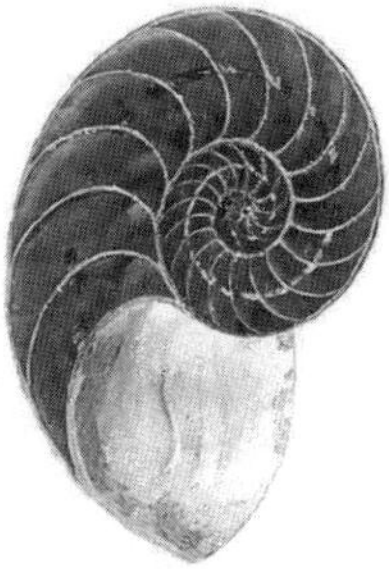

PART SEVEN

The Conclusion

13 Constitutional Case Studies

- A Case of Vata Imbalance
- A Case of Pitta Imbalance
- A Case of Kapha Imbalance
- An Ayurvedic Case Study: Pitta Prakruti Woman with Insomnia & Vata Vikruti

13.1 A Case of Vata Imbalance

A 76-year-old male patient came to our clinic for his dizziness, headaches and irregular heartbeat. He had been experiencing excessive flatulence and constipation. His physical build was tall and thin, his skin was dry and cool, and his pulse was irregular and weak. Mentally, he was anxious and very worried about his state of health.

His routine had been disturbed while he was on vacation and his erratic schedule continued after he returned home. His meal time was different everyday, he ate mostly steamed vegetables

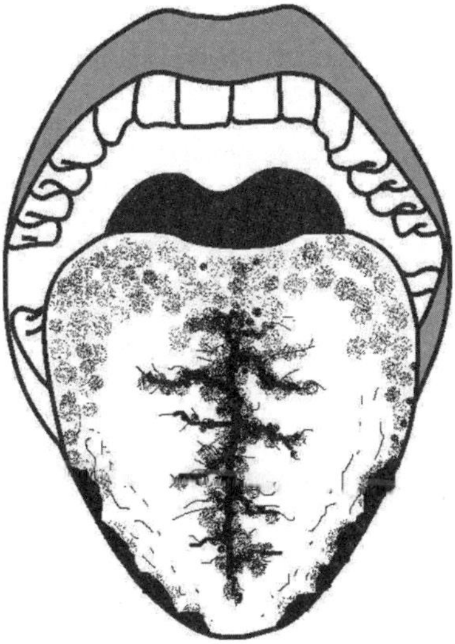

and some rice and beans. He was drinking two to three cans of carbonated drinks a day and his sleep was light and interrupted.

TONGUE DIAGNOSIS	
Prakruti- Body Color:	Pale with slightly reddish at sides
Prakruti-Body Shape:	Deep central crack extending to the tip, numerous other cracks radiating outward from it, swollen along central crack, tooth marked
Vikruti- Tongue Coating:	Dry, thin, grayish and murky appearance

This is a typical case of a Vata imbalance. This person's physical and mental characteristics and symptomatology fit into the Vata type. The irregularity in his diet and sleep, as well as his diet and carbonated drinks disturbed his Vata constitution. In Ayurvedic medicine, constipation is the result of blocked Apana vayu (downward Vata energy). This blockage results in energy moving upward, cause irregular heartbeats, headaches and dizziness.

Recommended Treatment Protocol

Dietary advice: Eat three meals regularly, at the same place and at the same time as often as possible. Chew food completely. Reduce the overly cooked vegetables, beans and carbonated drinks, which create excess flatulence. Eat warm, fresh juices, green leafy vegetables, sprouted and warmed mung beans and vegetable soups. These foods are warming and easily digestible. Drink plenty of water.

Lifestyle: Create regularity in sleeping and daily activities. Stay warm. Take a warm bath. Get plenty of rest and exercise daily in the great outdoors such as walking or swimming.

Cleansing technique: Retention enema with sesame oil. The colon is a seat of Vata energy, so a warming enema relieves excess Vata. Every morning, drink hot water with freshly squeezed lemon and a little honey and salt to stimulate the colon and relieve constipation.

Ayurvedic remedies: The balancing tastes for the Vata constitution are Sweet, Sour and Salty, so the Ayurvedic remedies that balance Vata contain foods, spices and herbs with these tastes. Drink Triphala tea daily to relieve constipation.

Results: After following this regimen for one week, the patient's constipation improved. His heart rate slowed down and became regular. He no longer experienced dizziness and headaches. The routine relaxation / meditation and spending time outdoors helped him relieve his anxiety and improve his sleep. Vata types need regularity in diet, lifestyle and sleep. Warm fluids, warm baths, calming exercise, movement activities and relaxation help keep Vata in balance.

13. 2 A Case of Pitta Imbalance

A 37-year-old female who was a workaholic executive manager complained of severe heartburn, which she had experienced for over a year. She has been to numerous health practitioners but with no relief. Her heartburn extended from her stomach to the throat. The symptoms were worse when lying down. She had previously taken numerous medications and antacids to relieve her symptoms, but they no longer helped and she was experiencing numerous side-effects from them. The heartburn was aggravated by fried oily foods and Sour, Pungent, and spicy food. She also had an unpleasant bitter taste in her mouth and moderately high blood pressure for the last six months.

Physically, she had a medium build with fair complexion. Her hair is a reddish-brown color and her eyes are greenish in color with a sharp intensity to them. She was very impatient and seemed to be irritated by the way her day was going. She kept complaining about numerous people who were present in her life. Her diet mainly consisted of fast food, including hamburgers, pizza, tacos, chili, french fries with ketchup, coffee and colas. She also smoked cigarettes on a regular basis, about half a pack a day.

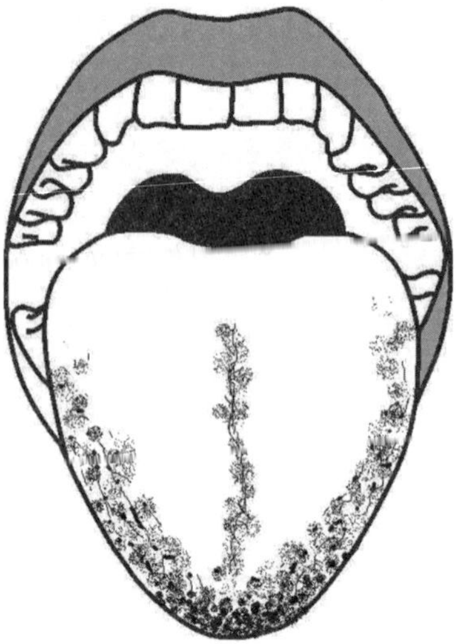

TONGUE DIAGNOSIS	
Prakruti- Body Color:	Red, tip redder and with red points
Prakruti- Body Shape:	Slightly swollen, especially in the front part, cracks on the edges
Vikruti- Tongue Coating:	Thick, sticky yellowish coating especially mid-central section

Impression: She was a fairly typical Pitta person, impatient and short-tempered. The food she was eating increased her Pitta, which was aggravated by Sour, Salty, Pungent and oily foods, and yet she kept eating them regularly. Her lifestyle was intense with no breaks for relaxing activities.

Recommended Treatment Protocol

Dietary advice: Eliminate coffee and cigarettes. Avoid heavy meals. Avoid acidic, Salty, Pungent-Spicy and oily food, and Sour fruits such as ketchup, citrus, lemon and grapefruits. Eat a bland diet: sprouted whole grains such as basmati rice, beans (except lentils), and plenty of fresh green leafy vegetables and vegetables juices. Balancing tastes for Pitta are Sweet, Bitter and Astringent. Use spices such as turmeric, coriander, and cilantro. Avoid eating fast and on the run or when in motion.

Lifestyle: Slow down; take a walk in nature. Listen to calming classical music. Avoid rushing and put limits on your schedule. Avoid becoming overheated. Cool showers or baths are helpful.

Cleansing techniques: Liver and hepatic herbs to support and relieve Pitta-dosha in the small intestine. She was advised to take the Triphala formula.

Results: Following this treatment plan the patient improved about 80 percent in two to three weeks. She realized the importance of eating nourishing food, altering her work habits, and adding leisure activities and rest to her daily routine.

13.3 A Case of Kapha Imbalance

A 16-year-old male came with his mother for the treatment of asthma and persistent allergies to numerous substances. His routine medications such as inhalers were not helping him. Very often he missed and skipped school. He had a sedentary lifestyle and was very stubborn in making changes in his life. His family and school situation were stressful. Physically he was tall and overweight. He had breathing difficulty, was usually congested and was coughing up thick white mucus. His lungs were congested and we could hear wheezing from his chest.

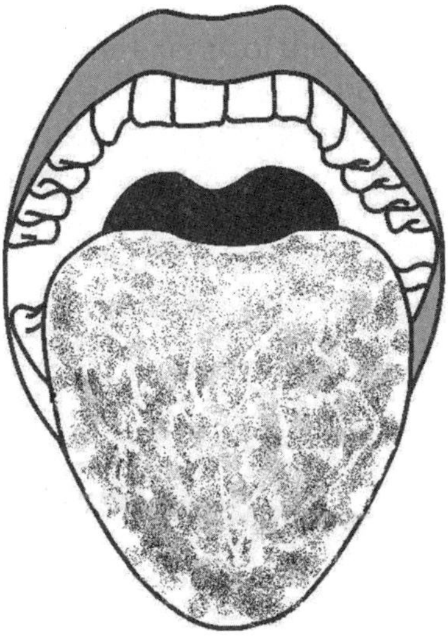

His diet consisted of shredded wheat cereal with milk and sugar, toast with jelly, sausage pizza, macaroni and cheese, peanut butter and jelly sandwich, bananas and Coca-Cola. This diet is highly Kaphic-mucus producing.

TONGUE DIAGNOSIS	
Prakruti - Body Color:	Pale
Prakruti - Body Shape:	Thick, swollen, tooth marked
Vikruti - Tongue Coating:	Sticky thick white coating especially in the front and back root area

Impression: This is a case of Kapha imbalance. Wheat, dairy, sweets, bananas and red meat create mucus. The boy's Kapha constitution was compounded by the Kapha-producing food, creating severe imbalance.

Recommended Treatment Protocol

Dietary advice: Reduce all mucus-producing food. Eat a diet of sprouted whole grains, such as, millet, buckwheat, mung beans, lentils, green leafy vegetables and fenugreek sprouts. Turmeric, ginger, garlic and pepper reduce mucus. Drinking plenty of water helps to loosen the mucus.

Lifestyle: Daily walking was recommended.

Cleansing technique: Daily nasal wash with neti pot to cleanse the upper nasal passages and improve the breathing. Upper wash (cleansing the stomach with Celtic sea salt water) was recommended, but he refused to follow the directions.

Results: This young man was not cooperative in following the recommended treatment; however, after changing his diet and incorporating some exercises, he improved significantly. In less than ten days, his breathing improved and he stopped using his inhalers. With consistent support and some counseling he is expected to improve slowly.

An Ayurvedic Case Study: Pitta Prakruti Woman with Insomnia and Vata Vikruti

A 37 year old woman came to me complaining that she has had sleeping problems for the last six months and that she does not feel as though she has as much energy as she used to. Prior to the last six months, her sleeping was light but restful. She had recently had a few nervous breakouts. She enjoys sex, however, intercourse has recently become painful as she does not lubricate as much as she used to. She also noticed that her hair appears to be drier and without sheen. Prior to six months ago, she recalls having healthier hair. Her history reveals that there have been no major illnesses or traumatic events that she can recall during her lifetime. She is presently taking no medications.

Further history reveals that her digestive system is healthy with occasional occurrences of flatulence and constipation over the last few years. She has always been a light sleeper and her appetite was always regular, but recently has become irregular. She consistently eats three meals a day but it's usually on the run and snacking has become much more frequent.

The emotional/psychological history reveals her to be a person who makes speedy decisions without much contemplation. In the past she would always finish what she started and always love a challenge. She doesn't have the urge or desire to take on a challenge anymore. Additionally, she appears to be fairly hard on herself as she accepts only her best and gets angry when she makes mistakes. Lately she has been making more mistakes than usual.

Upon examination of her routines, she enjoys physical sports and has been fairly active duing the past 10 years. In addition, she wakes up around 7:30 am and goes to bed around midnight. This has always been her waking/sleeping pattern.

Physical exam reveals a very slim woman with moderate bone density. She is 5′9″ and weighs just 117 pounds. She has lost over 15 pounds in the last 12 months and enjoys her petite figure. Her skin is moderately thick. Her hair is dry and fine. Her face is angular and her eyes are deep set and penetrating. She has excellent musculature.

13.4 An Ayurvedic Case Study

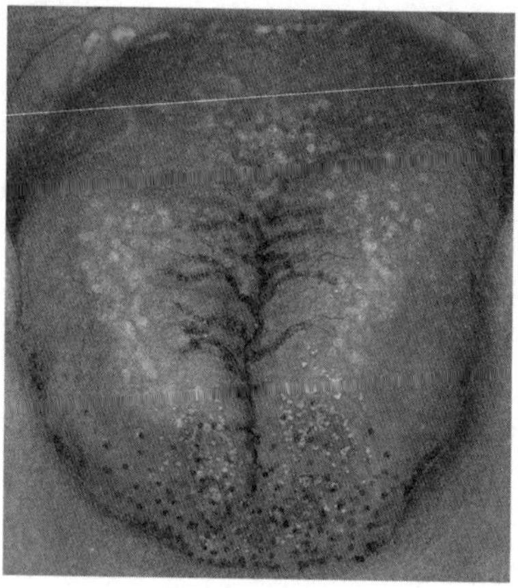

TONGUE DIAGNOSIS	
Prakruti - Body Color:	Redder in the front, red points in the center with slightly reddish-pale spots at sides
Prakruti - Body Shape:	Medium shaped with a slight point at the tip, deep central crack extending to the tip numerous other cracks radiating outward from it; swollen along central crack, concave, tooth marked
Vikruti -Coating:	Thin, quite white coating throughout, slight orange discoloration on the sides
Vikruti - Moisture:	Very dry
Vikruti - Movement:	Quivering and shaking rapidly

Her tongue is moderate in size and it has a light yellowish coating. She has a few medium cracks. This woman's complaints of insomnia, anxiety and a feeling of exhaustion clearly denote a deficiency of her fire, in this case of both the stomach and kidneys. The slight orange discoloration on the sides suggests a severe, long-standing blood deficiency. The dryness in this case derives from deficiency of her Prana, which is unable to move the fluids. The concave, pale red spots indicate cold in the interior of the body. The tooth marks denote deficiency of spleen energy, while the coating reflects the retention of food resulting from low Agni. The tongue moving rapidly and quivering indicates the nerves and mind are restless, another high Vata sign. In summary, this patient suffers from a severe and long-standing deficiency irregularity fire of the digestive organs, leading to blood stagnation and internal low fire.

The first step we need to take to move her toward balance is to determine her Prakruti and Vikruti. Also, remember this is a simple case showing just a few aspects of Ayurvedic assessment and tongue diagnosis and healing protocol. There are many more levels that would be attended to in an actual case.

Determining Her Prakruti Constitution

The first step is to determine her Prakruti, her basic constitution. To do this, we look at those aspects of her that are slow to change, like her body, bones, face, and tendencies she has carried her whole life. The following table lists the signs along with notes: The columns for VPK indicate it is an indication for Vata, Pitta, and Kapha dosha.

0= describes me not at all.

1= describes me a little.

2= describes me well.

3= describes me the most.

Indicator Signs	V	P	K	Dosha Signs
Moderate to light skeletal density	2	3		Pitta gives moderate skeletal bone density, Vata is light boned
5' 9"		2		Pitta- average size
Skin is slightly thick.	1	2		Pitta gives moderate skin thickness
Sleeps Well		2	1	Pitta or Kapha individuals can sleep well
Regular Appetite	1	2	1	Pitta or Vata individuals can have regular to irregular appetites
Eats three meals a day consistently		3	1	Pitta needs a lot of fuel, Kapha is consistent
Occasionally snacks	1	2		Pitta people need to snack
Quick decisions		2	1	Pitta gives a quick sharp mind
Critical of others		1		Pitta tends to make you critical

Indicator Signs	V	P	K	Dosha Signs
Enjoys Sex		2		Pitta gives passion, though all can enjoy Sex
Enjoys a Challenge		2	1	Pitta gives the passion to overcome challenges
Finishes what she begins		2		Pitta and Kapha can finish things
Nice ordinary hair		1		Pitta and Kapha tends to have the thickest and healthiest hair
Her face is angular		2		Pitta sign
Eyes are deep set and penetrating		3		Pitta sign
She has excellent musculature	1	2	1	Pitta gives good muscle tone
Her tongue is thin to medium in size	1	2		Pitta sign
Rises at 7, sleeps at 1		2		Pitta can stay up till midnight with no problem

Prakruti Constitution:

Vata 7

Pitta 37

Kapha 6

Her Prakruti is: Vata, 14%, Pitta, 74%, Kapha 12%

This woman has a dominant Pitta Prakruti constitution with a balanced Vata and Kapha ratio.

Determining her Vikruti Present Terrain Constitution

Next step is we have to find her present Vikruti constitution. To do this we look many of the aspects of her being that are in flux over the last few months or years. The following table lists these.

0= describes me not at all.

1= describes me a little.

2= describes me well.

3= describes me the most.

Indicator Signs	V	P	K	Dosha Signs
A 37 year old		3	2	Pitta is the dosha of mid-life
Complaining		3		Complaining is often a Pitta event
Irritable and sensitive	3			A typical Vata symptom when nerves are depleted
Low energy	3			Usually caused by low Prana
Thinning Hair	3	2		Can be Vata or excessive heat in head
Excessive flatulence	3			Too much Vata
Occasional constipation	3			Deranged Vata constipated
Crusty grayish vaginal discharge	3			Crusty (dry) and gray are both classic indicators of Vata
Painful intercourse	3			Vata brings pain
Dry vagina	3			Excessive Vata tends to dry
Being absentminded	3			Excessive Vata can make you forgetful
Lack of Concentration	3			Vata can move your mind disabling concentration
Very Slim, losing weight	3			She is losing weight, a sign of Vata
Enjoys her petite figure	3			Could be normal, could be Vata induced insecurity
Dry, thin skin and thinning hair	3	2		All signs of high Vata
Thick grayish-yellow coat-ing on tongue	3			The grey indicates Vata type toxins and Ama, low Agni
Cracks		2		Indicates Vata is disturbed
Scallops on tongue		3		Indicates digestion has been poor and sluggish
Excessive motion, moving too fast	3	3		Vata provoking when doing too much or too fast

This woman has a Vata Vikruti imbalance.

Vikruti Constitution:

Vata 45

Pitta 18

Kapha: 2

Her Vikruti is: Vata 90% Pitta, 36%, Kapha 4%

This woman has a dominant Pitta Prakruti constitution with a balanced Vata and Kapha ratio.

This woman has a dominant Vata Vikruti constitution with an imbalanced Pitta and Kapha ratio.

Constitutional Balance			
Her Prakruti is:	Vata, 14%	Pitta, 74%	Kapha 12%
Her Vikruti is:	Vata 90%	Pitta, 36%	Kapha 4%
Total Imbalance	+ 76	-38	-8%

The conclusion is that her Pitta dosha fire has burned out, thereby leaving her Air element high. Her unchecked Vata is creating a nervous system disorder and is further drying her up. She has been both physically and mentally hot and exhausting herself, literally burning and drying up her little bit of Kapha that she had. So given the symptoms and tongue diagnosis we have been given, our conclusion would be:

Her Vikruti is excessive Vata leading to deficient Pitta and deficient Kapha, which is almost all used up:

The first step is to still her Vata, cool her Pitta and build her Ojas, which is the essence of Kapha. An important thing to remember is that you don't want to build doshas themselves, but minimize them. You want to build the subtle doshas of Prana, Tejas and Ojas, which are the purified and stable aspects of Vata, Pitta and Kapha, correspondingly. So in this case we want to build Ojas, not Kapha.

Determining Which Subdoshas are Affected

Each of the doshas is divided into five subdoshas. Since she has a Vata Vikruti, we will only look at Vata subdoshas. The table below lists these subdoshas and the clues as to which ones are out of balance. Apana definitely has to be treated first.

Prana Vayu	Low energy, loss of concentration, and irritation
Udana Vayu	By association with the other vayu's, Udana will be affected
Samana Vayu	Yellowish coating on tongue, poor digestion
Vyana Vayu	Tongue quivering and moving rapidly, excessive motion and moving too fast
Apana Vayu	Tongue cracks, irregular digestion and constipation, excessive flatulence, dry vagina, dry & unhealthy hair, excessive motion

Determining Which Dhatus are Affected

To treat this woman, we must know which tissues are affected. The following table lists the seven dhatus and the body signs and dosha signs that indicate which dhatus are affected by her Vikruti.

Rasa Dhatu	**Gray tongue, dry skin and hair.**
Rakta Dhatu	Yellowish tongue coating on tongue indicates blood is sluggish and toxic.
Mamsa Dhatu	Tongue was quivering and shaking, excessive movement, weight loss.
Medas Dhatu	Weight loss and thin skin.
Asthi Dhatu	Dry brittle thinning hair indicates her bones are deficient.
Majja Dhatu	All her anger and irritability likely has made her nerves fragile.
Shukra Dhatu	The fact that her other dhatus are compromised indicate her shukra is compromised. Also, she seems to have low ojas, which can result from low shukra.

Determining Which Srota are Affected

The Srotas are the channels within the body. There are 16 of them in women, and 14 in men. The following table lists these srotas and the clues that indicate that the srota is affected by her Vikruti.

Pranavaha srota	Excessive flow - she is feeling absentminded and can't focus
Annavaha srota	A coated tongue, indicates sluggish flow of energy
Ambuvaha srota	Blocked flow - her Rasa is depleted, could possibly be from an obstruction in the water channel
Rasavaha srota	**Her Rasa is depleted**
Raktavaha srota	Dissatisfied and discouraged, has a lot of toxins having a difficulty being released
Mamsavaha srota	Has good muscles, but is losing mass and strength
Medovaha srota	Deficient flow - she has too little tissue mass to support her Pitta constitution
Majjavaha srota	**Too much uncontrolled Vata moving around in the body**
Asthivaha srota	Hair and skin is in poor condition which indicates problems with the flow in the bone channel, usually relates to low Agni.
Shukravaha srota	**Low concentration and focus, low energy**
Mutrivaha srota	No indication here
Purishavaha srota	Blocked flow - lots of flatulence and constipation, brittle, thinning hair, Ama on tongue
Svedavaha srota	An indication that points to an overall dry body
Manovaha srota	A burnt out feeling, mind is spacey, losing her center, frequently irritated
Lactation srota	No indication
Menstruation srota	**Main indicator, likely some sort of block in this srota channel**

Determining the State of Her Agni

As mentioned earlier, Agni is a very significant key in determining and understanding the health of an individual. It is the digestive power of the body, it determines how well it can transform food and all thought and sensory input into something pure and utilizable for the individual. With an excellent functioning Agni, you can care for and avoid most disorders and diseases. There are four states of Agni as listed in the table below.

Balanced	No indication
Slow	Low Agni is indicated by the fact that she has toxic grey discharges on her tongue and numerous drying-like symptoms and nerve and emotional disturbances.
Sharp	The fact that her appetite and digestion were good in the past, indicates that her Agni was strong. However, because that has changed and her Agni is no longer as strong, her body now has Ama.
Variable	The fact that it shows signs of slow and sharp indicates it is likely variable.

Determining the State of Her Subtle Doshas

The three subtle doshas are Prana, Tejas and Ojas. The table below lists these three with explanations of what is occurring.

Prana	Her Prana is basically out of control, it has lost its Ojas, which is essential to nourish and support Prana. Prana is in constant motion moving here and there and races around the body drying up her body and digestive system, burning out the digestive fire-Agni, burning more fuel than is there.
Tejas	Tejas is the source of her problem. Her Pitta became far too hot and burned out the Ojas and now Prana is totally running out of control, with no rhyme or reason. Tejas is now being moved left, right and center by Prana, making her unable to concentrate or focus, causing her to be absentminded, making it difficult for her to make even the simplest of decisions.
Ojas	The Ojas are just about all gone. She needs some deep nourishing to all the tissues and some deep loving and embracing of who she really is. And, of course, then sound and deep sleep and rest.

Determining the State of Her Gunas

The three Gunas are Sattva, Rajas and Tamas. The table below lists these three with my take on their state.

Sattva	Her challenge and her goal needs to be to break through her Rajas and move into Sattva in all aspects of her life from her personal to her food choices.
Rajas	Her constant action all the time is bringing her turmoil. Her irritation and judgment of others and situations is creating more Rajas within her body, mind and emotions. Her Prakruti wanting an active mind and life is following her deep desire, but she has over done it. Working so hard, but never being good enough in her own eyes.
Tamas	If she keeps going in this direction, she will experience Tamas very soon. She will not have any more fire to burn, she will be flat out on her feet and she will not be going too far or moving too fast.

Determining the Disease Pathways

The three pathways of disease are Inner, Outer and Central. The table below lists these three.

Inner	Her Ama being high and her digestion being irregular and constipated is enough of an indication to reveal that the inner channel is blocked quite a bit.
Outer	Her outer two doshas, rasa and rakta, are definitely affected by the symptoms of her outer body: skin, hair, etc.
Central	Her imbalance and the fact that her hair is affected indicates her bones are involved, but also the other signs and symptoms are stacking up.

Determining the Prognosis

The prognosis is actually excellent. Although all three pathways are affected, the Vikruti and Prakruti are not the same and her Ojas, although very low, still has some substance. Her biggest advantage is her age and willingness to make some dramatic changes in her diet, activity regime and lifestyle choices. By following a healing program to bring her to balance, within three to six months she should be at a different place in life. Working energetically with her physical body will bring her into a balanced and harmonious state. Since her Vata is not balanced, the hardest thing for her will be to stick with the program. The main goal is to keep her on the path with lots of encouragement and regular support.

The Tongue Progress

The main thing to monitor is the tongue coating. It should become less coated and the color and shape return to its natural vibrant state. This should show up within a few short months. If she decides to change her diet and do an "Agni: Restocking the Fire Program" there will be changes within a few weeks. Once again, that is the beauty of tongue diagnosis; you can see progress in a very short time.

What Kind of Dietary Approach to Take

Since she has a Pitta Prakruti and Vata Vikruti, and the Ojas are low, the key part of the dietary approach is to increase her Oja foods and stock her fire back up, which will naturally increase Kapha and Pitta and decrease her Vata. The following tables list the six tastes and the foods that would support her best.

TASTES	
Sweet	Using fresh whole living carbohydrates from root vegetables and simple sugars to increase Ojas
Sour	Some fresh sour fruits and berries, with a little fermented foods to deal with the Vata
Salty	A small amount of sea vegetables and celery will be excellent in helping to restore her digestive fire as well as provide those trace minerals
Pungent	A little, such as ginger root, to get the blood flowing and to move the blocks
Bitter	Very little, a small amount would help clear her liver and purify her stagnant blood
Astringent	Very little, a few greens and sprouts to keep her light and provide those nutrients to keep things balanced

HEALTHY FOOD CHOICES	
Grains	Organic sprouted whole grains: Buckwheat groats, Basmati Rice, Oatgroats, Kamut berries
Fruits	In Season and Organic: Apricots, Avocado, Bananas, Berries, Coconut, Dates, Figs, Grapefruit, Kiwi, Lemons, Limes, Mangos, Melons, Papayas, Peaches, Pineapple, Plums, Rhubarb, Tamarind, Tangerines
Vegetables	In Season and Organic: Artichoke, Asparagus, Carrots, Daikon, Leeks, pumpkin, Sweet potatoes, Summer squash, Winter squash, Watercress
Nuts & Seeds	Organic Raw and Soaked: Almonds, Brazil, Cashews, Chestnuts, Filberts, Macadamia, Pecans, Pine Nuts, Pistachios, Poppy seeds, Pumpkin seeds, Sesame Seeds, Sunflower, Walnuts
Oils	Organic: Increase Agni while decreasing Vata and stabilizing Pitta, Almond, Sesame, Sunflower
Legumes	Organic: Adzuki, Mung,
Sweeteners	Organic: Stevia, Yacon Root Syrup, Raw Carob, Raw Cacao and Dark Agave Nectar, Dates, Figs, unheated Honey, Maple Syrup, Raw Sugarcane
Herbs/ Spices	Organic: Anise, Hing, Basil, Bay Leaf, Black Cumin, Black Pepper, Caraway, Coriander, Dill, Fennel, Garma Masala, Kudzu, Mint, Orange Peel, Peppermint, Saffron, Sandalwood Chips, Spearmint, Tamarind, turmeric, Vanilla
Seaweeds	Wildcrafted Sea Vegetables: Arame, Dulse, Hiziki, Kelp, Kombu, Wakame
Beverages	Organic: Apricot Juices, Young Coconut Milk, Date or Fig shakes, Sweet fruit juices
Teas	Organic: Cardamom, Chamomile, Elder Flower, Fennel, Hops, Lavender, Lemon Balm, Lemon Grass, Peppermint, Rose Flowers, Rosehips, Spearmint

Healthy Lifestyle Recommendations

She needs to replenish her vital juices and restock the internal fires again.

Her goal is become more fluid in all aspects of her life, to open her heart and embrace the love of the world around her, to be calmer with fewer struggles and less anger and more ease and contentment. To learn how to move from a rajasic lifestyle towards a Sattvic way of living; from an active frenzied whirlwind toward balance and peace. She needs to move from a state of irritation and impatience to one of contentment in her life and her mind; to replace judgment with acceptance, hate with love, and anger with forgiveness. Moving her mind in this direction will bring her peace of mind and heart.

She needs to replace her running here and there with casual strolls through the forests and beaches. Her constant motion is one of her main causes of the imbalance. She should minimize sweating as to not sweat out all her juice, all her rasa dhatu, her sweating also causes her to lose energy, vitality and her fire. Sweating causes loss of her internal fire - this is burnout from within.

Instead of sleeping from midnight to 7:30 a.m., she should sleep from 10:00 p.m.to 6:00 a.m. This will be more Sattvic and also give her liver a rest at midnight and help ease her Pitta emotions that are aggravated by staying up through liver regeneration time around midnight.

Herbal Recommendations

She should take one to two grams of Triphala with warm water every night as she goes to bed at 10:00 p.m. for at least a month or two. This will gently normalize her Apana, remove the constipation, clean the blood and liver, build the Ojas, activate her period, nourish her heart and balance all three of her doshas. Triphala will have other great effects as well, but these are the main ones for her. Using Triphala alone will not treat her completely but it's a good start to bring change to her emotional heart and support her changing emotions. The other formula to bring in is Trikatu to increase her internal digestive fire. For treating her insomnia a few useful herbs are:

Vikruti Insomnia Herbs

Herb	Taste	Dosha	Actions
Skullcap 'Scutellaria spp.'	Bitter	PK-Vo	Nervine, antispasmodic
Oatstraw 'Avena sativa'	Sweet	VP-K+	Nervine tonic, nutritive, antispasmodic
Lemon Balm 'Melissa officinalis'	Pungent, Bitter	KP-Vo	Nervine tonic, demulcent, expectorant
Lady's Slipper 'Cypripedium pubescens'	Sweet, Pungent, Bitter	VK-Po	Nervine tonic, hypnotic, antispasmodic
Ashwagandha 'Withania somnifera'	Astringent, Bitter, Sweet	VK-P+	Adaptogen, nervine tonic, rejuvenative, aphrodisiac

Prakruti Pitta-Agni Herbs

Herb	Taste	Dosha	Actions
Basil 'Ocinum spp'	Pungent	VK-P+	Nervine, diaphoretic, febrifuge
Calamus (Sweet Flag) 'Acorus calamus'	Pungent, Bitter	VK-P+	Nervine tonic, rejuvenative, stimulant
False Unicorn 'Helonia dioica'	Bitter, Sweet	VK-P+	Emmenagogue, aphrodisiac, diuretic
Blue Cohosh 'Caulophyllum thalictroides'	Bitter, Sweet	KV-P+	Emmenagogue, antispasmodic
Damiana 'Turnera aphrodisiaca'	Pungent, Bitter	K-VoP+	Aphrodisiac, stimulant
Gotu Kola 'Hydrocyle asiatica'	Bitter	VPK+	Rejuvenative, nervine tonic, alterative

To treat her Vata Vikruti, we want to nourish her with warming, soothing unctuous demulcent tonic herbs and tone her Agni without increasing her Pitta, and we want to feed her Ojas. The following formula can be taken for at least one month before re-evaluating her situation. Then it could change or she could continue it depending on her response and compliance. This formula can be made and taken as a powder as described below.

A Vata Balancing and Agni, Kapha,Ojas Building/ Dietary and Herb Program

Herb	Herbal Actions	Energetics & Tastes	Dosage/Ratio
Rose Petals	Tridoshic, Sattvic, emmenagogue, alterative, nervine, induce Love, Feed Ojas	Cooling: Sweet, Pungent, Bitter, Astringent	Use as rose water in base
Blue Cohosh Root	Emmenagogue, antispasmodic, carminative, clears and dispels Vata, warms uterus	Heating: Sweet, Bitter	1 part in formula
Ashwagandha Root	Sattvic, Tonifies and rejuvenates nerve exhaustion, an excellent aphrodisiac, feeds Ojas	Heating: Bitter, Sweet, Astringent	1 part in formula
Sassafras	Sattvic, Vata Tonic, alterative, diaphoretic, rejuvenative,	Heating: Pungent	1 parts in formula
Angelica Root	A good warming Rasayana herb which has a emmenagogue, carminative and diaphoretic action	Heating: Sweet, Pungent	1 part in formula
Shatavari Root	Demulcent, Female Vata Tonic, Calming, feed Ojas	Cooling: Sweet, Bitter	1 part in formula
Licorice Root	Harmonize formula, demulcent, balance hormones, feed Ojas	Cooling: Sweet, Bitter	1 part in formula
Ginger Root	Activate formula, assimilate formula, increase Agni, universal tonic, Vata tonic, move blood, activate ovulation	Heating: Sweet, Pungent	½ part in formula

Herb	Herbal Actions	Energetics & Tastes	Dosage/Ratio
Gotu Kola Leaves	A Sattvic, Tridoshic, slightly cooling blood purifier, alterative, nervine stimulant, to remove her 'dizziness' and rebuild and purify her nerves.	Cooling: Bitter, Sweet	1 part in formula
Aloe Juice Gel	Sattvic, Tridoshic, emmenagogue, alterative, tonify Agni without increasing Pitta, nutritive, rejuvenative, feed Ojas	Cooling: Bitter, Sweet, Pungent, Astringent	2-4 ounces in base

DIRECTIONS: Add herbs to a base of Aloe Juice Gel, 2-4 ounces in 2-4 ounces of rose water.

Exercise Recommendations

Calming type of exercises would be recommended so as not to excite her Pitta or excessively move her Vata causing more imbalance. Instead of running and racing against others and the clock and stressing over whether she is going to get hit by that car or twist her ankle on that curb, she can be calm and hike in nature with calm loving friends, taking in good Prana or she can do some calming exercises in a calm, cool, friendly, loving environment.

14 Conscious Living: Bringing Peace to the Seven Aspects of Being

The purpose of this book has been to help you achieve your fullest potential in healthful living through the art and science of Ayurvedic tongue diagnosis, and, as well, offering you healing protocol through the healing tastes and a Sattvic approach to diet. In Ayurveda, we recognize that the fulfillment of health and happiness is reached through finding peace with the seven aspects of being. The first is peace with the body. A body that is vibrant and healthy is the foundation for the other aspects of oneself to flourish. When we experience harmony within our body, peace with mind, the emotions / family, community, culture, ecology and God / Goddess can follow with grace and ease.

As members of a global family, we have a beautiful responsibility to care for and love the body we have been gifted with. In learning to read the language and messages of the body, the laws of nature are revealed to us. We discover the wholeness of life and our part within this web of existence. We come home to our roots, our beginnings.

The practical and esoteric teachings of Ayurveda help us to achieve the unified peace we all seek. Tongue diagnosis is but one of the methods that can support us in achieving our goal to live conscious, beautiful lives in harmony with nature.

Conscious Living: Peace with the Seven Aspects of Being

Peace with the Body

We begin with the body. When the body is nourished by nature's seven healers: (1) organic, living foods; (2) fresh air; (3) adequate sunlight; (4) pure water; (5) exercise; (6) rest and (7) emotional, mental and spiritual nutrition, we experience a natural state of health and harmony. The body is honored as the manifestation of the laws of life and the cosmos. Through the study of the body is revealed the "keys" to the universe, and how to heal oneself.

Peace with the Mind

Peace with the mind involves creating a peaceful mind on three levels: the individual mind, the planetary mind and the cosmic mind. The mind's individual function is to utilize the power of thought to lovingly guide our feelings and actions. The planetary function is to contribute noble and uplifting thoughts to the planetary thinking body, thus connecting one with the cosmic ocean of thought from which all inspiration and truth comes. Through this most powerful force of thought one has the ability to achieve anything to which one aspires that is in harmony with the Cosmic Law.

Peace with the Family/Emotions

Peace with the family is concerned with harmony in the feeling body, harmony in the emotions. Divine love is the great cosmic power. It is the law of the body, but is expressed most powerfully through the feeling body. The key is to love oneself unconditionally. This gives one the strength to interact with family, friends and associates with unconditional love. The feeling body can be the most powerful capacity for creating health and vitality

Peace with Community

Peace with community is the ultimate result of a shift in individual consciousness to the awareness of global unity. To do this, we must heal the illusion of separation. The more we live in harmony with natural and divine laws the more we are likely to experience our true state of oneness with all of creation. From nature and each element we receive education and pleasure. Through meditation, study and nature we learn peace with community.

Peace with Culture

Peace with culture refers to the utilization of the masterpieces of wisdom from all ages, including the present. Humanity can take its rightful place in the universe by absorbing the great spiritual teachings given to us. The three approaches to spiritual evolution include: the intuitive path of the mystic, the path of studying nature, and the path of studying the works of the great masters of literature and art.

Peace with Ecology

Peace with the Earthly Mother is the foundation of our physical and spiritual existence. Our health, vitality and well-being requires an ability to attune ourselves to our inner nature so that we may know nature as an extension of our Self. As we re-sensitize ourselves to nature, we learn to co-operate with her laws and discover them as a natural expression of who we are.

Peace with God

Peace with God is total peace. Through this peace one becomes united with the highest values of the universe. It is the totality of the six other aspects of peace. As we attune with cosmic consciousness we unify with Universal Divine Law, synergistic with God as co-creator. Through this peace is awakened the inner intuition of Truth and Love resulting in great joy and love filling every aspect of one's life.

Final Thoughts

I give you this book to support you in discovering ways that you can take charge of your health and create the lifestyle that suites your uniqueness and potentiality. . We started our exploration of Ayurvedic tongue diagnosis to find out the type of seed we were born as; we then explored where you are now and how you got there. With this knowledge, we are able to re-create dietary and lifestyle practices that support every aspect of being. You are a unique and beautiful creation of life. May this book support you in the unfolding of your great potential.

Impressions – Expressions

Through Ayurveda tongue diagnosis we have been observing how the impressions of life experiences show up the tongue. Through years of impressions that we have experienced in only a matter of time they begin to be seen as expressions of health or disease. May we all learn on how to walk and be connected to our heart and to live with joy and compassion for ourselves and all life. As Dr. Frawley so beautifully stated *"trying to mediate without controlling our impressions puts our subconscious against us and prevents the development of inner peace and clarity."* We are an accumulation of our impressions; let us choose wisely of which impressions we take in, so we can express our true divine self – which is pure love.

By implementing the teachings of the tongue and the constitution, you are embracing the vital energy of the elements. Vital energy is the most primordial force of nature, driving the universe toward conscious awareness of its own existence. To be overflowing in vital energy is to be aligned with the creative power of life.

Ayurveda is learning about who you are and how to live consciously. Through observation of the tongue on a regular basis you can chart your journey back to wholeness. The most essential journey is the one that carries you back home, restoring your relationship with the source of what nourishes you. Life is a sacred journey to attain harmony above separation. The closer we approach the source, the greater access we have to vital pure energy.

Know that you started your life as a sacred seed.
Know that you are a sacred being.
Know that you are on sacred ground.

Peace be with you!

Walter 'Shantree' Kacera

15 Constitutional Questionnaires and Diagnostic Worksheet

- Prakruti Questionnaire
- Vikruti Questionnaire
- Tongue Diagnosis Worksheet

Prakruti Constitutional Questionnaire

What you came in the world with and characteristics that don't change or what you felt like at your healthiest stage in life.

The following questionnaire is to help determine the unique constitution that you came into the world with. It shows where we started constitutionally and where we may need to return to "feel ourselves."

The following characteristics are the ones that do not change, they reveal our Prakruti. The choices that you pick here reveal your original metabolic type. This is the body type that you were born into that you were meant to experience the world in. As we go through life, our lifestyle, diet, climate, etc., can, and will, shift you from this but the results will be compromised immunity and health. The distribution of your answers may reveal you to be predominantly one type or a mixed type, and this basic configuration VPK is where your health lies. The result of this questionnaire is compared to that of your Vikruti questionnaire.

To find out what your true body / mind type was at birth, take the following questionnaire, answering the questions NOT as you are now, but as you were at the peak of your health.

If you are under 20 and are in very excellent health, it may be necessary to do this only once.

0= describes me not at all.
1= describes me a little.
2= describes me well.
3= describes me the most.

Prakruti Constitution

15.1 Prakruti Questionnaire

Dosha Element Taste/Rasa		**Vata** Air & Ether Astringent, Bitter		**Pitta** Fire & Water Sour, Pungent		**Kapha** Water & Earth Sweet, Salty
ATTRIBUTES		Dry, Light, Cold, Clear, Rough, Subtle, Mobile		Hot, Sharp, Light, Oily, Liquid, Spreading		Heavy, Slow, Viscous, Cloudy, Smooth, Damp, Oily
BONES		Light, Small Bones		Medium Bones		Heavy Large Bones
BODY FRAME STRUCTURE		Small or tall, thin, underdeveloped		Medium build, moderate Muscular physique, Balanced & proportional		Thick, Tall or short, Large curved structure
JOINTS		Irregular, protruding		Regular		Large, Fleshy
FINGERS & TOES		Long & Tapering		Medium Length		Short & Large Fingers
HANDS & FEET		Small		Medium		Square & Thick Toes
NAILS		Cracked, brittle, Hang nails		Red nail bed, Nails bend		Thick & Strong Nails
LIPS		Thin, Small, Irregular		Medium, Red, Pink		Large, Full
EYEBROWS & LASHES		Thin, small		Medium		Thick, bushy

15.1 Prakruti Questionnaire (cont'd)

EYE SIZE		Small		Medium		Large
EYE COLOR		Dark Brown		Green, Amber, Mixed		Blue, Black, Chocolate
EYE MOVEMENT		Active, unsteady, Dry, jumpy		Sharp, penetrating, Light sensitive		Calm & steady, Liquid, moist
SCLERA COLOR		Gray		Red		White
TEETH		Small, Crooked, Uneven, Buck Teeth, Sensitive to heat & cold may need braces		Medium, Uniform, Even in Size		Large, Even, Gleaming
APPETITE USED TO BE		Variable, at times no interest in food & skipped meals		Excellent when hungry, Used to get Irritated & Angry		Good, Could easily skip a meal, but usually didn't
GENERALLY ATE FOOD WAS......		Quick & Small Meals, Warm, Moist & Oily		Moderately fast, Cool or Cold		Slowly but a lot, Warm & Dry
GAINS WEIGHT		Around Waist		Deposits fat evenly		In the rear & thighs
BODY HAIR		Scanty, or Over abundant, Tends to be Dark, Coarse & Curly		Light body hair, Fine texture, Straight & Soft		Moderate amount of body hair, Thick, Wavy, Soft
HAIR COLOR		Light or Medium Brown		Reddish Blonde		Dark Brown to Black
HEAD		Small, Thin, Unsteady		Medium		Large
FOREHEAD		Small		Medium with folds & Receding hairline		Large
NOSE		Uneven shape, Deviated septum, Crooked, Thin, Small		Long pointed, Reddish Nose tip, Medium size		Short rounded nose, Button nose, Large, Wide, Thick

15.1 Prakruti Questionnaire (cont'd)

CHIN & JAW		Receding, Small, Pointing		Medium		Thick, Large
NECK		Small, Thin, Unsteady		Medium		Thick, Large, Sturdy, Steady
SHOULDERS		Narrow, Thin		Medium balance		Thick, large, Sturdy, Steady
CHEST		Narrow, Twisted, Pigeon or Concave		Medium balance		Large, Broad
HIPS		Narrow		Medium		Large
COMPLEXION RELATIVE TO YOUR FAMILY		Dark, Tans easily		Fair skin, Burns easily, Freckles & Moles		Pale, White, Tans evenly
SKIN TENDS TO BE		Dry, Rough, Tough		Oily, Sensitive, Delicate		Smooth, Thick, Oily
SKIN THICKNESS ON FOREARM		Thin, Less than 1 cm.		Medium, 1-2 cm.		Thick, More than 2 cm.
BELLY BOTTOM		Small, Irregular, Herniated		Oval, superficial		Big, Deep, Round, Stretched
HAIR TENDED TO BE...		Kinky, Curly, Dry, Fine		Fine, Light, Straight, Early Graying		Wavy, Thick, Shiny
HAIR COLOR		Medium to Light Brown		Blond, Reddish		Black Brown to Black
AMOUNT OF HAIR		Average amount		Thin to Balding		Full, Thick
CHILDHOOD WEIGHT		Thin as a child, Difficulty gaining weight		Med. build, Periods of gaining & Losing weight		Large or Chunky build, Gains weight easily
SLEEP		Very light, Easily Interrupted, (Usually 4-6 hours)		Sound, Moderate (Usually 6-8 hours)		Very deep, Difficult to wake up (Usually 8-10 hours)

15.1 Prakruti Questionnaire (cont'd)

ENERGY LEVEL		Erratic, Up & Down		Moderate to High		Pretty good & Steady
STAMINA & FOLLOW THINGS TO COMPLETION		Variable, At times go for long periods other times not		Very good, Go for long Periods with much intensity, Always more to do		Excellent, Could outlast most people if motivated, Rather be relaxing
HEALTHY ATTRIBUTES & BEHAVIORS SEEN IN YOURSELF		Upbeat, Cheerful, Spontaneous, Flexible, Sensitivo, Exhilarating, Imaginative, Optimistic, Life-of-the party, Alert, Stimulating, Resilient, Active-Mind, Adaptable, Enthusiastic		Energetic, Intelligent, Joyous, Practical, Fiery, Enthusiastic, Resilient, Self-Developed, Sweet, Enterprising, Forceful, Friendly, Methodical, Confident, Strong, Fair, Exuberant, A Leader, Just, Efficient, Pleasant		Compassionate, Peaceful, Loving, Sympathetic, Courageous, Forgiving, Affectionate, Committed, Generous, Down-to-Earth, Forgiving, Patient, Quiet, Unshakeable, Steady, Serene, Humble
UNHEALTHY ATTRIBUTES & BEHAVIORS SEEN IN YOURSELF		Nervous, Insecure, Difficulty, Concentrating, Worried, Complaining, Unpredictable, Spacey, Unfocused, Apathetic, Fearful, Depressed, High Strung, Chaotic, Quick to burn out, Failure to complete projects		Angry, Frustrated, Hostile, Self-Criticizing, Irritable, Critical of others, Hurtful, Intolerance of others, Argumentative, Insecure, Outburst of Temper, Hot headed, domineering, Tyrannical, Impatient, Intolerant to delays		Stagnant, Possessive, Stubborn, Passive, Stuck, Tendency to mothering, Manipulative, Clinging, Unable to accept change, Procrastinator, Inactive, Caring to extremes, Quiet, Stagnant, Over-attached, Greedy, Insecure, Inflexible, Unwanted, Unloved, Withdrawn, Hopeless
TOTAL		**VATA**		**PITTA**		**KAPHA**

Vikruti: Your Current State of Balance & Health

The following descriptions may describe where you are presently, as within the recent past or so. This questionnaire will help show you where your present state of consciousness and imbalance are. This is a useful questionnaire to do on a regular basis. It's a good indicator to show which areas you need to give your attention to and which foods, herbs, exercises, breathwork and meditations would support you on your spiritual path.

0= describes me not at all.

1= describes me a little.

2= describes me well.

3= describes me the most.

Vikruti Constitutional Questionnaire

15.2 Vikruti Questionnaire

Dosha Elements		**Vata** Air & Ether		**Pitta** Fire & Water		**Kapha** Water & Earth
			PHYSICAL BODY			
WEIGHT		Difficulty gaining, gains around belly		If puts mind to it, gains evenly		Gains easily with exercise, Gains around hips & busts
JOINTS		Painful, Unsteady, Cracking or Stiff		Hot, Swollen, Burning		Loose, Aching, Watery, Swollen
WEATHER		Craves warmth, Dislikes Wind, Cold & Dryness		Craves Cool, Dislikes Fire, Heat & Sun		Craves Dryness, Dislikes Water, Dampness, Humidity & Clammy
ODOR		Astringent		Sour, Sharp		Sweet, Pleasant
LIPS		Chapped & Cracked		Cold Sores & Fever Blisters		Full & Moist
GUMS		Receding		Inflamed, Bleeding Gums		Thick

15.2 Vikruti Questionnaire (cont'd)

Dosha Elements		**Vata** Air & Ether		**Pitta** Fire & Water		**Kapha** Water & Earth
TONGUE		Dry, Thin		Red Inflamed		Swollen, thick and curled along the edges.
TONGUE COLOR		Grayish		Yellowish-Orange Red		Whitish Coating
EYES		Dry & Scratchy		Sclera has red-dish or Yellowish ting, Sites		Tendency toward Eye Puffiness
HAIR		Dry, Luster-less, Splits		Oily, Early Gray, Easily Thinning		Thick, Slightly Wavy & Oily, Lustrous
WHEN ILL		Nervous disorders, Sharp Pains, Backaches		Fevers, Rashes, or Inflammation		Swelling, Fluid, Retention, Con-gestion, Mucous
TOTAL		**VATA**		**PITTA**		**KAPHA**

The Body Systems

NERVOUS SYSTEM						
NERVOUS DISORDERS		Pain in the joints, Giddiness, Trem-ors, Insomnia, Anxiety, Paralysis or Paresis of the Muscles		Wrong perception of sensations of temperature, Fainting		Lack of Motivation
DIGESTION SYSTEM						
APPETITE		Variable		Strong, Exces-sive		Steady, Slow
BOWEL MOVE-MENTS		Irregular, Hard, Dry or Consti-pated		Loose, more than twice dai-ly, Tendency to Diarrhea		Large, Full move-ments, Once daily, Mucus, Itching

The Body Systems (cont'd)

DIGESTION SYSTEM						
DISORDERS		Gas formation, Nausea, Parasites, Constipation, Pain in the colon, Vomiting, Hemorrhoids		Pain or Burning Sensation in the gastric region, Diarrhea, Colitis, Vomiting with blood, Blood in the Stool, Bacillary Dysentery		Sluggishness, Heaviness, Parasites
MUSCU-SKELETAL SYSTEM						
DISORDERS		Muscular Pain		Muscular Inflammation, Warts		Sloughing of flesh, Oily, Heavy and greasy skin, Tumors, Gangrene in the Muscles
REPRODUCTIVE SYSTEM						
DISORDERS		Sterility or Impotency, Disturbances, Irregularity		Excessive Bleeding, Extreme Hot Flashes, PMS, Night Sweats		Enlargement of Prostrate, Hydrocele
WOMEN DISORDERS		Deficient milk supply, Painful Menstruation		Impure Milk		Breast Tumors, or Abscesses
URINARY SYSTEM						
THIRST		Irregular		Strong, Excessive		Slight
URINE		Scanty, Cloudy		Profuse, Yellow		Moderate
DISORDERS		Painful Urination		Urinary Tract Infection		Edema, Diabetes. Urinary Tract Stones
CIRCULATORY SYSTEM						
CIRCULATION		Colds Hands & Feet		Skin Warm to the Touch		Skin cool but not Cold
SWEAT		Scanty		Profuse		Moderate

The Body Systems (cont'd)

CIRCULATORY SYSTEM						
DISORDERS		Disinclination for food, Anemia, Acne, Deficient Sweating, Hardening of the Blood		Imbalanced digestive fire, Skin Rashes, Stomatitis, Blood in the urine or feces, Rectum Inflammation, Jaundice, Excessive Sweating, Hypertension, Heart Diseases		Abscesses, Tumors, Bluish-Black Skin Spots, Leucoderma
IMMUNITY SYSTEM						
DISORDERS		Tendency to acute Allergies		Prone to Infections		Tendency to Chronic Conditions
RESPIRATORY SYSTEM						
DISORDERS		Lack of strength, Shortness of breath, Wasting away of tissues, Dehydration, Tuberculosis, Hay fever		Severe Infectious Disease, Bronchitis, Allergic Rhinitis		Accumulation of Mucous Colds, Flus, Sore Throat, Swollen Glands, Asthma, Pneumonia
TOTAL		**VATA**		**PITTA**		**KAPHA**

The Seven Tissues

LYMPH/ PLASMA (RASA)		Dry Skin, Colds hands & feet, Numbness or Discoloration of Skin, Eczema, Psoriasis, Dry Cough		Fever, Acne, Bronchitis, Increased Sweating & Thirst, Sensitive eyes, Sore Throat, Psoriasis, Eczema		Water Retention, swollen Joints, Frequent Colds, Bronchial Congestion, Loss of Ap-petite, Lethargy
BLOOD (RAKTA)		Hypertension, Heart Disease, Palpitation, Dry Eczema, Gout, Varicose Veins, Bruises Easily, Heart Palpitation, Anemia		Dermatitis, Inflammation, Inflammations, Flushing of the Skin, Rashes, Hot Flashes, Burning Sensations in hands & feet		Congestion of Liver, Poor Circulation, High Cholesterol, Gall Stones, Anemia
MUSCLE (MAMSA)		Muscle pain, Spasm, Atrophy, Lack of Coordination, Twitching, Decreased Flexibility		Inflammation of Muscles, Bursitis, Tendon		Swelling, Rigidity in Mus-cles, Increased Nasal Mucus, Difficulty Moving, Lethargy
FAT (MEDAS)		Dry Skin, Cracking of Joints, Increased Thirst, Diabetes, Low Backache		Kidney Infections, Profuse Sweating, Cellulites, Excess Urination		High Cholesterol, Obesity, Pancreas & Spleen Disorders, Fatigue
BONE (ASTHI)		Bone & Joint, Arthritis, Rheumatoid Arthritis, Weakening of bone tissue, Fractures, Osteoporosis, Dental Caries, Infections		Redness of Joints, Burning Pain in Joints, Inflammatory Arthritis, Early &/ or Graying Hair		Swollen Joints, Bone Spurs
NERVE & MARROW (MAJA)		Memory loss, Nerve Pain, Weakened Nervous System, Paralysis, Dizziness, Anemia, Feeling Emptiness, & Fear, Sciatica, Neuralgia, Fainting, Lack of Coordination, Insomnia, Ringing in Ears, Tremors		Headaches, Dizziness, Anger, Irritability, Neuritis, Nervous System Sensitivity overly Sharp & Painful Perception		Dullness of Senses, Dull Aching Pain, Cracking Joints & Pain

The Seven Tissues (cont'd)

REPRODUCTIVE TISSUE (SHUKRA)		Decreased Vitality, Fear, Irregular Hormonal Cycle, Low Sexual Desire, Anxiety, Painful Menstruation		Painful Menstruation, Reproductive Tissue Inflammation, Uterine Bleeding, Swollen & Inflamed Prostrate		Low Energy, Infertility, Poor Resistance to Colds, Flus, Lack of Motivation, En-larged Prostrate Impotency, Endometriosis
TOTAL		**VATA**		**PITTA**		**KAPHA**

The Emotions

The emotional characteristics of each type have both positive and negative aspects. As you go through this section, take note to where you are emotionally: are you manifesting negative or positive aspects, are you in alignment with your Prakruti, your Vikruti, or have you developed characteristics outside of your dosha. This emotional questionnaire will show that if our depressing or negative emotions match your "dosha imbalance", they need to be taken care of by appropriate lifestyle and dietary regimes. If, however, they fall out of pattern, they are associated with a different dosha (VPK). Specific herbs to reduce those emotions can be applied.

EXPERIENCES		Fear, Anxious, Nervous, Secretive, Communicative, Practices, Dynamic, Sneaky, Flexible, Takes Change Well, Self- Destructive		Anger or Hate, Irritable, Angry, Caring, Perceptive, Manipulative, Tolerant, Accepts things when no other choice, Can be Vindictive, Destructive		Apathy, Attached, Desirous, Loyal, Devoted, Harmonious, Greedy, Enjoys possessions, Patient, Accepts all, Can be Uncaring, Feels Victimized
FEELINGS		Feelings & Emotions Change Easily		Aggressive about options & feelings, Gives Options even if not asked for		Avoids giving options in difficult situations
DREAMS		About flying, Running, Restless nightmare		In color, Passion, Conflicts, Speed & Moving Fast		About Romance, Often Involves Water

The Emotions (cont'd)

HEALTHY ATTRIBUTES & BEHAVIORS THAT YOU SEE IN YOURSELF		Upbeat, Cheerful, Spontaneous, Flexible, Sensitive, Exhilarating, Imaginative, Optimistic, Life-of-the party, Alert, Stimulating, Resilient, Active-Mind, Adaptable, Enthusiastic		Energetic, Intelligent, Joyous, Practical, Fiery, Enthu-siastic, Resilient, Self Developed, Sweet, Enterprising, Forceful, Friendly, Methodical, Con-fident, Strong, Fair, Exuberant, A Leader, Just, Efficient, Pleasant		Compassionate, Peaceful, Loving, Sympathetic, Courageous, Forgiving, Affectionate, Committed, Generous, Down-to-Earth, Patient, Quiet, Unshakeable, Steady, Serene, Humble
UN-HEALTHY ATTRIBUTES & BEHAVIORS THAT YOU SEE IN YOURSELF		Nervous, Insecure, Difficulty concentrating, Worried, Complaining, Unpredictable, Spacey, Unfocused, Apathetic, Fearful, Depressed, High Strung, Chaotic, Quick to burn out, Failure to complete projects		Angry, frustrated, Hostile, Self-Criticizing, Irritable, Critical of others, Hurtful, Intolerance of others, Argumentative, Insecure, Outburst of Temper, Hot headed, domineering, Tyrannical, Impatient, Intolerant to delays		Stagnant, Possessive, Stubborn, Passive, Stuck, Tendency to mothering, Manipulative, Clinging, Unable to accept change, Procrastinator, Inactive, Caring to extremes, Quiet, Stagnant, Over-attached, Greedy, Insecure, Inflexible, Unwanted, Unloved, Withdrawn, Hopeless
WHEN YOU SEE YOURSELF AS HEALTHY & BALANCED, YOU SEE YOUSELF AS BEING		Knowledgeable, Good Communicator, Positive, Active, Enterprising, Acute, Awareness, Lively, Energetic, Adaptable, Good Comprehension, Initiator		Intelligent, Rational, Independent, Warm, Clear Thinker, Bright, Friendly, Intellectual, Courageous, Perceptive, Leadership Qualities, Discriminating, Enlightened		Peaceful, Compassionate, Calm, Forgiving, Loyal, Faithful, Steadfast, Firm, Stable, Receptive, Nurturing, Content, Devoted, Supportive

The Emotions (cont'd)

WHEN YOU SEE YOURSELF AS OUT OF BALANCE, YOU SEE YOUSELF AS BEING		Indecisive, Nervous, Disruptive, Agitated, Unreliable, Distressed, Superficial, Anxious, Restless		Angry, Manipulative, Vain, Ambitious, Aggressive, Willful, Impulsive, Proud, Dominating, Critical		Materialistic. Greedy, seeking Luxury, & Comfort, Sentimental, Very Controlling, Covetous, Over-Attached
WHEN YOU SEE YOURSELF AS UNHEALTHY, YOU SEE YOUSELF AS BEING		Addictive, Fearful, Self-Destructive, Secretive Depressed, Suicidal, Dishonest, Harmful		Angry towards others, Contemptible, Paltry, Base, Hateful		Dispassionate, Unemotional, Apathetic, Insensitive, Listless, Lethargic, Dull
TOTAL		**VATA**		**PITTA**		**KAPHA**

The Mind

The mind of each metabolic type demonstrates favorable and unfavorable characteristics. By understanding and knowing how you think can save you much discomfort. This understanding as to which of the Elements are most predominant, may make you much happier in your day-to-day activities. The mind questionnaire reveals to us our mind's potentials with our gifts and challenges we may face. Taking time to understand our mental nature can assist us in choosing an occupation that works and suits our innate abilities and avoid those activities that do not suit us.

MIND		Restless, Active, Likes Motion		Enjoys Completion, Aggressive Actives		Calm & Relaxed, Leisure Actives
CONCENTRATION		Short-term Memory, Forgets Quickly		Long-term Memory, Logical, Rational Thoughts		Excellent Memory, Takes time to Learn
ORGANIZATION		Dislikes Structure		Likes Planning		Well Organized

The Mind (cont'd)

DECISION MAKING		Changes Mind Easily, Difficult Deciding		Sees things Easily, Rapid Decision-Making		Slow in Making Decisions, Sticks with Decision
THINKER		Creative		Organized		Follows Plan of Action
PROJECTS		Takes on many projects all at once		Proceeds in an orderly way, Constantly Organizing		Resists Change & New Projects, Enjoys Simplicity
FRIENDS		Few close friends, Knows a lot of people		Creates warm friendships but very selective, & makes enemies easily		Loyal with many friends
FINANCIAL		Spends quickly & Impulsively, Doesn't save, Money is used		Plans spending, Saves but big spender, money is for Achieving Purpose		Spends reluctantly, Saves regularly, Accumulates Wealth, Likes to Save
SPEECH		Fast talker, rapid, Changes subjects		Sharp, Fluid, Orderly, Serious		Slow, Thoughtful, Melodious
VOICE		High pitch & fast		Moderate Pitch, Clear		Low Pitch, Deep, Resonating
TOTAL		**VATA**		**PITTA**		**KAPHA**

These questionnaires show us where we are operating physically, mentally and emotionally at this present moment. After initiating therapies, diet, herb, and lifestyle changes to balance your doshas, you can retake these three parts and see a shift. Your Prakruti will always remain the same and so is not included in the total, nor is it necessary to retake that questionnaire.

15.3 Prakruti – Vikruti Consitutional Results

Prakruti Constitution Results						
PRAKRUTI TOTAL		Vata		Pitta		Kapha
Vikruti Constitution Results						
THE PHYSICAL BODY						
PHYSICAL BODY TOTAL						
THE BODY SYSTEMS						
NERVOUS						
DIGESTIVE						
MUSCU-SKELETAL						
REPRODUCTIVE						
URINARY						
CIRCULATORY						
IMMUNE						
RESPIRATORY						
BODY SYSTEMS TOTAL						
THE SEVEN TISSUES						
LYMPH & PLASMA						
BLOOD						
MUSCLES						
FAT						
BONE						
NERVE & MARROW						
REPRODUCTIVE TISSUE						
SEVEN TISSUES TOTAL						
THE EMOTIONS						
EMOTIONS TOTAL						
THE MIND						
MIND TOTAL						
VIKRUTI TOTAL						

Tongue Diagnosis Results						
PRAKRUTI		**VATA**		**PITTA**		**KAPHA**
Tongue Vitality						
Tongue Body-Color		Pale/ dull		Red/purplish/ yellow		Pale/white
Tongue Body Shape/Size		Thin/black		Yellow		White/mucus layer
PRAKRUTI TOTAL						

VIKRUTI		**VATA**		**PITTA**		**KAPHA**
Tongue Coating-Color		Back zone-Brownish-dark		Mid zone-Reddish-yellow		Front zone-White to dirty white
Tongue Coating-Thickness		Light coating		Some coating		Thick shiny coating
Tongue Coating-Location		Back zone-large colon area		Mid zone-small intes-tines area		Front zone-stomach area
Cracks in Tongue Body		Back zone-crack(s) in large colon area, the deeper and more number of cracks		Mid zone-crack(s) in small intestines area, usually midline crack		Front zone-crack(s) in stomach area, shallow and few cracks
Teeth Marks		Back zone-teeth marks back side of tongue, usually heavy		Mid zone-teeth marks mid side of tongue, usually slight marks		Front zone-teeth marks front side of tongue, usually slight markings
Spots on Tongue		Back zone-dark spots in the back of the tongue		Mid zone-or both sides in-dicating liver imbalance		Front zone-whitish spots towards the front or front side of tongue
Tongue Moisture		Back zone-on the dry and dull in appearance		Mid zone-moderate moisture with a reddish tone		Front zone-thick moist throughout tongue espe-cially towards the front
Tongue Moisture		Cracks-midline		Sores/fever blisters		Foamy/lungs
VIKRUTI TOTAL						

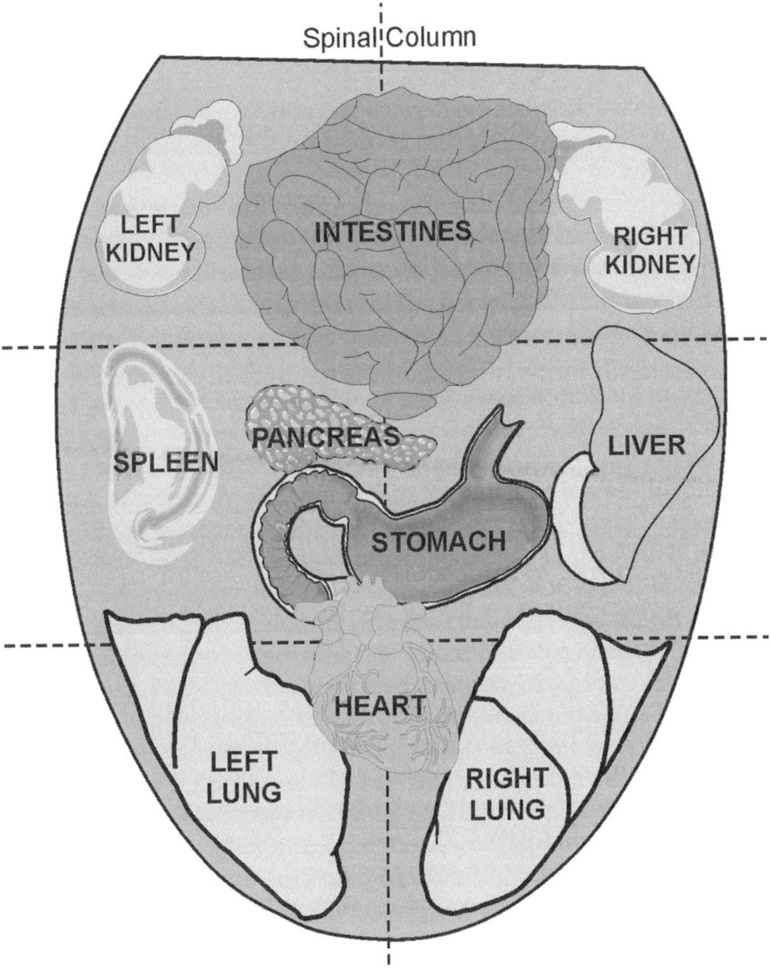

Prakruti Constitution Results						
PRAKRUTI TOTAL		Vata		Pitta		Kapha
Vikruti Constitution Results						
VIKRUTI TOTAL		Vata		Pitta		Kapha
Constitution Results						
TOTAL %		Vata		Pitta		Kapha

Comments & Suggestions:

Elements:

Tastes:

Body Systems:

Tissues:

Attributes:

Actions:

Herbs & Spices:

Dietary Recommendations

Herbal Glossary of Terms

ALTERATIVES - agents that gradually and favorably alter the condition of the body; cleanses and purifies the blood; alters existing nutritive and excretory processes gradually restoring normal body function.

ANALGESIC - relieves pain.

ANODYNE - plants that have action of pain relief.

ANTHELMINTIC - stimulating plants that work against parasitic worms that may be present in the digestive system.

ANTICATARRHAL - plants that eliminate or counteract the formation of mucous.

ANTILITIC - plants that have the ability to remove or prevent formation of stones or gravel in the urinary system.

ANTIMICROBIAL - plants used to rid the body of microorganisms that have invaded it or act on the skin.

ANTIPLASTIC - plants that have the specific action of inhibiting and combating the development of tumors.

ANTIPYRETIC - plants that dispel heat, fire and fever.

ANTIRHEUMATIC - herbs with a reputation for preventing, relieving and curing rheumatic problems.

ANTIPLASTIC - plants that have a constricting or binding effect (used to prevent or counteract the growth of disease germs).

ANTISPASMODIC - herbal remedies that rapidly relax nervous tension that may be causing digestive spasms of colic.

AROMATIC - oils of aromatic herbs that will penetrate into muscles, increasing circulation.

ASTRINGENT - substances that have constricting or binding effects; aid in breaking down secretions.

BITTER - plants in small amounts stimulate and promote appetite, aid digestion and otherwise help regulate fire in the body.

CARMINATIVE - herbs and spices taken to relieve gas and griping.

CATHARTIC - herbs that have a laxative effort.

CHOLAGOGUE - promotes the flow and discharge of bile into

the small intestine.

DEMULCENT - soothing substances taken internally to protect damaged tissue.

DIAPHORETIC - herbs used to induce sweating.

DIURETIC - herbs that increase the flow of urine.

DYSMENORRHEA - condition of menstruation accompanied by cramping pains that may be incapacitating in their intensity.

EMMENAGOGUE - herbs that promote menstruation.

EMETIC - induce vomiting.

EMOLLIENT - soothes, softens and protects the skin.

EXPECTORANT - promotes the discharge of phlegm and mucus from the lungs and throat.

FEBRIFIGE - reduces fever.

HEMATOSTATIC - plants that stop the flow of blood; a type of astringent action that stops the flow of internal bleeding.

HEPATIC - plants that strengthen tone and stimulate secretive functions of the liver.

LAXATIVE - plants that promote bowel movements.

NERVINE - herbs used to ease anxiety and stress and nourish the nerves.

NUTRITIVE TONIC - increases weight and density and nourishes the body.

PURGATIVE - plants that promotes bowel movement and increased intestinal peristalsis.

RUBEFACIENT - herbs that, when applied to the skin, stimulate circulation in that area.

REFRIGERANT - plants that reduce body temperature and relieve thirst.

REJUVENATIVE - prevents decay, postpones aging, revitalizes the organs.

SEDATIVE - plants that calm the nervous and lowering functional activity of organ or body part.

STIMULANT - increases internal heat; dispels internal chill and strengthens digestion, metabolism and circulation.

STOMACHIC - strengthens stomach function.

STYPTIC - plants that cause capillaries to contract and thus stop superficial hemorrhage

bleeding.

TONIC - herbs that promote the functions of the systems of the body.

VASODILATOR - causes relaxation of blood vessels.

VERMICIDAL - kills parasites in the intestines.

VERMIFUGE - herbs taken to kill worms in the intestine.

VULNERARY - plants that assist in the healing of wounds by protecting against infection and stimulating cell growth.

Ayurvedic Tongue Diagnosis Glossary

ABSORPTION - is the process by which nutrients move from the intestine into the blood.

AIR ELEMENT - is one of the lightest of the five elements. Its properties are cold, light, clear, fine and rough. Its effect both in the body and the external world is purifying, drying, loosening, and promoting movement. Its taste is classified as astringent and bitter.

AGNI - the Latin word "ignis" from which the English word "ignite" is derived, has a common root with the Sanskrit word "Agni." Agni means that which ignites, which is Fire.

Bodily fire, particularly digestive fire, biological fire governing metabolism and everything that is heat in the body (temperature, sight, and heat); its function is transformation, absorption, elimination and discrimination. It is the essential form of fire and heat, the basis of good digestion.

ANABOLIC - the construction or building-up of body tissues; building phase of metabolism, referring to all chemical changes by which simple substances are used to manufacture complicated substances.

ANNA – food.

AMA - matter that is generated internally and/or results from poor assimilation, toxins, undigested food or unlimited waste materials.

ANTIOXIDANT - a substance that delays or prevents oxidation, a normal part of the respiration process (energy production in the cells) which produces potentially harmful free radicals.

AROMATHERAPY - therapeutic use of essential oils from plants.

ASTHI- bone and cartilage tissue is one of the seven components and the bone tissues that support the body by giving it protection, shape, nourishment and longevity.

ATTRIBUTES- the inherent qualities or properties of a substance

AURA - light, color emanating from living beings, usually visible only to those gifted in the perception of such things.

AYURVEDA- the 5,000-year-old science of medicine from India, knowledge of life, Vedic science of health.

BIOACTIVE - live, organic foods that are fully matured, add energy to the human being, and have a positive effect on the human mind and body.

BIOCIDIC - a category of cooked foods that are stale, processed, adulterated, and/or commercially grown with herbicides, insecticides and pesticides; foods which have a deleterious effect on the body and mind when eaten.

BIOGENIC - live, organic foods that are not fully grown and are filled with regenerative energy; they add more energy and have a positive effect on the human body and mind than any other food category.

BIOSTATIC - a category of cooked foods or minimally processed foods, as well as foods that are raw but no longer fresh, they are life-sustaining on the short –term but are gradually life-force depleting on the long-term

CARCINOGENENS - substances that initiate or promote the development of cancer.

CATABOLIC - the destruction or breakdown process of body

tissue; tearing down phase of metabolism, refers to all chemical reactions by which complex substances are further broken down to simpler components.

CEREMONY - respectful performance of a ritual.

CIT – consciousness.

CHAKRA - wheel; seven energy centers of consciousness in the body; they are responsible for the different levels of consciousness, they correspond physiologically to the nerve plexus centers.

CHARAK- great Ayurvedic physician who wrote one of the classic medical texts of Ayurveda: *Charak Samita.*

CHARAKA - an Indian herbal or pharmacopoeia.

CHLOROPHYLL - the green pigment of plants; it represents hemoglobin in structure except it has a magnesium in it instead of iron; it collects sunlight energy and converts CO_2 and water into carbohydrates.

CONSCIOUSNESS - the state of being, characterized by sensation, emotion, volition and thought; the quality or state of being aware, especially of something within oneself; the state of being conscious of an external object, state or fact.

CONSTITUTION - the basic genetic psychological and physiological blueprint a person is born with.

DECOCTION - a plant extract made by gently warming the plant parts (usually seeds, roots or bark) for a few hours or over night in water.

DENATURE - to change the nature or natural qualities, to render unfit to eat or drink without destroying some usefulness, to cause the tertiary structure of (a protein) to unfold, as with heat, alkali or acid, so that some of its original properties, especially its biological activity, are diminished or eliminated; any foods which have been heated to a high-temperature, processed, "pesticided" or "herbicided," microwaved, irradiated or genetically engineered.

DENATURED- to deprive of natural qualities, change the nature of **a)** to make unfit for drinking without impairing usefulness for other purposes, **b)** to modify the molecular structure of (as a protein or DNA) especially by heat, acid, alkali, or ultraviolet radiation so as to destroy or diminish some of the original properties and especially the specific biological activity, **c)** referring to protein that has been heated and lost the required molecular shape needed to function properly; in essence, having its nature destroyed.

DETOXIFIERS - foods and herbs or healing substances that help the body discharge toxins.

DHATU - literally, "that which supports the body," a dhatu is one of the seven body tissues which, when well nourished, nourishes the whole individual; the basic nutritional and structural factors of the body; literally, to support or to nourish; there are seven dhatu (tissues) in the body; the seven bodily tissues are *rasa, rakta, mamsa, meda, asthi, majja* and *shukra*.

DOCTRINE OF SIGNATURES - a doctrine of medieval herbalists to the effect that the appearance, fragrance and taste of a plant provides the clues that resemble its curative influence.

DREAMTIME - a sacred time realm in Aborigine belief that is entered through sounding, chanting and dancing ceremonies.

DIGESTION - is the breaking down of complex substances into simple substances.

DISEASE - is a condition in which one or more body parts impair the performance of the vital functions and thus bring the absence of ease. Desire is considered to be the root cause of all diseases. It is said that desires pull the individuals from awareness and affection and this creates imbalances.

DOSHA - Sanskrit for humor; "that which will imbalance," a dynamic factor in human function in Ayurvedic system of thought. There are three doshas: Vata / air, Pitta / fire and Kapha / water. These three basic types of biological humors determine an individual's constitution; a dosha is one of the three forces that bind the Five Great Elements; is that which is "neither retained nor eliminated." It is a fault, meaning it defies the definition of Dhatu tissue, which is retained within the body, and Mala, waste product that is eliminated from the body.

EARTH ELEMENT - a basic element of life. Earth is the densest of the five elements. Earth promotes growth and stability. Its attributes are heaviness, stability and coarseness. It is solid with a downward movement energy. Its taste is classified as sweet and astringent.

ELEMENT - is a basic component of reality. Ancient sciences used it to designate fundamental building blocks of a multilevel universe- spanning the physical, the energetic and consciousness. Modern materialistic science uses the term to apply to atomic variants.

ELIXIR - usually a liquid concoction that is used as a medicine; also a "sovereign" or outstanding remedy that gives long or everlasting life.

ENZYME - a biologically, chemically, and energetically active protein complex that is made by a living organism that accelerates metabolic processes, digests food, helps to detoxify the body and protects it against free radicals; any of numerous proteins or conjugated proteins produced by living organisms and functioning as biochemical catalysts.

ESSENTIAL AMINO ACIDS - those amino acids that the body cannot produce on its own and must take in by the diet.

ESSENTIAL FATTY ACIDS - those fatty acids that the body cannot produce on its own and must take in by diet.

ETHER ELEMENT - is also called space, the unmanifested space of the universe. Its properties are subtle, smooth and soft. Its effect is softening and unblocking. Its taste is difficult to describe, but since it is cold and expansive it has the qualities of bitter and astringent.

FAST OXIDIZER - a metabolic body type that rapidly metabolizes carbohydrates.

FERMENTED FOODS - foods predigested by the enzymatic action of bacteria; these ferments are not only easier to digest but contain lactic acid produced by the bacteria that is healthy for the body.

FIRE ELEMENT - The fire element is the hottest and lightest of the five elements. Its properties are hot, dry, fine, light, rough and clear. Its effect both in the body and the external world is radiant and purifying with an upward movement. Its taste is classified as sour and salty.

FIVE ELEMENTS - the five states of material existence: mass, liquidity, transformation, movement and the field in which they function; also called: Earth, Water, Fire, Air and Ether.

FLAVONALS - fresh live food components that enhance health.

FLOWER ESSENCE - the healing energy of a flower, transmitted to dew that has settled on the blossom or to pure water in which it has been steeped.

FOOD - is anything that nourishes and sustains the body. It may be in the form of solids, semi-solids or liquids. It is essential for life as it contains substances which perform important functions in our body. These essential substances are called nutrients. Food also contains energetic factors such as aromas, tastes and natural coloring substances.

FREE RADICAL - is a highly reactive molecule made inside the body. Free radical molecules are one electron molecule short (electrons are usually paired), so they grab an electron from another molecule, disturbing the chemical balance by making this molecule one electron short, thus setting up a chain reaction. Free radicals are produced constantly in the body as a part of normal functions. They need to be dealt with immediately because they can damage D.N.A. resulting in premature aging.

FRESH - having its original qualities unimpaired, full of or renewed in vigor.

KAPHA - one of the three doshas or dynamic factors in human functioning, as conceptualized in Ayurvedic medicine, it has to do with the more solid and substantial aspects of the person and is made up of the Elements of Water and Earth; is related to the fluids and mucus in the body; one of the three dosha; the water humor; the extra cellular and intracellular fluid playing a vital role in the nutrition and existence of cells and tissues in the body.

GREENING - the medieval herbalist and mystic Hildegard of Bingen talked of Viridatas, the greening power. This greening power is the vital energy that is life, the Spirit of the Earth, the Earth Gaia in action that heals and transforms humanity. The natural healing that comes to us so freely and abundantly from the plant realm is indeed a greening of the human condition.

GUNAS - the prime quality of nature (Prakruti), the subtle medical science of qualities or attributes are also called Gunas.

HEALTH - is a state of complete physical, mental and social well being and not merely the absence of disease or infirmity.

HERBALISM - one of the oldest natural healing arts and sciences of the world; the usage, administration practices and working with plants and trees.

HERBALIST - one who has studied and applied the usage and practice of administering healing plants to support healing.

HOMEOSTATSIS - the maintenance of a steady balance in the individual by coordinated physiological processes in the body.

HUMORS - according to Ayurveda there are three primary life forces in the body, or three biological humors. These are called in Sanskrit Vata, Pitta and Kapha.

INFUSION - a tea made by gently steeping plant parts in warm water to preserve the life force and essential oils of the plant.

LIFE ESSENCE - the distinct energy of a living being, whether plant or animal.

LIVE FOODS - are foods that have not been denatured, cooked to a high-temperature, processed, pesticided or herbicided, microwaved, irradiated or genetically engineered. They are whole, fresh, sun-ripened, enzyme-rich, organically-grown plants. They still contain their full potential of Prana, Tejas and Oja qualities of the life-giving elements.

OJAS - life sap, the prime energy of the body, the subtle essence of all vital fluids, the essence of food; perfected essence of all tissues (dhatus) of the body; the basis of the immune system; responsible for health, harmony and spiritual growth, when bodily system is in excellent order; glow of health; it means the life sap or the essence of immune system and spiritual energy. Ojas is a protoplasmic substance called the albumin and globulin that is formed during the biosynthesis of bodily tissues and strengthens the tissues.

OXIDATION - the process in which oxygen is combined with other substances. When another molecule is oxidized, it may go on to produce free radicals. Oxidation therefore increases the demand for antioxidant nutrients.

OXIDATIVE DAMAGE - a condition in which free radicals are formed in excess of the body's ability to remove them, resulting in damage to body cells and to tissues.

MACRO-NUTRIENTS - most of the weight of the food is due to the nutrients of carbohydrates, proteins, fats and water.

MANDAGNI - weakened state of digestive fire.

MAJJA - one of the seven bodily constituents, mainly the bone marrow and its metabolism.

MALAS - wastes that must be excreted from the system, but which serve the body between creation and their excretion, for example, sweat, urine and feces.

MAMSA - one of the seven bodily constituents, mainly muscle and its metabolism.

MEDIA - one of the seven bodily constituents, mainly fat and metabolism of fat, carbohydrates, and hormones.

MEDITATION - a contemplative process that releases us from our everyday thoughts, has the ability to lead an individual to altered states of consciousness and enhanced powers of perception.

METABOLISM - the sum of all the biophysical and chemical processes through which living organisms function and maintain life. The transformation of ingested food by which energy is made available for the use of the organism, refers to all the chemical changes that take place in the cells, after the end products of digestion are absorbed.

MICROCOSM - a diminutive representative world; a system more or less analogous to a larger system.

NADI - literally, a river; the river of life as expressed through the pulse; the pulse; channel systems of subtle body.

NATURE - the material world and its phenomena, the elemental forces and processes that produce and control all the phenomena of the material world; the laws of nature, the world of living things and the outdoors, a primitive state of existence, untouched and uninfluenced by civilization or artificiality, the essential characteristics and qualities of a person or thing, the fundamental character or disposition of a person; temperament, the processes and functions of the body.

NIRAMA - conditions without Ama, non-clogging (no Ama)

digestive system.

NUTRITION - is the term used for the scientific study of food and how it is utilized by the body. It is the science of foods, the nutrients and other substances and their actions, interaction and balance in relation to health / disease. It is the processes such as ingestion, digestion, absorption, transportation, utilization of nutrients and disposal of end products. The social, economic, cultural and psychological implications of food and eating.

PANCHA KARMA - the Five Traditional Purification Methods and Rebalancing Practices that are used to rid the body of excess doshas; they are enemas, purging, emesis, nasal medication and bloodletting.

PACHAMAMMA - sacred Earth Mother in numerous south American cultures.

PITTA - one of the three doshas or dynamic factors in human functioning, as conceptualized in Ayurvedic medicine, it has to do with the fiery aspects of the human and is central to digestion, intelligence, and transformation.

PLANT SPIRIT MEDICINE - remedy inspired by the spirits of healing plants.

PRAB HAVA - the specific action of an herb or substance.

PRAKRUTI - according to Ayurveda, an individual's inherited constitution; inborn tendencies that influence personality; the dynamic energy of consciousness; natal constitution; primal nature; biological constitution.

PRANA - Pra=before, ana=breath; life-breath, another name for energy or life force, which activates the body and mind often associated with breath, but can refer to cosmic energy; Prana is responsible for the higher cerebral functions and the motor and sensory activities; that which governs inhalation and swallowing.

PRANAYAMA - a method of breath control used to regulate the mind and Prana and thereby physical and mental health.

PRESENCE - a state of consciousness characterized by awareness, simplicity, openness and the ability to be fully present in the moment; presence means bringing the resonant field of one's total being into the field of the present moment.

PSYCHOPHYSIOLOGY- that which pertains to the functioning of the body and mind.

PSYCHOSOMATIC COMPLEX - that which pertains to connection between mind and body.

PURUSHA - pure consciousness, spirit.

RAJAS/RAJASIC - quality of energy, turbulence and distraction, activity or aggressive force of creation; a diet and lifestyle that leads to an outgoing and/or aggressive activity; one of the three Gunas.

RASA - taste, especially the Six Tastes of Ayurveda initial taste in the three stages of taste; emotion, literally, "external beauty," or "maturity" or "essence,"; plasma; the first of the seven dhatus, rasa is derived from the digested food and after absorption it circulates in the entire body by specific channels; its main function is to provide nutrition to each and every cell of the body; the plasma dhatu.

RASAYANA - rejuvenation therapy that includes foods and herbs that supports immunity, regenerates body-mind, prevents decay, postpones aging; that which causes Ojas to be produced.

RISHI - literally "seer": a seer, ancient Rishis seers created Ayurveda out of compassion for the sufferings of humanity; a seer, one who sees the reality of life as described in the Veda and Vedic literature, one that is able to perceive hidden realities and manifest those realities in a way comprehensible to humans.

RESONANCE- the congruent mutual response elicited in the bodies of similar structure and frequency, as when the sound of one tuning fork causes another to vibrate with a similar tone, or the spirit of one person awakens that of another.

SADHANA - wholesome activity practiced with presence of mind in harmony with nature; helps to revive ancient memory.

SAMA - with Ama, coated tongue due to Ama in the digestive system.

SAMADHI - absorption, bliss.

SANSKRIT - Vedic and mantric language.

SATTVA/ SATTVIC - literally means, that what possesses the same nature as truth or reality. It is the cosmic force of balance and contentment, a diet and lifestyle that supports a spiritual life; central aspect of the three Gunas, essence; the spiritual principle of prime matter, one of the three Gunas.

SATTVIC DIET- a diet that promotes Sattva; mild, calming and nourishing foods; Buddhist dietary doctrine.

SHAMAN - literally means, "to know," one who is skilled in accessing realities not apparent to ordinary people in order to communicate with conscious entities there and / or make adjustments that will result in healing on this plane.

SHAMANISM - a spiritual practice of Asian countries, India and Native American Indians of Central, South and North America, in which a medicine man (the shaman) can influence spirits for the benefit of human beings' health and good fortune.

SHANTI- Peace.

SHUKRA - one of the seven bodily constituents, mainly the ova and their supportive tissue.

SOMA - Nectar; the most subtle essence of Ojas and Kapha; the essence energy of the mind and nervous system.

SROTAS - pathway; a subtle or gross channel made up of dhatus (tissues) that carry substances or energies from place to place in the body; one of the innumerable special systems in the body. Each channel has a root, which is a governing organ or area of the body, a pathway, and an opening or outlet. Srotas are a channel system used in Ayurvedic medicine.

SROTO AGNI - is the fire component of a specific bodily srotas. Located in the root of the srotas, it maintains the function of that channel.

STRUCTURED WATER - water that has the highest energy; usually found in fresh herbs, fruits and vegetables.

SUBDOSHA - subdivision of a dosha; each dosha has five subdoshas that carry out different functions in the body.

SUTRA - the Sanskrit word sutra literally means "thread" but it also means an idea expressed as a concise, clear statement. The sutra texts, express a variety of world views.

SYNERGISTIC - working together to create an effect.

STNERGISTIC EFFECT - combined effect which is greater then the effect of a substance on its own.

SYNERGY - combining different parts into a unified pattern in which the whole is greater than the sum of its parts.

TAMAS/TAMASIC - inert aspect of creation; a diet and lifestyle that creates a negative, lethargic, anti-social attitude and mind; one of the three Gunas.

TANTRA - the web of life; practices to become aware of the spiritual nature of all things.

TASTE - the beginning of the therapeutic actions of any substance on and in the body.

TEJAS - cool, refined essence of universal fire; subtle, fire of the mind; controls the mind's digestion and is transmitted via Ojas into the digestive system, one of the three Gunas; the superfine essence of Pitta; one of the five elements Fire; its characteristics are: light, illumination, luster, brilliance, and majesty.

TRIPHALA -"Three Fruits," a purifying and rejuvenating compound that is composed of Amalaki, Haritaki and Bibhitaki, usually in equal proportions.

TRIDOSHA - the three bodily organizations: Vata/Air, Pitta/Fire and Kapha/Water- which govern the psychosomatic activity of daily living, the doshas in a state of balance; the three humors, Vata, Pitta, and Kapha are counted both as constituents and as doshas, or morbid substances; the human body is the combination of these three primary essential factors; the three doshas are responsible for maintaining the integrity of the human body; they govern the entire physical structure and function in a living being.

UNNATURAL - not being in accordance with nature or consistent with a normal course of events, in violation of a natural law; inconsistent with an individual pattern or custom; contrived or constrained; artificial.

UPADHATU - a tissue which is nourished by dhatu but which does not itself nourish any dhatu, a final destination of tissue that is being nourished, a secondary tissue that supports the main tissue.

WATER ELEMENT - this is the moistest and most fluid of the five elements. Its properties are cold, oily, inert, mobile, soft and gelatinous. Its effect is moistening, binding, lubricating, cooling and solvent. Its taste is sweet, salty and slightly sour and astringent.

UPADHATU - The superior by-product that results from the formation of a dhatu.

UPANISHADS - Vedic philosophical texts.

VAIDYA - an Ayurvedic physician.

VAKRUTI - the constitution of the moment.

VATA - one of the three doshas in the Ayurvedic system, Vata is responsible for motion and nearly synonymous with "wind." It is made up of the Elements of Air and Ether.

VEGAN - a person who eats neither flesh foods nor eggs nor uses any product from an animal

VEDAS - the most ancient of the Hindu Indian scriptures of knowledge presenting the spiritual science of awareness; first knowledge on earth; the oldest extant literary composition of the human race. The word Veda is derived from a Sanskrit root meaning "knowledge," and the Vedas are verily the seeds of universal knowledge that have bloomed into Indian culture. Thousands of years ago the Rishis of India addressed the problem of eternal life, writing their answers to this conundrum in the four Vedas, the collections of hymns which are the oldest existing literary compositions of the human race. A famous Vedic prayer states: "Lead me from darkness into light; lead me from untruth into truth; lead me from mortality into immortality." We lay emphasis on the last clause of this prayer in our study of medicine, for Ayurveda's purpose is the systematic transformation of a mortal human into an immortal being."

VEDANTA - Vedic philosophy of Self-knowledge.

VEDIC - belonging to the Vedas.

VEDIC SCIENCE - integral spiritual science of the Vedas.

VIKRITI - disease or disorder nature, current dosha imbalance; deviation from nature; as differentiated from Prakruti or life constitution; modification; the pathological condition of the psychological condition of the psychosomatic apparatus; imbalance; disease.

VIPAKA - post-digestive taste and effects of foods, herbs or any substance has on an organism after it has been digested and assimilated into the system (sweet, sour and pungent).

VIRIDATAS - The medieval herbalist and mystic Hildegard of Bingen talked of Viridatas, the greening power. This greening power is the vital energy that is life, the Spirit of the Earth, the Earth Gaia in action that heals and transforms humanity.

VIRYA - the "energy" of a food, medicine or poison; potency, vigor, the enhancing or depressing effect a substance has on an individual organism's digestive power; energetic effects of foods and herbs as heating or cooling.

VITAL-FORCE - it is the equivalent to the Asian concepts of Chi, or Ki, or Prana in Ayurvedic terms.

VYANA VATA - a subdivision of Vata dosha that governs all circulation and is associated with moisture balance and sensation in the skin.

YANG - associated with heat, moisture, activity of mind and body. It is usually identified with the masculine principle in the universe and sun energy.

YIN - associated with cold, dryness, quiet mind and body. It is usually identified with the feminine principle in the universe and moon energy.

YOGA - Union; from the root yuj, "to join," a methodology of the practical, psycho-physical practices and coordinated application of knowledge; spirituality; the science of self-realization, aimed at self-knowledge.

Bibliography

Ayurveda

Atreya, *Perfect Balance: Ayurvedic Nutrition for Mind, Body & Soul,* Avery, 2001

Ballentine, Rudolf, M.D. *Diet & Nutrition,* Honesdale, PA, Himilayan Publishers, *1978,* Harmony Books, 1999

Ballentine, Rudolf, M.D. *Ayurveda and Aromatherapy, Radical Healing,* Harmony Books, 1999

Caraka Samhita, tras, Dr. Bhagwan, and Dr. R.K. Sharma, Varanasi, India: Chowkamba Series Office, 3 Vols., 1992

Chopra, Deepak, *Perfect Health,* New York, Harmony Books, 1990

Das, B., *Fundamentals of Ayurvedic Medicine,* Delhi: Bansal & Co., 1978

Frawley, Dr. David, *Ayurvedic Healing: A Comprehensive Guide, 2nd Revised and Enlarged Edition,* Lotus Press, Twin Lakes, WI, 2000

Dondeb, Yeshi, *Health Through Balance: An Introduction to Tibetan Medicine,* Snow Lion Publications, Ithaca, New York, 1986

Heyn, Birgit, *Ayurvedic Medicine,* publ. by Thorsons 1987

Gerson, Scott, M.D. *Ayurveda: The Ancient Indian Healing Art,* Element Press, 1993

Gerson, Scott, M.D. *The Ayurvedic Guide to Diet & Weight Loss: The Sattva Program,* Lotus Press, Twin Lakes, WI, 2002

Lewanski/Zuraw, *Health Force,* Taoist Publ., 1983

Joshi, Sunil V., M.D., *Ayurveda & Panchakarma,* Lotus Press, Twin Lakes, WI, 1997

Lad, Dr. Vasant, *Ayurveda: The Science of Self-Healing,* Lotus Press, Twin Lakes, WI, 1984

Lad, Dr. Vasant, *The Textbook of Ayurveda: Fundamental Principles,* Ayurvedic Press, 2002

Lad, Dr. Vasant, *The Art of Ayurvedic Pulse Diagnosis*, The Ayurvedic Press, 1996

Miller, Light and Miller, Bryan, D.C., *Ayurveda & Aromatherapy*, Lotus Press, Twin Lakes, WI, 1995

Warrier, Gopi & Deepika Gunawant, M.D., *The complete Illustrated Guide to Ayurveda*, Element 1997

Sachs, Melanie, *Ayurvedic Beauty Care: Ageless Techniques to Invoke Natural Beauty*, Lotus Press, Twin Lakes, WI, 1994

Simon David, M.D. *Vital Energy*, John Wiley & Sons, Inc. 2000

Svoboda, Dr. Robert, *Prakriti: Your Ayurvedic Constitution, Revised Enlarged Second Edition*, Lotus Press, Twin Lakes, WI, 1998

Svobada, Dr. Robert, *Ayurveda, Life, Health and Longevity*, New York, Penguin Books, 1992

Svoboda, Dr. Robert and Lade, Arnie, *Tao & Dharma: Chinese Medicine & Ayurveda*, Lotus Press, Twin Lakes, WI, 1995

Tarabilda, Edward, *Ayurveda Revolutionized, Integrating Ancient & Modern Ayurveda*, Lotus Press, Twin Lakes, WI, 1997

Tierra Michael, *The Way of Herbs*, New York, NY: Washington Square Press, 1983

Tierra, Dr. Michael, *Planetary Herbology*, Lotus Press, Twin Lakes, WI 1988

Tirtha Sada Shiva , *Ayurveda Encyclopia*, The AHC Press, 1998

Tiwari. Maya, *Ayurveda: A Life of Balance*, Rochester, VT, Healing Arts Press, 1995

Tiwari, Bri. Maya, *Ayurveda, Secrets of Healing*, Lotus Press, Twin Lakes, WI 1995

Vinod Verma, *Ayurveda: A Way of Life*,

Chinese Medicine & Tongue Diagnosis

Kirschbaum, Barbara *Atlas of Chinese Tongue Diagnosis*, Eastland Press, 2000

Maciocia Giovanni, *Tongue Diagnosis in Chinese Medicine*, Eastland Press, 1987

Pitchford, Paul, Healing With Whole Foods, Berkeley, CA: North Atlantic, 1993

Tierra, Michael and Tierra, Leslie, L.Ac., OMD., A.H.G., *Chinese Traditional Herbal Medicine, Volumes I & II*, Lotus Press, Twin Lakes, WI, 1998

Veith, Ilza, *The Yellow Empor's Classic of Internal Medicine*, University of California Press, 1949

Constitutional Medicine & Natural Healing

Coghill, Roger, *The Healing Energies of Light*, Charlie Journey Editions, 2000

Farida Sharon, MD (MA), ND, MH, FBRI, *Iridology: Complementary Medical Textbook*, Thorsons Publ., 1989

Johnson, Denny Ray *What the Eye Reveals*, Rayid Publication, 1995

Pitchford, Paul, *Healing with Whole Foods*, North Atlantic Books, 2002

Ryrie, Charlie, *The Healing Energies of Water*, Journey Editions, 1999

Wolf, Harriet, *The Iris and the Constitution*, self-published 1991

Wolf, Harriet, *Applied Iridology- Volume I*, self-published 1989

Zadok, Clifford, *Clinical Iridology: Neuro-Optic Reflex Analysis*, self published in 1988

Herbal Energetics

Frawley, Dr. David and Lad, Dr. Vasant, *The Yoga of Herbs: An Ayurvedic Guide to Herbal Medicine, Second Revised and Enlarged Edition*, Lotus Press, Twin Lakes, WI, 2001

Holmes, Peter, *The Energetics of Western Herbs- Vol. I-II*, Atemis Press, 1989

Tierra, Leslie, *The Herbs of Life*, The Crossing Press, Freedom, CA. 1992

Tierra, Michael, Dr. *The Way of Herbs*, New York, NY: Washington Square Press, 1983

Tierra, Dr. Michael, *Planetary Herbology*, Lotus Press, Twin Lakes, WI, 1988

Wood, Matthew, *The Book of Herbal Wisdom: Using Plants as Medicines*, North Atlantic Books, 1997

Nutritional Medicine

Cousens, Gabriel, M.D., *Rainbow Green Live-Food Cuisine*, North Atlantic Books, 2003

Cousens, Gabriel, M.D., *Conscious Eating*, North Atlantic Books, 2000

Cousens, Gabriel, M.D., *Spiritual Nutrition and the Rainbow Diet*, Cassandra Press, 1986

Diamond, Harvey and Marilyn, *Living Health*, New York, Warner Books, 1987

Elson M. Haas, *Staying Healthy with Nutrition*, Celestial Arts, Berkeley CA, 1992

Howell, Edward, *Enzyme Nutrition*, Garden City Park, NY, Avery Publishing Group, 1985

Howell, Dr. Edward, *Food Enzymes for Health & Longevity*, Lotus Press, Twin Lakes, WI, 1994

Klapper, Michael, *Vega Nutrition: Pure and Simple*, Umitilla, Florida, Gentle World, Inc., 1987

Levine, Stephen A., and Kidd, Paris M, *Antioxidant Adaptation: Its Role in Free Radical Pathology*, San Lea

Marc, David, *Nourishing Wisdom: A New Understanding of Eating*, Marc David, Bell Tower, 1991

Jensen, Bernard, Ph.D. *The Healing Power of Chlorophyll from Plant Life*, Bernard Jensen Enterprises, 1973

Jensen, Bernard, Ph.D. *The Chemistry of Man*, Bernard Jensen Enterprises, 1983

Jensen, Bernard, Ph.D. *Food Healing for Man*, Bernard Jensen Enterprises, 1983

Robbins, John, *Diet for a New American*, Walpole, NH: Stillpoint Publishing, 1987

Robbins, John, *Reclaiming Our Health,* Tiburon, CA: HJ Kramer, Inc, *1996*

Szekely, Edmond Boreaux, *The Essene Way: Biogenic Living,* U.S.A., International Biogenic Society, 1989

Szekely, Edmond Boreaux, *Scientific Vegetarianism,* U.S.A., International Biogenic Society, 1989

Wolf David, *Sunfood Diet Success System,* Maul Brothers Publishing Company, 1996,

Kulvinskas, Viktoras, M.S. *Survival Into the 21st Century,* Fairfield, Iowa, 21st Century Publishing, 1975

Kulvinskas, Viktoras, M.S. *Love Your Body,* Fairfield, Iowa, 21st Century Publishing, 1972

Nutritional Medicine

Howell, Edward, *Enzyme Nutrition,* Garden City Park, NY., Avery Publishing Group, 1985

Howell, Dr. Edward, *Food Enzymes for Health & Longevity,* Lotus Press, Twin Lakes, WI, 1994

Lopez, D.A., Williams, R.M., and Miehlke, K. Enzymes: The Fountain of Youth, Munchen, Germany, The Neville Press, 1994

Santillo, Humbart, Food Enzymes: The Missing Link, Prescott Valley, Arizona, Hohm Press, 1987

About Spirit of the Earth, 'The Living Centre' (TLC) & Living Arts Institute (LAI)

Founded in 1983, The Living Centre (TLC) and Living Arts Institute (LAI) is one of North America's foremost educational centers offering the highest quality leading edge education in wholistic living through a Sevenfold Path to Peace.

The centre offers a wide range of perspectives and philosophies on healing and lifestyle practices drawn from ancient and present day cultures. These include: Ayurvedic Medicine, Living Nutrition, Therapeutic, Practical and Shamanic Herbalism, Fasting & Rejuvenation Retreats, Constitutional Iridology, Movement-Sound-Breath Therapies, Meditation, Vibrational Healing, Emotional and Psycho-Spiritual Counseling.

The educational approach to study and learning is to provide an academic, theoretically based study program which includes equal time in experiential hands-on learning. The Sevenfold Path to Peace forms the basis of the training program. This model offers an integrated approach to health, embracing all aspects of one's life – physical, mental, emotional, purpose, cultural, ecological and spiritual. Drawing on the laws of nature to motivate and guide the individual, the programs are designed to bring about positive personal and planetary change.

Located on 50 acres of pristine, organic land in fertile southwestern Ontario, Canada, this beautiful part of Earth Mother is a natural sanctuary and teaching site. The dynamically alive energy of this land and wide range of wild life are all a part of what makes this a safe haven for growth and learning. A unique circular medicine wheel garden with over 500 medicinal herbs, organic fruit and vegetable gardens, the teaching lodge surrounded by a 1000 sq. ft. Earthship solar greenhouse, a pear orchard, fields of wildflowers, a tranquil pond, meandering stream and a magical forest have provided an enlivening space for thousands of healing sessions, workshops, retreats and celebrations.

The vision of the Centre and Institute is to serve and provide people of all faiths and spiritual paths a direct experience of what it means to live a vital, joyful and purposeful life. The commitment is to the healing and awakening of consciousness within the individual and the world community. A spiritual sanctuary whose primary purpose is to support personal growth and offer educational programs that inspire and empower each person to live their passion and become the change that they desire.

Spirit of the Earth, 'The Living Centre' and Living Arts Institute in Canada and Costa Rica. Directors: Walter 'Shantree' Kacera, D.N., Ph.D. and Lorenna Bousquet-Kacera.

Please visit us online at www.thelivingcentre.com

Spirit of the Earth, 'The Living Centre' and
Living Arts Institute
5871 Bells Rd.
London, ON., Canada N6J 3P9
1-519-652-0230 or 1-519-652-9109

Offered at the Centre

- Conscious Living Workshops & Retreats
- Purification & Rejuvenation Retreats
- Spiritual Fasting Retreats
- Ayurvedic Living Foods Nutrition Intensives
- Transitioning into Vegetarianism & Live Foods
- Living Movement Workshops & Retreats
- Healing with Breath & Sound workshops
- Emotional Bodywork & Body Reflexology
- Sacred Relationship Workshops
- Earth Wisdom: Deep Ecology
- The Sacred Journey Retreats
- Sweat Lodges

(all of the above offered as a private or group experience)

Correspondence & Apprenticeship Certification Programs

- Herbal Energetics & Plant Spirit Medicine
- Ayurvedic Constitutional Medicine
- Living Nutrition: Vital Energy for Life
- Clinical Transformational Iridology
- Conscious Living: The SevenFold Path
- Earth Wisdom Teachings

• Practical & Therapeutic Herbalism

Celebrations

• Full Moon & Equinox & Solstice Gatherings
• YES! To Life Festival

Private Consultations & Healing Sessions

Walter 'Shantree' Kacera, D.N., Ph.D.

Shantree is an Ayurvedic Educator and Live-Food Nutritionist, Therapeutic & Shamanic Herbalist, and Constitutional Iridologist with over 30 years experience in the Natural Healing Arts. He is the founder and co-director of Spirit of the Earth, The Living Centre and Living Arts Institute, an Eco-Spiritual Educational Retreat & Sanctuary, founded in 1983. He uses the modalities of the Natural Healing Arts with spiritual awareness, in the healing of body, mind and spirit.

Since receiving his doctorate in Nutritional Medicine and becoming a Herbal Practitioner he has written and teaches courses on Constitutional Ayurvedic Medicine, Living Nutrition and Herbal Wisdom. Presently Shantree is writing a book on 'The Healing Tastes' which will be a workbook and exploration of the healing essence of tastes on body, mind, and emotions.

Through his private practice and certification courses he has empowered thousands of people on their journey to health and spiritual awareness. He has also educated and trained over thousand students in the Natural Healing Arts through his certification courses.

Shantree is dedicated to providing an integrated preventative approach to well being, applying the healing wisdom of the East and West. He formulates and dispenses his own herbal preparations - HerbSpirit Botanicals. His deep spiritual connection to the Earth has drawn him to an involvement with ancient shamanic and earth wisdom practices, as well as Rain Forest preservation and studies. He now offers his services as an educator, with his wife in Costa Rica and at their home in London, Ontario. He is an internationally celebrated visionary, author, lecturer, and nutritional researcher, and world peaceworker.

Index

D

E

F

G

H

P

Q

R

S

T

U

V

W

Y

Z